NOVEL TREATMENT OF EPILEPSY

Edited by **Humberto Foyaca- Sibat**

Novel Treatment of Epilepsy
Edited by Humberto Foyaca- Sibat

Published by InTech

Janeza Trdine 9, 51000 Rijeka, Croatia

Publishing Process Manager Dragana Manestar

Technical Editor Teodora Smiljanic

Cover Designer InTech Design Team

Additional hard copies can be obtained from orders@intechopen.com

Novel Treatment of Epilepsy, Edited by Humberto Foyaca- Sibat
p. cm.
ISBN 978-953-307-667-6

For EU product safety concerns:
IN TECH d.o.o., Prolaz Marije Krucifikse Kozulić 3, 51000 Rijeka, Croatia,
info@intechopen.com or visit our website at intechopen.com.

Meet the editor

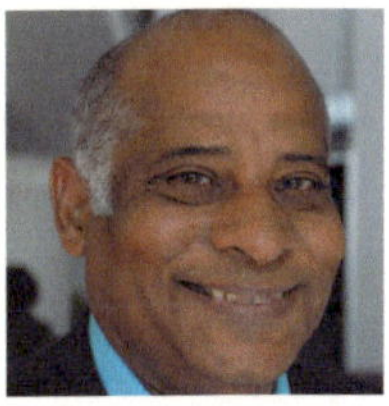

Prof. Humberto Foyaca Sibat, born on May 03, 1948 in Havana City, Republic of Cuba, graduated as a Medical Doctor in Havana University in 1971, soon after he assessed his first epileptic patient. He became specialist in neurology in 1975 and higher level specialist in 1984. He is married and has three daughters and one son; his one daughter tragically passed away in 1979. Currently Dr. Foyaca has been an Associate Professor of Walter Sisulu University for more than 14 years, and he is also Master in Sciences and Associate Investigator of Cuban Academy of Sciences. He is a member of 15 Medical Societies from all over the world; he presented more than 350 papers in different scientific events and he published more than 70 manuscripts in peer-review journals. He is the Chief-Editor of The Internet Journal of Neurology. He received and delivered many short training courses and organized many National and International conferences.

Contents

Preface

Epilepsy continues to be a major health problem throughout the planet affecting millions of people, mainly in developing countries where parasitic zoonoses are more common and cysticercosis, as a leading cause, is endemic. There is epidemiological evidence for an increasing prevalence of epilepsy throughout the world, and evidence of increasing morbidity and mortality in many countries as a consequence of higher incidence of infectious diseases, head injury and stroke.

At the present moment, the number of available books about the treatment of epilepsy is quite big. Then, why did we decide to edit another one?

We decided to edit this book because we identified another way to approach this problem covering aspects of the treatment of epilepsy based on the most recent technological results "in vitro" from developed countries, and the basic treatment of epilepsy at the primary care level in rural areas of South Africa. Therefore, apart from the classic issues that cannot be missing in any book about epilepsy, we introduced novel aspects related with epilepsy and neurocysticercosis as a leading cause of epilepsy in developing countries. Of course, the publication of this book could not have been possible but for the ungrudging efforts put in by a large number of individuals working in the field of epilepsy and many people from many countries, ethnic, religious and socioeconomic groups that coincidentally confluence in this publication.

In this book we focus on novel antiepileptic drug (AED) as zonisamide and lacosamide, and the role of mithocondria in epilepsy.

Because of the fact that the adverse metabolic effects of AEDs are probably currently underestimated, and thus represent an area of legitimate concern, we dedicated one chapter to the adverse metabolic effects of antiepileptic drug treatment.

Another chapter is dedicated to antiepileptic drugs targeting cerebral presynaptic ion channels reduced cerebral excitability decreasing the Glu release. Nevertheless, the higher potency and efficacy of vinpocetine as the most effective antiepileptic drugs to inhibit presynaptic Na^+ and Ca^{2+} channels permeability is described and we suggest that vinpocetine should be considered as a potential third generation AED for a better seizure control in patients presenting refractory epilepsy. The role of cell therapy and the cell transplants in epilepsy is also analyzed.

Diagnosing pregnancy in an epileptic woman is something of frequent occurrence in everyday medical practice and scientific societies have not given us any decisive recommendations about such cases, which makes any risk/benefit assessment uneasy. Therefore in this book we bring all our readers up to date with the impact and the latest development of antiepileptic drugs in regard to pregnancy, and we suggest a proper use of such drug in this situation.

The chapter related to treatment of epilepsy and epileptic seizures secondary to neurocysticercosis, is addressed to health professionals working in the more disadvantage places and offers another difference between this book and similar other ones.

Finally we discuss another way of non-pharmacological treatment of epilepsy throughout selected topics related to brain stimulation, presurgical assessment, corpus callosotomy, neuromodulation, surgical treatment and vagus nerves stimulation with update information and wise guidelines and recommendations.

Some chapters and the edition job were entirely made in a rural setting and this edition is aimed at health care professionals including general practitioners, family doctors, internists, neurologists, epileptologists, neurosurgeons, psychiatrists, medical students, nursing students, and students of the professions allied to medicine among others.

More than 150 abstracts were submitted for review from different parts of the world; about 50 % were selected for the first phase of this editorial process, some were considered for other books and unfortunately some were rejected. All material for this first edition has been thoroughly revised, and updated. Many specialists have provided expert advice on changes in their field and their help has been invaluable to us in our efforts to keep the relevance of the book for our readership community. All chapters were revised by each author twice after submission; the final version was peer-reviewed by two experts and recommendations were made. Nevertheless, some advices of contributors may differ from the approach of the editors or can be even different from the neurological community. However, we kept and supported it as a part of our policy of respecting all scientific criteria, mainly for that work which still remains controversial. The future will decide who was wrong. On the other hand, we also encouraged each author as an expert in the field, straight from the beginning to report their personal experience, expertise, and obtained results.

Knowing that authors from many countries may have different experience and scientific results, in order to achieve a high degree of scientific content with a standard level of acceptance, we took a detailed overview of all important novel information. We all tried to keep the high prestige of our Editorial Company as a main priority and we declare our happiness in writing this book in the electronic era with a full-text website allowing us to display our scientific messages to an even larger global readership, apart from all benefits of print format.

Our aim has been to produce a reference book in which this information would be presented in an integrated and rapidly accessible format.

In regard to pharmacological treatment, many agree that treatment of epilepsy should be driven by "evidence-based" neurology approach, and although this type of evidence is mainly possible through well designed and ethically approved randomized clinical trials, we did not exclude any "experience-based" approach from expert contributors and from the disadvantaged regions.

Every effort has been made to check the drug dosages given in this book. Despite dosages from all medication were double checked, it is important for our readership to scrutinize last information sheets about new dosages, side-effects, contraindications before administering any of the drugs listed.

We all attempted to bring in valuable updated information about the treatment of epilepsy and other related problems to our readership.

ACKNOWLEDGEMENTS

We sincerely thank to INTECH Open Access Publisher that initially put forth the idea of writing this book and support this initiative. Special thanks should be given to my editorial process managers and beautiful friends Ms Dragana Manestar and Natalia Reinic for their kind attention, great inspiration, constant encouragement, and professional support which is highly appreciated.

For understanding my long nights at the computer, I'd like to thank my wife Lourdes de Fátima, who was worked with me on this project; to my first daughter Zayra Susana who died in 1979 but continues inspiring me from wherever she is; to my second daughter Lorna Maria who is a good lawyer and encourages me all the time to continue moving forward, and to my children Fatima Susana Adolfina (2 years old) and Thabo Humberto Jorge (3 years old) for helping me to find peace of mind, persistence and hope every time I needed. My father, my sisters, nephews, nieces, aunts, uncles, cousins and almost all members of my family contributed to this project in one way or another - to all of them: a great Thank You indeed.

Many thanks also to family, relatives, and friends of all the collaborators for their patience and tolerance of the lost evenings, nights, weekends, and holidays.

In the end, I extend my deepest sense of appreciation to Dr. Roberto Gonzalez Martin Vice-Minister of the Cuban Ministry of Health (CMH), Dra Luisa Maria Diaz National Director of Postgraduate (CMH) and Dr. Jorge Delgado Bustillo Deputy Head of National Unit of International Collaboration (CMH), Prof. PhD Nereyda Cantelar del

Castillo, Dr. PhD Reinaldo Menendez and Lic Maribel Chao from the National Institute of Tropical Medicine "Pedro Kouri", Prof. MM Balintulo Vice-Chancellor and Principal of Walter Sisulu University (WSU) in Mthatha, South Africa, Prof CL Obi Deputy Vice Chancellor, Academic Affairs and Research, Prof. G Buijs Deputy Chancellor, Planning, quality Assurance and Development, Prof. KJ Mammen Director, Directorate of Post Graduate Studies, Prof. GE Ekosse Director: Research Development (WSU); Prof K Mfenyana Executive Dean of Faculty of Health Sciences (WSU), Prof JE Iputo Director of the School of Medicine (WSU), Prof. A Awotedu Chairman of the Department of Medicine (WSU) , Dr. C Xamlashe CEO and Dr. TM Madiba Head: Clinical Governance of Mthatha Hospital Complex and to all my friends, colleagues and collaborators.

Prof. Humberto Foyaca- Sibat
Walter Sisulu University, Mthatha
South Africa

Part 1

Pharmacological Treatment of Epilepsy

1

Drug Discovery in Epilepsy: A Synthetic Review

Raul SanMartin* and Fátima Churruca
Department of Organic Chemistry II,
Faculty of Science and Technology,
University of the Basque Country,
Spain

1. Introduction

Although recurrent unprovoked seizures or epilepsy has been known for more than three thousand years, and even considering pivotal contributions like that of Hypocrates (*circa* 400 BC) establishing epilepsy as a brain disease instead of a religious or evil phenomenon, it was not until the 20th century that the first relatively effective antiepileptic drugs were discovered. Starting from phenobarbital and phenytoin almost 100 years ago, much research has been devoted to the development of new, more active drugs to treat such a broad category of symptom complexes (Krasowski, 2010). A chronological overview of the aforementioned development would provide interesting information about trial and errors in antiepileptic therapy, but from a chemical point of view (drug discovery) a classification according to structure is by far more useful. That is the aim of this review, thus covering the most relevant literature concerning synthetic approaches to the main anticonvulsant drugs. More detailed, comprehensive reviews on some of the main anti-epileptic drugs (AEDs) have been reported so far (Carril et al., 2007; Kraus et al., 2010), in some cases describing also aspects like pharmacokinetics, medicinal uses, approval for commercialization, etc. The present review intends to give a concise outlook at the most significant strategies employed in the synthesis of a good number of AEDs. Currently marketed drugs and some others in development will be briefly examined. Finally, a slightly more profound coverage has been given to some sections (i.e. carbamazepine, oxcarbazepine and eslicarbazepine acetate) on the basis of the relevance, therapeutic importance or promising applications of some AEDs over other ones occasionally employed or with a narrower application spectrum.

2. Results

2.1 First generation AEDs and related

2.1.1 Carbamazepine, oxcarbazepine and eslicarbazepine acetate

Despite the obvious similarity between these three compounds, which share a *N*-carbamoyldibenzo[*b,f*]azepine framework, their chronological appearance as antiepileptic drugs has been delayed for more than 30 years. Indeed, carbamazepine was first marketed as a drug to treat trigeminal neuralgia in 1962 and then started to be used as an anticonvulsant in the UK in 1965 and approved in the US by 1967 (Schlinder, 1958). Oxcarbazepine was first synthesized in 1965, just a few years after its precursor carbamazepine, but it was not until 1990 that it was approved to treat epileptic seizures in Denmark, the rest of the EU (1999) and US (2000). Geigy (now part of Novartis) was the company that discovered both carbamazepine and oxcarbazepine drugs and commercialized them under the trade names of Tegretol® and Trileptal® respectively. The last member of this family, eslicarbazepine acetate, which has been developed by Bial, has been approved in Europe as an adjunctive therapy for adults with refractory partial-onset seizures and is in review for US approval (Chung, 2010).

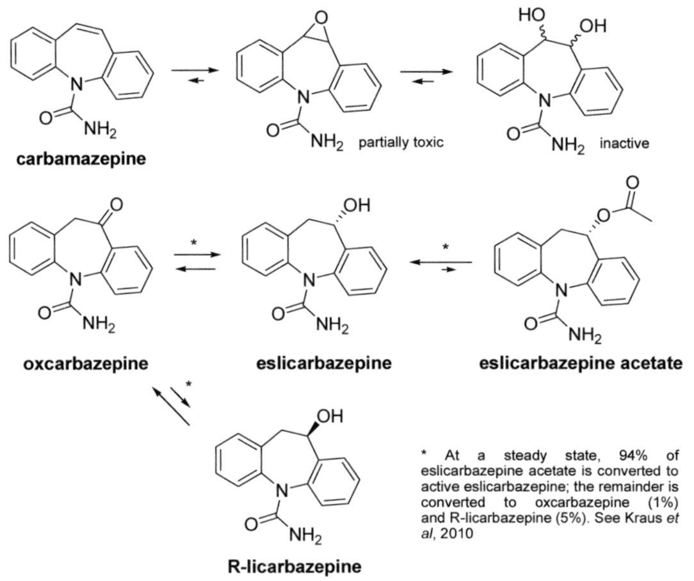

Scheme 1. Summary of metabolic paths concerning carbamazepine, oxcarbazepine and eslicarbazepine acetate.

Scheme 1 shows a summary of the metabolic paths and connections between these drugs. Both oxcarbazepine and eslicarbazepine acetate are considered prodrugs of eslicarbazepine or S-licarbazepine, the most active and selective (towards preferential modulation of inactivated voltage-dependent sodium channels more than sodium channels in the resting state) metabolite. The also active (and toxic) carbamazepine-10,11-epoxide is generated by metabolic oxidation of carbamazepine, but this compound and the *R*-isomer of licarbazepine (R-licarbazepine, generated in a approximate 5% proportion from eslicarbazepine acetate and 25% from oxcarbazepine) result to be less active and selective. Finally, trans-10,11-dihydroxy-10,11-dihydrocarbamazepine is an inactive metabolite which is excreted in the urine mainly in an unconjugated form. One of the advantages of oxcarbazepine over carbamazepine is a clear reduction of the impact on the liver and prevention of the serious forms of anemia or agranulocytosis occasionally associated with carbamazepine. A tolerability improvement has been also observed when comparing oxacarbazepine with the third generation drug eslicarbazepine acetate. (Kraus et al., 2010).

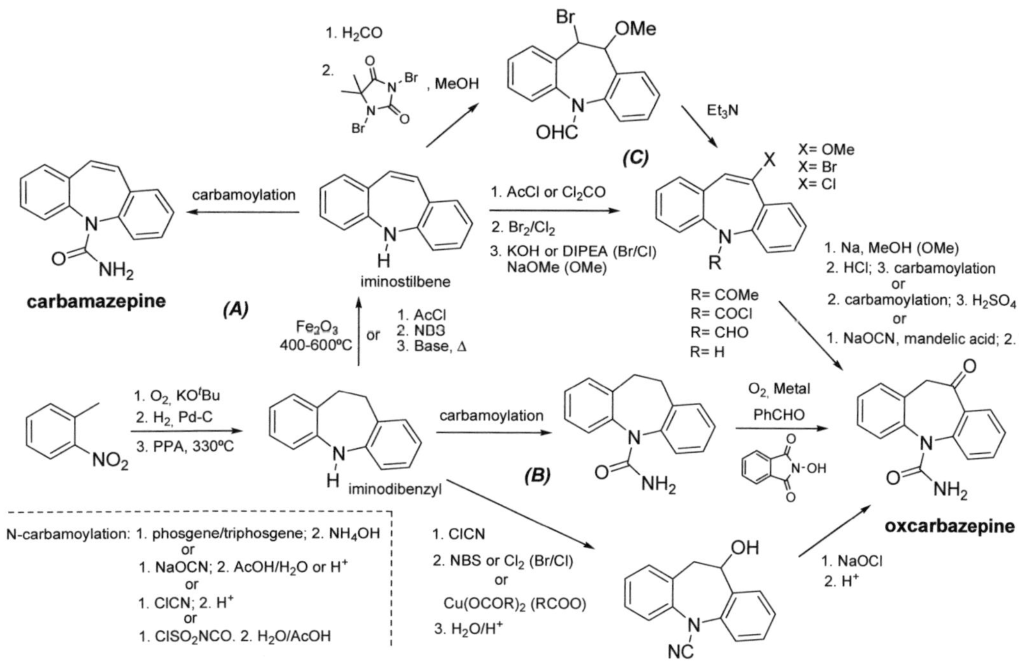

Scheme 2. A first selection of the reported approaches to carbamazepine and oxcarbazepine.

Both carbamazepine and oxcarbazepine have been crucial milestones, reference drugs in the therapy of epilepsy for a long time, and eslicarbazepine acetate looks like a suitable candidate for the future. Due to the aforementioned importance of carbamazepine and oxcarbazepine, a good number of synthetic strategies have been developed for the access to both dibenzoazepine drugs. Moreover, most of the existing methodologies share common substrates and intermediates in such a way that it can be said they are interconnected, as shown in schemes 2 and 3, and many alternative protocols have been developed for the same step or transformation. In fact, some of the publications or patents claim overall yield improvements by slight modifications in the procedures for just one or two steps of the whole sequence. One of those common intermediates is 10,11-dihydro-5*H*-dibenzo[*b,f*]azepine, also known as iminodibenzyl, obtained by an initial oxidative coupling of *o*-nitrotoluene, reduction of the nitro groups and PPA-promoted cyclization (Method A). After oxidation to dibenzoazepine ring, a carbamoylation step (see alternative procedures for this transformation) renders carbamazepine (Aufderhaar et al., 1980). A relatively straightforward approach to oxcarbazepine from iminodibenzyl involves benzylic direct or stepwise (Method B) oxidation after a suitable *N*-functionalization (carbamoylation, cyanation, etc.). Another well-established strategy relies on the preparation of 10-methoxy or 10-haloiminostilbene derivatives by a *N*-protection/halogenation/elimination sequence (Karusala et al., 2009) or alternatively by a dehydrohalogenation of a halomethoxy intermediate obtained by using 1,3-dihalodimethylhydantoin (Method C). Demethylation or hydrolysis and carbamoylation steps provide target oxcarbazepine (Gupta et al., 2007).

Scheme 3 displays another set of synthetic strategies towards oxcarbazepine. Carbamazepine, though a final product itself, has been employed as intermediate for the synthesis of oxcarbazepine. Epoxidation of the former and rearrangement by iodide salts or hydrogenation/oxidation (Method D) provided target compound (Heckendorn et al., 1982). Other interesting approaches from iminostilbene involved the use of 10-nitro derivative intermediates and, in some cases, of the corresponding oximes. Iron-catalyzed reduction and acidic hydrolysis (Methods E and F) were the key steps in these synthetic sequences (Aufderhaar, 1981; Eidenhammer et al., 2000). The latter approaches are related to the originally employed industrial procedure at Novartis (Fuenfschilling et al., 2005).

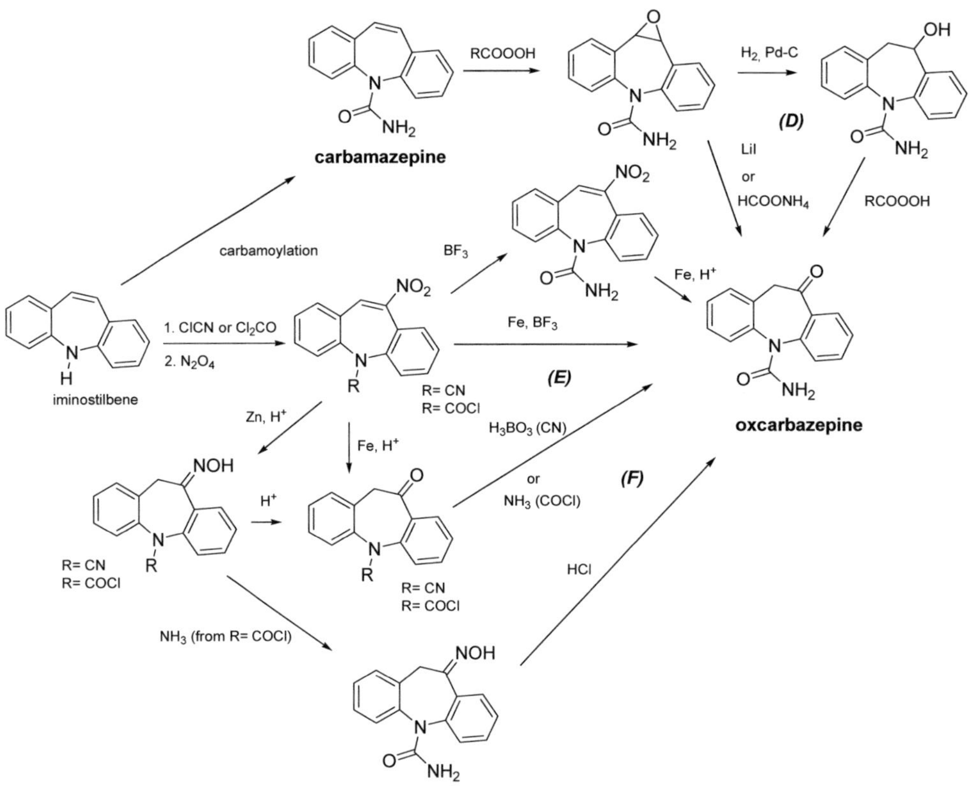

Scheme 3. Other synthetic sequences leading to carbamazepine and oxcarbazepine.

In the last years more innovative entries to oxcarbazepine have been reported. As shown in Scheme 4, an intramolecular Friedel-Crafts acylation performed at a 2-carboxymethyldiarylamine intermediate provides 10-methoxyiminostilbene, which upon carbamoylation and hydrolysis (Method G) provides target compound (Kaufmann et al., 2004). A tandem remote metalation/cyclization was applied to 2-carboxamido-2′-methyldiarylamines (Method H), thus affording the corresponding dibenzoazepinones which were finally *N*-deprotected and carbamoylated, or alternatively transformed into the aforementioned 10-methoxyiminostilbene and carbamoylated/hydrolysed (Lohse et al., 2001). A straightforward, efficient approach to oxcarbazepine, based two palladium-catalyzed *N*-arylation reactions, was recently reported (Scheme 5). The scope of the latter strategy was expanded by the synthesis of a series of analogs which incorporated different substituents in the arene or heteroarene rings (Carril eta al., 2005, 2007).

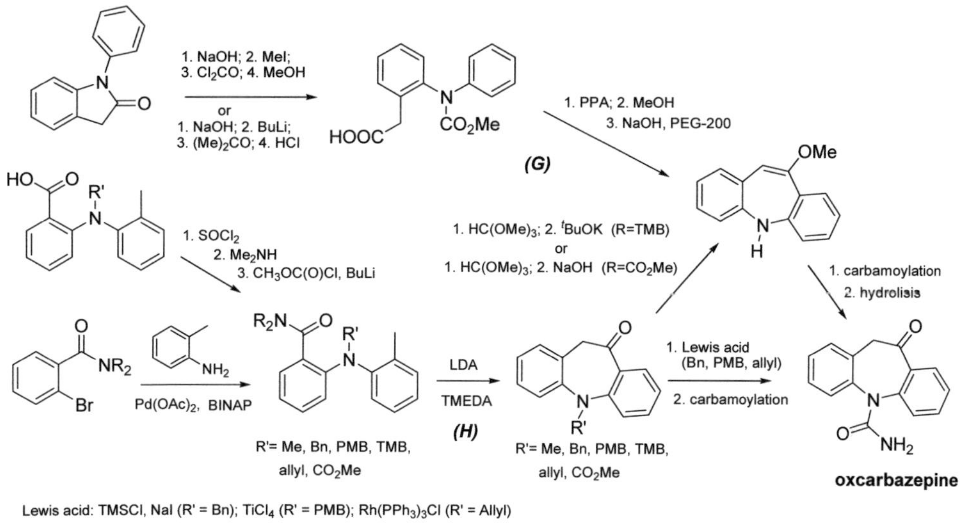

Scheme 4. Remote metalation/cyclization and intramolecular F-C acylation as key steps for the synthesis of oxcarbazepine.

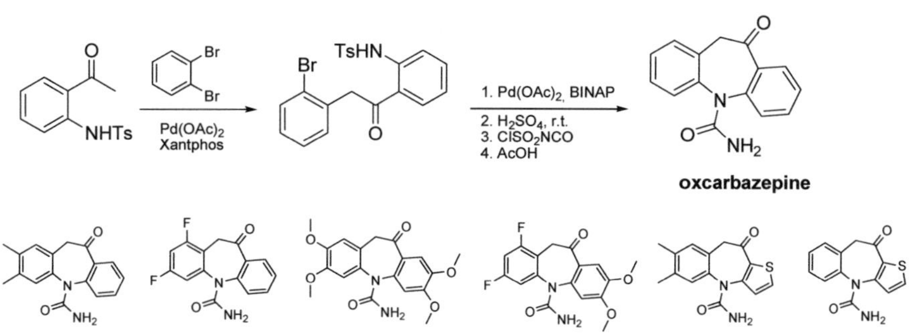

Scheme 5. Palladium-catalyzed sequential *N*-arylations for the synthesis of oxcarbazepine and several structural analogs.

Considering the above metabolic paths and the commercial availability of oxcarbazepine, all the synthetic approaches to eslicarbazepine acetate start from the former AED, as displayed in Scheme 6. A chiral resolution of the reduction products of oxcarbazepine under standard conditions, the racemic mixture of 10-hydroxyderivatives, can be performed by means of either menthoxyacetic acid chloride or L-(+)-tartaric acid acetic anhydride (Method I). Eslicarbazepine would be obtained in this way and then transformed into eslicarbazepine acetate by acetylation (Benes et al., 1999; Learmonth, 2002). A more efficient approach to eslicarbazepine implies an stereoselective reduction of oxcarbazepine (Method J) using formic acid derivatives and a chiral ruthenium catalyst with *p*-cymene and sulfonamide (S,S)-TsDAEN ligands (Learmonth et al., 2007). Finally, an asymmetric catalytic hydrogenation catalyzed by Rh((*SSRR*)-TangPhos)(COD)BF4 complex also afforded highly enantiopure eslicarbazepine acetate (Method K), this time from achiral 10-acetoxyiminostilbene, readily prepared from oxcarbazepine (Yu et al., 2007).

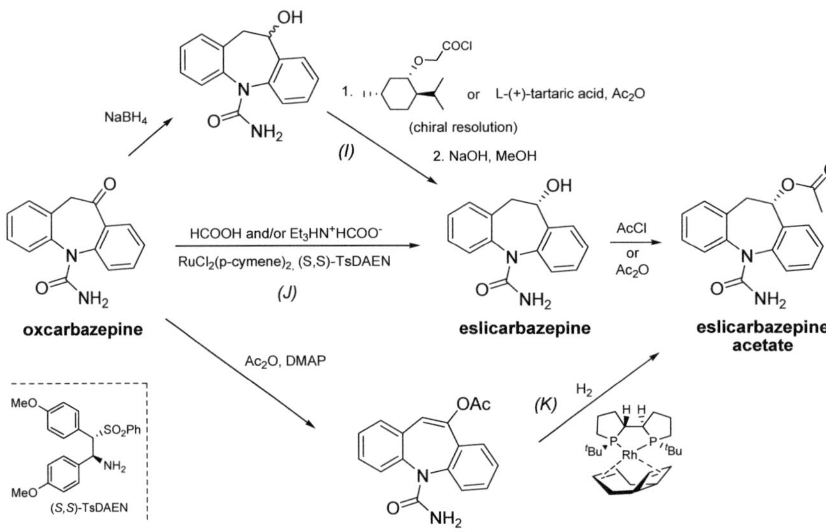

Scheme 6. Synthesis of eslicarbazepine acetate from oxcarbazepine.

2.1.2 Phenobarbital, primidone, phenytoin and phosphenytoin

Phenobarbital (PHB, Luminal®) is one of the first discovered AEDs and still remains as effective as more modern drugs in a wide variety of seizures (Kwan & Brodie, 2004). PHB acts directly on $GABA_A$ receptors by modulating chloride currents through receptor channels, as well as inhibits glutamate induced depolarizations. Similar mechanism of action is shared by primidone (Mysoline®), another AED related to the barbiturates, which is partly metabolized to PHB in the body (Gallagher et al., 1972). Currently they use is limited because of their adverse effects but in developing countries, PHB is still widely employed for the treatment of all types of seizures except absence due to its low cost.

Since its early discovery and introduction in 1938, phenytoin (PHT, 5,5-diphenylhydantoin, Dilantin®) has become one of the most commonly used drug in adjunctive treatments for partial and generalized seizures as well as various epileptic syndromes (Tunnicliff, 1997). The primary site of action appears to be the motor cortex where, by blocking voltage-sensitive sodium channels in neurons, the spread of seizures is reduced and the development of maximal seizure activity is limited. PHT is a highly effective and economical AED but the complications in its administration associated to its physicochemical properties led to the development of a better tolerated and safer derivative, fosphenytoin (Cerebyx®), a phosphate ester containing PHT prodrug (Luer, 1998).

Despite their differences, the chemical structure of these four derivatives is related. Among the variety of approaches reported in literature for their synthesis (Roth & Kleeman, 1988), there are two general and common methods for the preparation of the heterocyclic cores (Scheme 1): the condensation of dicarbonyl derivates with urea under basic conditions (method A) and the treatment of β-diamido/β-aminoamido compounds with phosgene (method B). Several related approaches have been developed in which alternative reagents to urea and phosgene are employed, such as guanidine (method C) and thiourea (method D), or formic acid (method E), respectively. In addition to these methods, modifications on the heterocyclic ring include the phenyl insertion, both under superacidic conditions (method F) (Klummp et al., 1998) and/or by using phenyllead(IV) compounds (method G)

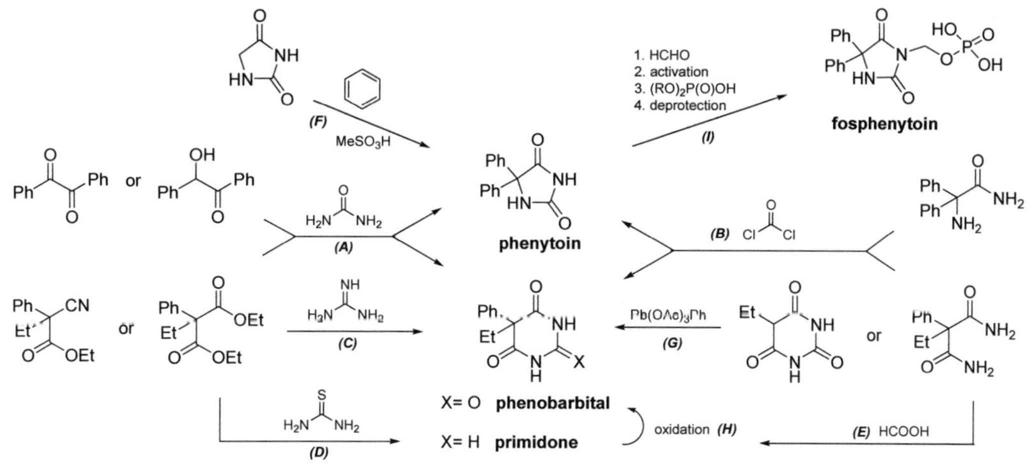

Scheme 7. General methods for the synthesis of phenobarbital, primidone, phenytoin and fosphenytoin.

(Pinhey & Rowe, 1980), and oxidation reactions (method H) (Mac Leod et al., 2008). Most of these classical methods suffer from general drawbacks, including long reaction times, low yield, and difficult operating conditions. However, by the application of new technologies or the use of newly developed heterogeneous reagents, their scope has been considerably extended. Thus, for example, the synthesis of PHT in almost quantitatively yield is accomplished using method A assisted by microwave irradiation (Safari et al., 2009).
Finally, fosphenytoin is readily available from PHT by its sequential treatment with formaldehyde and, after activation of the so-obtained aminoalcohol, with the corresponding phosphoric acid. The recently reported use of an *in situ* prepared tertiary ammonium phosphate as phosphorylating reagent has resulted in a considerably improvement regarding reaction yield and steps, affording fosphenytoin in an overall 82% yield (Grassi & Volante, 2005).

2.1.3 Valproate and valproic acid

Valproic acid (VPA, Depakote®, Depakene®) and sodium valproate (Depacon®, Epilim®), are a broad spectrum AEDs very effective for generalized seizure types. With an unknown mechanism of action, VPA has the shortest half life (10-15 h) among the all existing AEDs (Badir et al., 1991), which results on a multiple daily dosing administration. Although clinically effective, its use is restricted because of rare but potentially severe life threatening side effects, such as teratogenicity and hepatotoxicity.

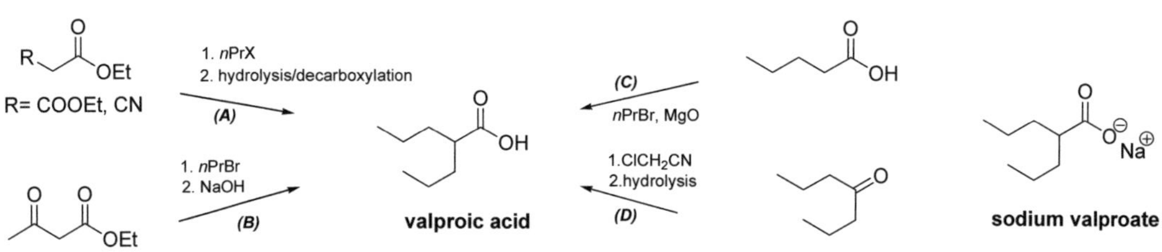

Scheme 8. General methods for the synthesis of valproic acid.

The alkylation of carboxy acid derivatives with *n*-propyl halides is the most general approach reported in literature for the synthesis of VPA and so far the most effective (Santaniello et al., 1998). Starting from diverse substrates, different variations of the method have been carried out, as the elimination-hydrolysis of 2,2-dipropyl acetoacetic ethyl ester via retroclaisen reaction promoted by NaOH (method B) or the monoalkylation of a soluble metalated magnesium carboxylate derived from valeric acid (method C). Among all, the classical alkylation β-activated carboxylic esters (method A) is still the better studied method. The optimization of the hydrolysis and decarboxylation steps had provided a one-pot, easy to operate and high yielding (84%) synthesis of VPA using methanesulfonic acid (Zeiler, 1994). Alternatively, the transformation of 4-heptanone into VPA has also received much attention. Recently, a novel approach has been described in which after addition of 2-chloroacetonitrile, the hydrolysis of the so-obtained epoxynitrile is successfully accomplished in presence of a phase transfer catalyst (method D), yielding VPA in an overall 71% (Nagarajan et al., 2009).

2.2 Second generation AEDs

2.2.1 Clorazepate and clonazepam

Benzodiazepines (BDZs) are a class of drugs that have long been employed to treat convulsive seizures as well as used as tranquilizers, sedatives and muscle relaxants (Ashton, 1994). Clonacepam (Klonopin®) was the first BDZ used for epilepsy and nowadays is a potent AED for the treatment of myoclonic seizures and subcortical myoclonus. Another important member of this family is Clorazepate (Traxene®), a prodrug for desmethyl diazepam and very rapidly produced as active metabolite. BDZs are partial agonist of the $GABA_A$ receptor which leads to increase the frequency of chloride ion channel opening and therefore to the inhibition of the synaptic transmissions across the CNS. Due to the development of tolerance and their sedative effect, BDZs are not appropriate for a long-term and adjunctive treatment of refractory epilepsy (Riss et al., 2008).

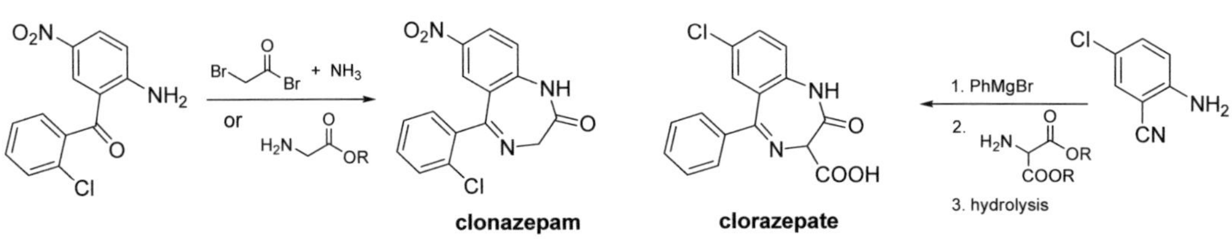

Scheme 9. Synthesis of clorazepate and clonazepam.

Two general approaches have been reported for the access of 5-aryl-1-4-benzodiazepines. The first method, which is the condensation of 2-amino benzophenone derivatives with bromoacetyl bromide and ammonia or glycine alkyl esters, has been successfully applied to the synthesis of clonazepam (Vardanyan & Hruby, 2006). The alternative method includes an additional step which consists of the Grignard addition to benzonitriles to afford benzophenone imine intermediate before condensation with the corresponding 2-aminomalonic ester derivate. Both approaches are high yielding and effective in the synthesis of benzodiazepines, therefore, the scope of their application has relied on the availability of starting materials. Thus, this second approach has been the method of choice for a straightforward and efficient access to clorazepate (Schmitt, 1970).

2.2.2 Gabapentin and pregabalin

Despite being GABA analogues and having been designed as GABA agonists, both gabapentin (GBP, Neurontin®) and its more potent successor pregabalin (Lyrica®) have shown to be inactive at GABA receptors. Nevertheless, they are effective in several neurological and psychiatric conditions and they are conventionally used in the treatment of partial epilepsies. GBP´s mechanism of action was recently discovered (Eroglu et al., 2009) and demonstrates that by binding to the alpha2delta-1 receptor on neurons, GBP avoids synapse formation. The main advantage of these AEDs is that both are relatively well tolerated although they have some adverse effects, particularly in high doses, but these usually are relatively minor. Compared to GBP, pregabalin is more potent, absorbs faster and has greater bioavailability (Bryans & Wustrow, 1999).

Two general approaches for the synthesis of geminally substituted aminomethyl acetic acid compounds are known (Johnson & Li, 2007): the transformation of geminal diacetic acids into suitable amido intermediates which rearrange to desired target (method A) and the reduction of saturated aminomethyl derivatives such as nitro-, cyano-, imino-, or oxime-containing geminal acetic acetates (method B). Method A constitutes the most straightforward procedure for the synthesis of GBP, which is efficiently accomplished in just 3 steps in a 80% yield through the Hofmann rearrangement of 3,3-pentamethylene glutarimide intermediate (Ferrari et al., 2004). Pregabalin, for other hand, contains a chiral centre and requires an asymmetric approach for its synthesis. Typically, a racemic mixture of pregabalin or its intermediates is synthesized and then processes involving racemic chiral or enzymatic resolution are applied (method C), but the effective throughput of the process is reduced by 50%. Much effort has been focused on the development of enantioselective routes. The employment of chiral auxiliaries and ligands has proven to be effective but also unsuitable for the high cost of the reagents. However, asymmetric organocatalysis has emerged as a very efficient and sustainable alternative for the synthesis of enantiopure intermediates via conjugated addition of cyanide or nitromethane to the corresponding α,β-unsaturated precursors (method D) (Bassas et al., 2009).

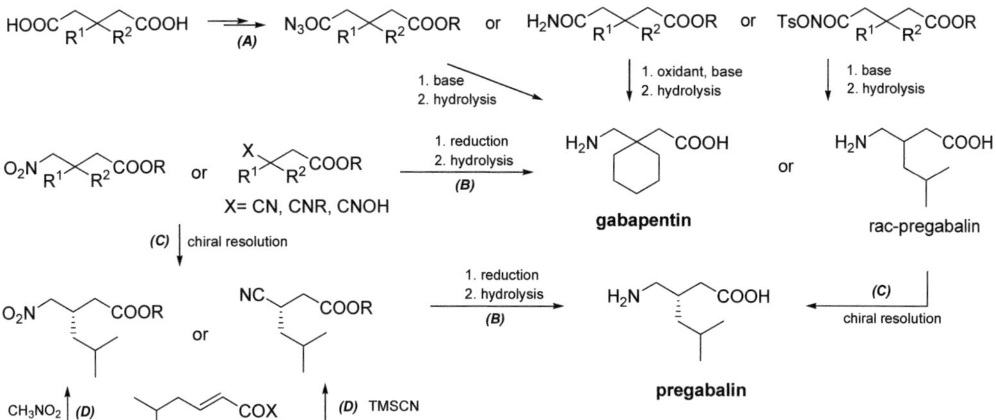

Scheme 10. General methods for the synthesis of gabapentin and pregabalin.

2.2.3 Felbamate

Felbamate (Felbatol®) was first marketed in the early 90s and reported as a potent anticonvulsant very effective against multiple seizure types (Pellock & Boggs, 1995). It is usually well tolerated but due to very serious side effects such as aplastic anemia and hepatic failure, its use is restricted to patients with severe refractory epilepsy or Lennox-Gastaut syndrome. Felbamate´s mechanism of action is not known, but it has been reported as an allosteric antagonist at the NR2B subunit of the NMDA glutamate receptor and also as $GABA_A$ receptor agonist.

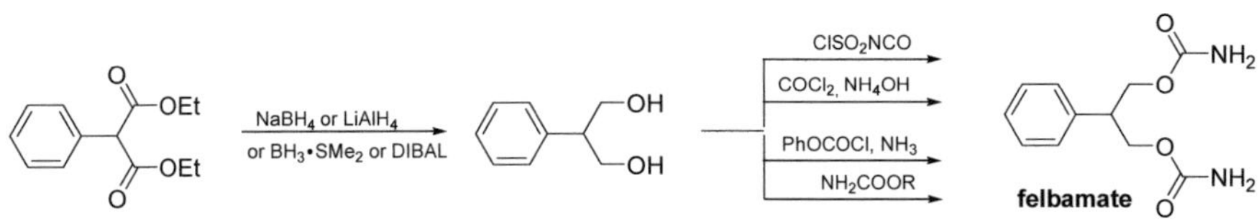

Scheme 11. General methods for the synthesis of felbamate.

The synthesis of felbamate involves a two step procedure, for which during these years, different reaction conditions have been developed. The reduction of commercially available diethyl phenyl malonate to diol intermediate has been carried out with several reagents, among which sodium borohydride has performed the best results regarding effectiveness and handeling-purification (Walker et al., 1994). Its subsequent transformation into the corresponding carbamate has been studied using phosgene, chloroformate as well as cyanate derivates, but still urethane exchange constitutes the best method for preparing felbamate (Walker et al., 1994).

2.2.4 Tiagabine

Tiagabine (TBG, Gabitril®) is a GABA uptake inhibitor primarily used in combination with other AEDs for the treatment of partial seizures (Schachter, 1999). The precise mechanism of action is not known but it modulates the excitatory synaptic currents by retarding the neuronal reuptake of GABA into the presynaptic terminal, which leads to the maintenance of the extra cellular concentration of GABA.

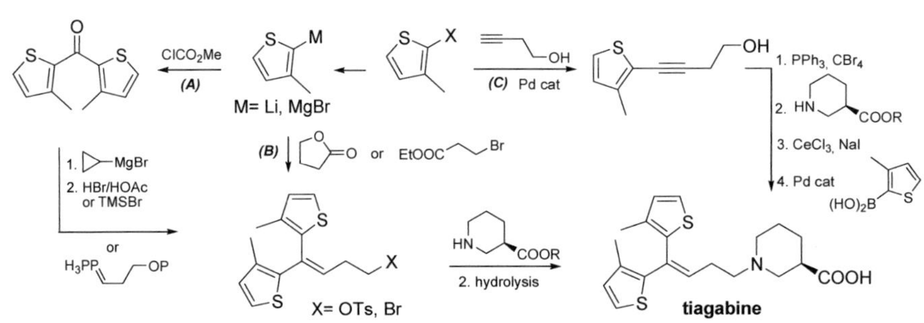

Scheme 12. General methods for the synthesis of tiagabine.

There is one general approach for the synthesis of TGB, which includes the Grignard addition of 2-metallo-3-methylthiofuran to different carbonyl electrophiles as common step (Andersen et al., 1993). When methylchloroformate is employed (method A), the resulting diarylketone can be transformed into the alkenyl precursor of TGB by reaction with cyclopropylmagnesium bromide and subsequent opening under acidic conditions or *via* Wittig olefination. However, the reaction of the Grignard with γ-butyrolactone or ethyl 3-bromopropanoate (method B) has resulted as a much more straightforward and effective method. Then, the synthesis of TGB is completed by the N-alkylation of the 4-bromo or 4-tosylbutene intermediate with the corresponding protected cyclic amino acid. Recently, an alternative method (C) based on palladium catalyzed Sonogashira and Suzuki reactions for new carbon-carbon connections and $CeCl_3$-NaI mediated diastereoselective hydroiodination of alkynes as key step has been published (Bartoli et al., 2010). Nevertheless, despite the synthetic importance of this newly developed methodology applied to the synthesis of TGB, still it lacks of practical and industrial extend.

2.2.5 Levetiracetam and brivaracetam

Levetiracetam (LEV, Keppra®) is a newly developed potent AED for the adjunctive therapy in the treatment of partial onset seizures in both adults and children. Even if its mechanism of action is not fully elucidated, it is known to target the synaptic vesicle protein 2A (SV2A) as well as high-voltage, N-type calcium channels. With a nearly ideal pharmacokinetics, LEV reveal a very good safety profile which makes it a very well tolerated AED and also efficient for different patient populations (Grosso et al., 2005). Brivaracetam (UCB 34714), the *n*-propyl derivate of LEV, possesses a ten-fold higher binding affinity for SV2A compared to LEV and it shows as a very promising new AED but still is under development (Malawka & Kulig, 2008).

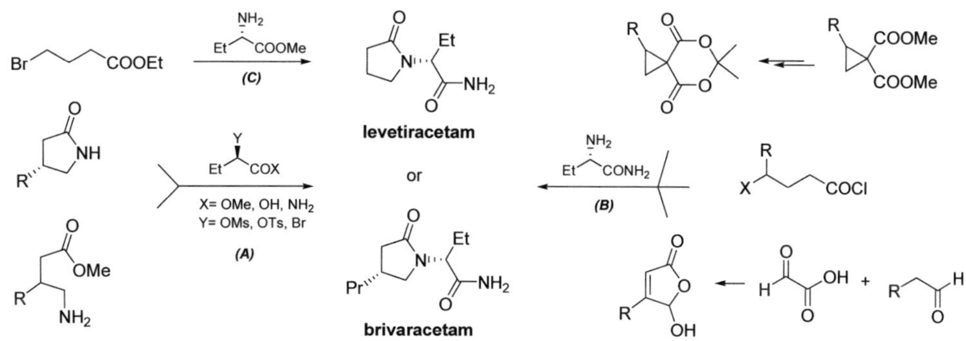

Scheme 13. General methods for the synthesis of levetiracetam and brivaracetam.

The main chemical disconnection of both LEV and brivaracetam occurs at the C-N-pyrrolidinone bond, which can be accomplished by the alkylation of N-pyrrolidinone or N-alkyl intermediate with an activated butyric acid derivative (method A) as well as by the construction of the pyrrolidinone ring from (s)-aminobutyramide or the methyl ester of (s)-aminobutyric acid as nitrogen source (method B and C, respectively) (Kenda et al., 2004). Enantiomerically pure (s)-aminobutyric acid derivatives are readily available from L-methionine and easier to obtain than the required butyric acid derivate in method A. Thus, by using method C, LEV has been successfully prepared in an overall 71% (Ates et al., 2003). However, the most efficient approach for the synthesis of brivaracetam consist of the palladium catalyzed diastereoselective reductive amination of aminobutyramide with a furan intermediate suitably prepared from butyric acid and glyoxalic acid (method B)(Surtees et al., 2005).

2.2.6 Lacosamide

The continuous search for new AEDs has lead to the discovery of a novel category of drugs labeled as Functionalized Amino Acids, among which lacosamide (LCM, Vimpat®) is the first-in-class. LCM is effective for the adjunctive treatment of partial-onset seizures in adults and it has a novel mode of action: a "novel dual mechanism" consisting of selective enhancement of sodium channel slow inactivation and modulation of CRMP-2 activity (Chung, 2009). It is generally well tolerated but still presents regular side effects such as dizziness, nausea and vomiting.

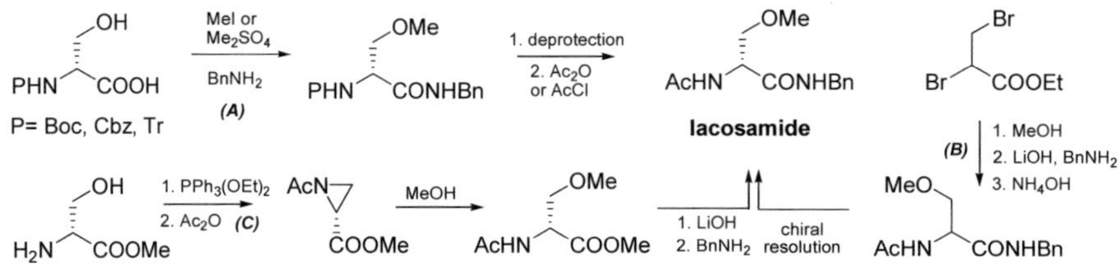

Scheme 14. General methods for the synthesis of lacosamide.

The synthesis of LCM is primarily based on the stepwise functionalization of L-serine, which starts in most of the cases with the protection of the free amine (method A). Then, after methylation of the hydroxyl group and amidation, the N-protecting group is removed and the amine acylated to afford LCM with high enantioselectivity and in good overall yield (Riedner & Dunne, 2008). Alternatively, and also starting from serine an elegant approach has been reported based on the selective ring opening of N-acetylazirine methylester (method C) (Morieux et al., 2008). For other hand, a new route beginning with ethyl 2,3-dibromopropionate has been published recently in which additional chiral resolution step is necessary to obtained enantiomerically pure LCM (method B) (Bouvi et al., 2010).

2.2.7 Topiramate and zonisamide

Topiramate (Topamax®) is a highly effective anticonvulsant for the treatment of primary and secondary generalized tonic-clonic seizures as well as the Lennox Gastaut syndrome (Perucca, 1997). It differs from other AED in its structure, which is derived from D-fructose and also contains an unusual sulfamate functional group. Topiramate´s mechanism of action is not fully elucidated, but it shows inhibitory effect on voltage-dependent sodium channels and AMPA subtype glutamate receptor, and enhances some of $GABA_A$ receptors.

Zonisamide (ZNS, Zonegran®, Excegran ®) is another sulfonamide containing AED, effective as adjunctive therapy in adults with partial onset seizures (Schulze-Bonhage, 2010). With an unknown mechanism of action, it is reported to block voltage-dependent sodium channels, which would lead to inhibit the spread of epileptiform activity, and the reduction of T-type calcium channel currents, or to inhibit the uptake of the inhibitory neurotransmitter GABA while enhancing the uptake of the excitatory neurotransmitter glutamate. ZNS is generally well-tolerated but also associated to various side effects such as drowsiness, loss of appetite, gastrointestinal problems and CNS toxicity. However, the rare occurrence of nephrolithiasis suggests a careful monitorization of patients.

Sulfonamide containing AEDs are prepared *via* amidation of the corresponding sulfonyl derivative as last step. Thus, topiramate is readily available from D-fructose by condensation with acetone and transformation of the pendant hydroxyl group into a sulfonate derivative before amidation. Among the different reagents described for the sulfamoylation step, chlorosulfonyl isocyanate is the one providing better results regarding safety and effectiveness (Arvai eta al., 2006). For other hand, the synthesis of ZNS has been accomplished following two general and complementary approaches: through a 1,2-benzisoxazole-3-acetic acid intermediate derived from 4-hydroxycoumarin (method A) and the conversion of methyl salicylate into 1,2-benzoxathiin-4(3*H*)-one-2,2-dioxide, which is reacted with hydroxylamine to afford the corresponding sulfonyl 1,2-benzisoxazole in a later step (method B)(Arava et al., 2007). Despite the similarities between these two routes, the application of method A using chlorosulfonic acid as sulfonylating reagent has offered a higher-yielding (65% overall yield) and cost-effective process (Nageib et al., 2008)

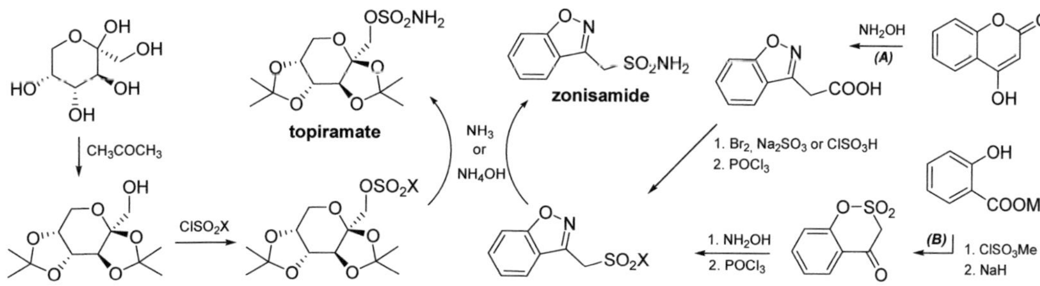

Scheme 15. General methods for the synthesis of topiramate and zonisamide.

2.2.8 Lamotrigine

In addition to being approved in 1994 as an adjunctive treatment of partial seizures in adults, lamotrigine (LTG, Lamictal®) has shown since then a broad spectrum of antiepileptic activity (Malik et al., 2006). It may stabilize neuronal membranes by inhibition of voltage-sensitive sodium channel, but still the mechanism of action is unknown. Alternative to VPA, LTG shows a better side effect profile and also an important safety record in pregnancy, which makes it as the AED of choice in pregnant women with epilepsy (Sabers & Tomson, 2009).

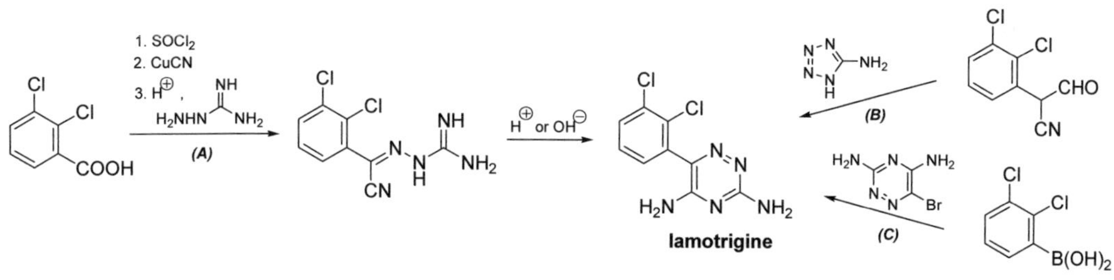

Scheme 16. General methods for the synthesis of lamotrigine.

The different methods for preparation of LTG can be classified according to the existing approaches for the formation of the triazine heterocyclic ring. The acid or base promoted intramolecular cyclization of aminoguanidine intermediates (method A) consists of the most studied and effective route so far, providing desired LTG product in moderate yield (52%) (Dalmasses Barjoan & Bessa Bellmunt, 2004). Alternatively, the synthesis of LTG has been also accomplished by using tetrazolamine instead of aminoguanidine (method B)(Ulomskii et al., 2005) or by the direct Suzuki coupling of a preformed diamino triazine halide with the corresponding boronic acid (method C) (Titirmare, 2007). But despite the potential applicability of these two approaches, the preparation of required intermediates as well as the poor reaction yields obtained limits considerably their scope.

2.3 New generation AEDs

Despite the continuous research and advances in the field, none of the currently available treatments for epilepsy accomplishes satisfactory control of seizures without causing important side effects. Therefore, ongoing studies towards the development of new AEDs regarding efficiency, tolerability and safety have been carried out and have lead to a new generation of AEDs, most of which have already undergone preclinical and clinical studies (Bialer et al., 2010; Stephen & Brodie, 2011). Some of these new candidates are optimized analogues of known AEDs, such as eslicarbazepine acetate (see section 2.11 for more details) or brivaracetam, but most of them are being developed with novel mechanisms and clinical characteristics compared with previous AEDs: Perampanel was designed as an AMPA-type glutamate receptor antagonist, retigabine modulates neuronal $K_V7.2$–7.5 voltage-activated K^+ channels while 2-deoxy-D-glucose acts on the NRSF-CtBP–dependent metabolic regulation of chromatin structure.

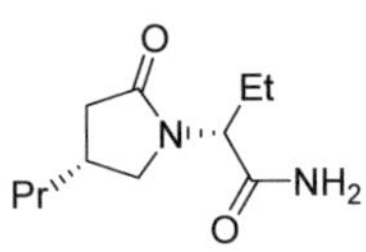

brivaracetam

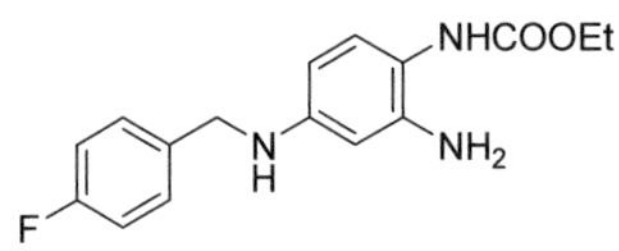

retigabine

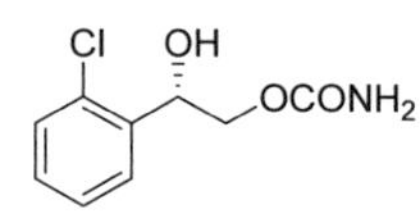

carisbamate

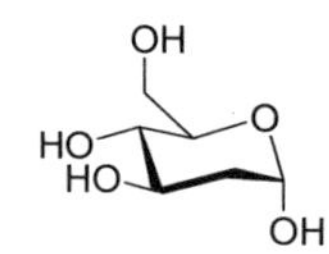

2-deoxy-D-glucose

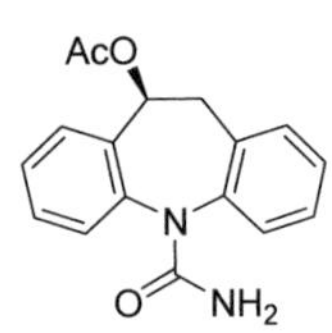

eslicarbazepine acetate

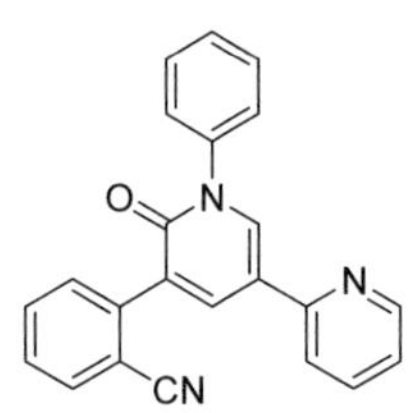

perampanel

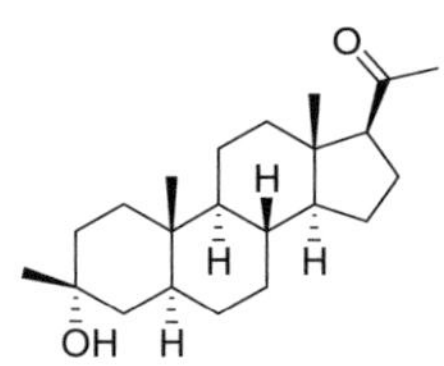

ganaxolone

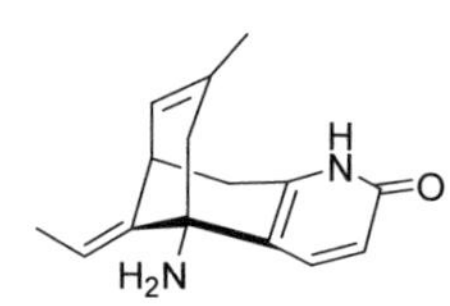

Huperzine A

Scheme 17. Chemical structures of the new generation of AEDs.

Given the heterogeneity of their functions, they show big differences on their chemical structures as well as their occurrence. Thus, Huperzine A is a natural sesquiterpene alkaloid and both 2-deoxy-D-glucose and ganaxolone are analogues and therefore easily available from D-glucose and progesterone respectively. Most of the new AEDs, nevertheless, are synthetic small molecules whose preparation processes are not yet reported or even with unknown structures as for ICA-105665, NAX 5055 or YKP3089 candidates.

3. Conclusion

To sum up, there is a broad spectrum of compounds active against several seizure types. In addition to the synthetic approaches patented by the pharmaceutical companies that discovered or marketed them, an acceptable (and in some cases overwhelming) number of preparation strategies to these AEDs have been reported, thus overcoming in some cases problems (low overall yields, long sequences, harsh conditions, etc.) encountered in the initial protocols. Since a variety of structural motifs (dibenzoazepines, imidazodiones, benzodiazepines, piperidines, triazines, isoxazoles, pyrrolidinones, etc.) has proved activity in antiepileptic therapy, a complete arsenal of synthetic tools has been required for their preparation. It becomes clear to the reader that a valuable evolution from classical transformations to modern (stereoselective, catalytic, more sustainable) procedures has occurred also in this field. However, only in a limited number of cases can be found whole approaches with an extensive scope, that is, applicable to the preparation of a reasonably diverse series of structural analogs that could provide more effective drugs and/or reduced side-effects. One of the main features of the aforementioned evolution in the future will be probably related to filling the latter gap.

4. Acknowledgment

This research was supported by the University of the Basque Country/Basque Government (Projects GIC10/52/IT-370-10 and Saiotek S-PC10UN10).

5. References

Andersen, K. E.; Braestrup, C.; Gronwald, F.C.; Jørgensen, A.S.; Nielsen, E.B.; Sonnewald, U.; Sørensen, P.O.; Suzdak, P.D. & Knutsen, L.J.S. (1993). The Synthesis of Novel GABA Uptake Inhibitors. 1. Elucidation of the Structure-Activity Studies Leading to the Choice of (R)-1-[4,4-Bis(3-methyl-2-thienyl)-3-butenyl]-3-piperidinecarboxylic Acid (Tiagabine) as an Anticonvulsant Drug Candidate. *J. Med. Chem.*, Vol.36, No.12, (June 1993), pp. 1716-1725, ISSN 0022-2623.

Arava, V.R.; Siripalli, U.B.R.; Nadkarni, V. & Chinnapillai, R. (2007). Novel base catalyzed rearrangement of sultone oximes to 1,2-benzisoxazole-3-methane sulfonate derivatives. *Beilstein J. Org. Chem.*, Vol.3, No.20, (June 2007), no pp. given, ISSN 1860-5397.

Arvai, G.; Garaczi, S.; Mate, A.G.; Lukacs, F.; Viski, Z. & Scheider, G. (2006). Process for the preparation of topiramate. *U.S. Pat. Appl.*, US 2006/0040874 A1, (23 February 2006), 10pp.

Ashton, H. (1994). Guidelines for the rational use of benzodiazepines. When and what to use. *Drugs*, Vol.48, No.1, (July 1994), pp. 25-40, ISSN 0012-6667.

Ates, C.; Surtees, J.; Burteau, A.C.; Marmon, V. & Caboy, E. (2003). Oxopyrrolidine compounds, preparation of said compounds and their use in the manufacturing of levetiracetam and analogues. *PCT Int. Appl.*, WO 2003/014080 A2, (20 February 2003), 48pp.

Aufderhaar, E.; Sprecher, K.; Zergényi, J. (1980). Process for preparing 5-cyano-5H-dibenz(*b,f*)azepine and 5H-dibenz(*b,f*)azepine-5-carboxamide. *Eur. Pat. Appl.*, EP0029409 A1, (24 October 1980), 16pp.

Aufderhaar, E. (1981). Processes for the preparation of an oxo compound, and intermediates required therefor. *Eur. Pat. Appl.*, EP0028028 A2, (6 May 1981), 42 pp.

Badir, K.; Haj-Yehia, A.; Vree, T.B.; Kleijn, E.V.D. & Bialer, M. (1991). Pharmacokinetics and anticonvulsant activity of three monoesteric prodrugs of valproic acid. *Pharm. Res.*, Vol.8, No.6, (June 1991), pp. 750-753, ISSN 0724-8741.

Bartoli, B.; Cipolletti, R.; Di Antonio, A.; Giovannini, R.; Lanari, S.; Marcolini, M. & Marcantoni, E. (2010). A convergent approach to (R)-Tiagabine by a regio- and stereocontrolled hydroiodination of alkynes. *Org. Biomol. Chem.*, Vol.8, No.15, (July 2010), pp. 3509–3517, ISNN 1477-0520.

Bassas, O.; Huuskonen, J.; Rissanen, K. & Koskinen, A.M.P. (2009). A Simple Organocatalytic Enantioselective Synthesis of Pregabalin. *Eur. J. Org. Chem.* No.9, (March 2009), pp. 1340–1351, ISNN 1099-0690.

Benes, J.; Parada, A.; Figueiredo, A.A.; Alves, P.C.; Freitas, A.P.; Learmonth, D.A.; Cunha, R.A.; Garrett, J. & Soares-da-Silva, P. (1999). Anticonvulsant and sodium channel-blocking properties of novel 10,11-dihydro-5*H*-dibenz[*b,f*]azepine-5-carboxamide derivatives. *J. Med. Chem.*, Vol.42, No.14, (July 1999), pp. 2582-2587, ISSN 0022-2623.

Bialer, M.; Johannessen, S.I.; Levy, R.H.; Perucca, E.; Tomson, T. & White, H.S. (2010). Progress report on new antiepileptic drugs: a summary of the Tenth Eilat Conference (EILAT X). *Epilepsy Res.* Vol.92, No.2-3, (December 2010), pp. 89-124, ISSN 0920-1211.

Bouvi, D.; Merschaert, A.; Pinilla, V.; Hamann, J.; Kanzler, J. & Thomas, A. (2010). Novel process for the preparation of amino acid derivatives. *PCT Int. Appl.*, WO 2010/052011 A1, (14 May 2010), 47pp.

Bryans, J.S. & Wustrow, D.J. (1999). 3-substituted GABA analogs with central nervous system activity: a review. *Med. Res. Rev.*, Vol.19, No.2, (March 1999), pp. 149-177, ISSN 1098-1128.

Carril, M.; SanMartin, R.; Churruca, F.; Tellitu, I. & Domínguez, E. (2005). An advantageous route to oxcarbazepine (Trileptal) based on palladium-catalyzed arylations free of transmetallating agents. *Org. Lett.*, Vol.7, No.22, (October 2005), pp. 4787-4789, ISSN 1523-7060.

Carril, M.; SanMartin, R.; Domínguez, E. & Tellitu, I. (2007). Sequential palladium-catalysed C- and N-arylation reactions as a practical and general protocol for the synthesis of the first series of oxcarbazepine analogues. *Tetrahedron*, Vol.63, No.3, (January 2007), pp. 690-702, ISSN 0040-4020.

Carril, M.; SanMartin, R. & Domínguez, E. (2007). Applications and synthesis of the antiepileptic drug oxcarbazepine and related structures. *Current Organic Chemistry*, Vol.11, No.15, (October 2007), pp. 1385-1399, ISSN 1385-2728.

Chung, S.S. (2009). Third-generation Antiepileptic Drugs for Partial-onset Seizures: Lacosamide, Retigabine, and Eslicarbazepine Acetate. *Eur. Neurol. J.*, Vol.1, No.1, (September 2009), pp. 1-12, ISSN 2041-8000.

Dalmasses Barjoan, P. & Bessa Bellmunt, J. (2004). Process for preparing a pharmaceutically active compound and for preparing its intermediate. *PCT Int. Appl.*, WO 2004/039767 A1, (13 May 2004), 17pp.

Eidenhammer, G.; Altreiter, J.; Schwendinger, K. (2000). Method of producing oxcarbazepine (=10,11-dihydro-10-oxo-5H-dibenz[*b,f*]azepine-5-carboxamide) and its intermediate products. *PCT Int. Appl.*, WO 2000/55138, (21 September 2000), 16pp.

Eroglu, C.; Allen, N.J.; Susman, M.W.; O'Rourke, N.A.; Park, C.Y.; Ozkan, E.; Chakraborty, C.; Mulinyawe, S.B.; Annis, D.S; Huberman, A.D; Green, E.M.; Lawler, J.; Dolmetsch, R.; Garcia, K.C.; Smith, S.J.; Luo, Z.D.; Rosenthal, A.; Mosher, D.F. &

Barres, B.A. (2009). Gabapentin receptor alpha2delta-1 is a neuronal thrombospondin receptor responsible for excitatory CNS synaptogenesis. *Cell*, Vol.139, No.2, (October 2009), pp. 380-392, ISSN 0092-8674.

Ferrari, M.; Ghezzi, M.; Belotti, P. (2004). Process for synthesis 1-(aminomethyl) cyclohexane acetic acid hydrochloride. *U.S. Pat. Appl.*, US 2004/063997 A1, (1 April 2004), 3pp.

Fuenfschilling, P.C.; Zaugg, W.; Beutler, U.; Kauffmann, D.; Lohse, O.; Mutz, J.-P.; Onken, U.; Reber, J.L. & Shenton, D. (2005). A new industrial process for oxcarbazepine. Org. Proc. Res. Dev., Vol.9, No.3, (May 2005), pp. 272-277, ISSN 1083-6160.

Gallagher, B.B. & Baumel, I.P. (1972). Primidone. Absorption, distribution, and excretion, In: *Antiepileptic Drugs*, Woodbury, D.M.; Penry, J.K. & Schmit, R.P., pp. 357-359, Raven Press, ISBN 089-0044-98-8, New York.

Grassi, S. & Volante, P. (2005). Process for preparation of 3-phosphoryloxymethyl-5,5-diphenylidantoin (fosphenytoin) by phosphorylation of 3-(chloromethyl) diphenylidantoin with tertiary ammonium phosphates formed in situ. *Ital. Appl.*, IT 2005/MI1145 A1, (17 September 2005), 10pp.

Grosso, S.; Franzoni, E.; Coppola, G.; Iannetti, P.; Verrotti, A.; Cordelli, D.M.; Marchiani, V.; Pascotto, A.; Spalice, A.; Acampora, B.; Morgese, G. & Balestri, P. (2005). Efficacy and safety of levetiracetam: an add-on trial in children with refractory epilepsy. *Seizure*, Vol.14, No.4, (June 2005), pp. 248-253, ISSN 1059-1311.

Gupta, N.; Singh, H.; Kumar, P. & Dubei, S.K. (2007). Process for producing oxcarbazepine via an 11-alkoxy-10-halo-dihydroxyiminostilbene intermediate. *PCT Int. Appl.*, WO 2007/141798 A1, (13 December 2007), 24pp.

Kaufmann, D.; Fünfschilling, P.C.; Beutler, U.; Hoehn, P.; Lohse, O. & Zaugg, W. (2004). A new synthesis of oxcarbazepine using a Friedel–Crafts cyclization strategy. *Tetrahedron Lett.*, Vol.45, No.27, (June 2004), pp. 5275-5278, ISNN *0040-4039.*

Karusala, N.R.; Tummalapally, U.S.S.; Talatala, A.R. & Datta, D. (2009). An improved process for the preparation of oxcarbazepine. *PCT Int. Appl.*, WO 2009/139001, (19 November 2009), 13pp.

Heckendorn, R.; Zergényi, J. & Ménard, E. (1982). Process for the transformation of 10,11-epoxi-10,11-dihydro-5H-dibenz[*b,f*]azepine in 10-oxo-10,11-dihydro-5H-dibenz[*b,f*]azepine. *Swiss Pat. Appl.*, CH633271 A5, (30 November 1982), 4pp.

Kenda, B.M.; Matagne, A.C.; Talaga, P.E.; Pasau, P.M.; Differding, E.; Lallemand, B.I.; Frycia, A.M.; Moureau, F.G.; Klitgaard, H.V.; Gillard, M.R.; Fuks,B. & Michel, P. (2004). Discovery of 4-Substituted Pyrrolidone Butanamides as New Agents with Significant Antiepileptic Activity. *J. Med. Chem.*, Vol.47, No.3, (January 2004), pp. 530-549, ISSN 0022-2623.

Klumpp, D.A.; Yeung, K.Y.; Prakash, G.K.; Surya; O. & George A. (1998) Superacid-activated condensation of parabanic acid and derivatives with arenes. A new synthesis of phenytoin and 5,5-diarylhydantoins. *Synlett*, No.8, (August 1998), pp. 918-920, ISSN: 0936-5214.

Krasowski, M.D. (2010) Therapeutic drug monitoring of the newer anti-epilepsy medications. *Pharmaceuticals* , Vol.3, No.6, (June 2010), pp. 1909-1935, ISNN 1424-4287.

Krauss, G.L.; Choi, J. & Tran, T. (2010). Third-Generation Antiepileptic Drugs for Treating Partial-Onset Seizures. *Eur. Neurol. J.*, Vol.2, No.2, (August 2010), pp. 1-8, ISNN 2041-8000.

Kwan, P. & Brodie, M.J. (2004). Phenobarbital for the treatment of epilepsy in the 21st century: a critical review. Epilepsia, Vol.45, No.9, (September 2004), pp. 1141–1149, ISNN *0013-9580.*

Learmonth, D.A. (2002). Method for the preparation of (S)-(+)- and (R)-(-)-10,11-dihydro-10-hydroxy-5H-dibenz[*b,f*]azepine-5-carboxamide. *PCT Int. Appl.*, WO 2002/092572 A, (21 November 2002), 29pp.

Learmonth, D.A.; Grasa, G.A. & Zanotti-Gerosa, A. (2007). Asymmetric catalytic reduction of oxcarbazepine. *PCT Int. Appl.*, WO 2007/012793 A1, (1 February 2007), 36pp.

Lohse, O.; Beutler, U.; Fünfschilling, P.; Furet, P.; France, J.; Kaufmann, D.; Penn, G. & Zaugg, W. (2001). New synthesis of oxcarbazepine via remote metalation of protected *N-o*-tolyl-anthranilamide derivatives. *Tetrahedron Lett.*, Vol.42, No.3, (January 2001), pp. 385-389, ISNN *0040-4039.*

Luer, M. S. (1998). Fosphenytoin. *Neurol. Res.*, Vol.20, No.2 (March 1998), pp. 178–182, ISSN 0161-6412.

Mac Leod, T.C.O.; Faria, A.L.; Barros, V.P.; Queiroz, M.E.C. & Assis, M.D. (2008). Primidone oxidation catalyzed by metalloporphyrins and Jacobsen catalyst. *J. Mol. Catal. A Chem.*, Vol.296, No.1-2, (December 2008), pp. 54-60, ISSN 1381-1169.

Malawska, B. & Kulig, K. (2008). Brivaracetam: a new drug in development for epilepsy and neuropathic pain. Expert Opin. Investig. Drugs, Vol.17, No.3, (March 2008), pp.361-369, ISSN 1354-3784.

Malik, S.; Arif, H. & Hirsch, L.J. (2006). Lamotrigine and its applications in the treatment of epilepsy and other neurological and psychiatric disorders. *Expert Rev. Neurother.*, Vol.6, No.11, (November 2006), pp. 1609-1627, ISSN 1473-7175.

Morieux, P.; Stables, J. P. & Kohn, H. (2008). Synthesis and anticonvulsant activities of N-benzyl (2R)-2-acetamido-3-oxysubstituted propionamide derivatives. *Bioorg. Med. Chem.*, Vol.16, No.19, (October 2008), pp. 8968–8975, ISSN 0968-0896.

Nagarajan, K.; Gupta, R.P.; Murugan, A. & Revanasiddhayya, S. (2009). A process for the preparation of valproic acid. *Indian Pat. Appl.* IN 2008/CH01148 A, (13 November 2009), 13pp.

Nageib, M.; Eckardt, W.; Weeratunga, C.G.; Rey, G.; Guntoori, A.W. & Reddy, B. Process for preparation of zonisamide and intermediates. *Can. Pat. Appl.*, CA 2578559 A1, (14 August 2008), 27pp.

Pellock, J.M. & Boggs, J.G. (1995). Felbamate: a unique anticonvulsant. *Drugs Today*, Vol.31, No.1, (January 1995), pp. 9-17, ISNN 1699-3993

Perucca, E. (1997). A Pharmacological and Clinical Review on Topiramate, a New Antiepileptic Drug. *Pharmacol. Res.*, Vol.35, No.4, (April 1997), pp. 241-256, ISNN 1043-6618.

Pinhey, J.T. & Rowe, B.A. (1980). The α-arylation of derivatives of mamnic acid with aryllead triacetates. New synthesis of ibuprofen and Phenobarbital. *Tetrahedron Lett.*, Vol.21, No.10, (March 1980), pp. 965–968, ISNN *0040-4039.*

Riedner, J. & Dunne, G. (2008). Synthesis scheme for lacosamide. *U.S. Pat. Appl.*, US 2008/027137 A1, (31 January 2008), 11pp.

Riss, J.; Cloyd, J.; Gates, J. & Collins, S. (2008). Benzodiazepines in epilepsy: pharmacology and pharmacokinetics. *Acta Neurol Scand.*, Vol.118, No.2, (August 2008), pp. 69-86, ISNN 0365-5598.

Roth, H.J. & Kleeman, A. (1988). *Pharmaceutical chemistry. Volume 1. Drug synthesis.* John Wiley and Sons, ISBN 047-0210-37-0, New York.

Sabers, A. & Tomson, T. (2009). Managing antiepileptic drugs during pregnancy and lactation. *Curr. Opin. Neurol.*, Vol.22, No.2 (April 2009), pp. 157–161, ISSN 1350-7540.

Safari, J.; Naeimi, H.; Ghanbari, M.M. & Sabzi Fini, O. (2009). Preparation of Phenytoin Derivatives under Solvent-Free Conditions Using Microwave Irradiation. *Russian J. Org. Chem.*, Vol.45, No.3, (March 2009), pp. 477-479, ISSN 1070-4280.

Santaniello, M.; Bagolini, C.A.; Uttaro, A. & Fontana, S. (1998). Process for producing valproic acid. *Eur. Pat. Appl.*, EP0835859 A1, (15 April 1998), 9pp.

Schachter, S.C. (1999). A review of the anti-epileptic drug tiagabine. *Clin. Neuropharmacol.*, Vol.22, No.6 (November-December 1999), pp. 312-317, ISSN 0362-5664.

Schindler, W. (1958). Methods for the synthesis of N-substituted azepines. *German Pat.*, DE1136707, (19 December 1958), 2pp.

Schmitt, J. (1970). 1,4-Benzodiazepine-2-ones having a carboxylic acid ester or amide group in the 3-position. *US. Pat.*, 3516988, (23 June 1970), 15pp.

Schulze-Bonhage, A. (2010). Zonisamide in the treatment of epilepsy. *Expert Opin. Pharmacother.*, Vol.11, No.1, (January 2010), pp. 115-126, ISNN 1465-6566.

Stephen, L.J.& Brodie, M.J. (2011) Pharmacotherapy of epilepsy: newly approved and developmental agents. *CNS Drugs*. Vol.25, No.2, (February 2011), pp. 89-107, ISNN 1172-7047.

Surtees, J. Lurquin, F. & Diouf, O. (2005). Process for preparing 2-oxo-1-pyrrolidine derivatives. *PCT Int. Appl.*, WO 2005/028435, (31 March 2005), 19pp.

Titirmare, S. (2007). Process for the preparation of lamotrigine. *Indian Pat. Appl.*, IN 2005/MU01166 A, (20 July 2007), 16pp.

Tunnicliff, G. (1997). Basis of the antiseizure action of phenytoin. *Gen. Pharmacol.*, Vol.27, No.7 (October 1997), pp. 1091-1097, ISNN 0306-3623.

Ulomskii, E.N.; Shestakova, T.S.; Deev, S.L.; Rusinov, V.L. & Chupakhin, O.N. (2005), A new approach to the synthesis of lamotrigine and other 3,5-diamino-1,2,4-triazine derivatives. *Russian Chem. Bull.*, Vol.54, No.3, (March 2005), pp. 726-732, ISNN 1066-5285.

Vardanyan, R. & Hruby, V. (2006). *Synthesis of essential drugs*. pp. 130-133. Elsevier Ltd., ISBN 044-4521-66-6, Amsterdam.

Walker, D. Babad, E.; Tann, C.-H.; Kwok, D.-L.; Belski, K.A. & Herczeg, L. (1994). Process for preparing felbamate, 2-phenyl-1,3-propanediol and intermediates. *PCT Int. Appl.*, WO94/06737 A1, (31 March 1994), 34pp.

Yu, B.; Li, W. & Learmonth, D.A. (2007). 10-Acyloxy-5H-dibenz[*b,f*]azepine-5-carboxamides and their asymmetric hydrogenation to the chiral 10,11-dihydro derivatives. *UK Pat. Appl.*, GB 2437078 A, (11 April 2007), 34pp.

Zeiler, A. G. (1994). Process for producing lower alkanoic acids. *U.S. Pat.*, US005344975 A, (06 September 1994), 6pp.

2

Different Mechanisms Underlying the Antiepileptic and Antiparkinsonian Effects of Zonisamide

Motohiro Okada[1] and Sunao Kaneko[2]
[1]Department of psychiatry, Brain science and animal model research center (BSAM), Graduate school of medicine, Mie University
[2]Department of neuropsychiatry, Graduate school of medicine, Hirosaki University, Japan

1. Introduction

Zonisamide (ZNS, 3-sulfamoylmethyl-1,2-benzisoxazole) was developed by Dainippon Pharma (Osaka, Japan: currently Dainippon Sumitomo Pharma) and is currently used as an antiepileptic drug (AED) in Japan, South Korea, USA and Europe (Seino, 2004; Seino & Leppik, 2007). Indeed, the wide antiepileptic spectrum of ZNS has been established (Brodie, 2004; Karceski et al., 2005; Seino, 2004; Seino & Leppik, 2007; Willmore, 2004). Several clinical studies have also reported the wide clinical spectrum of ZNS against psychiatric and non-epileptic neurological disorders, including mood disorders (Ghaemi et al., 2008; Ghaemi et al., 2006; Kanba et al., 1994; McElroy et al., 2005), essential tremors (Bermejo, 2007), and its protective effects against ischemic cerebral damage (Willmore, 2004) and Parkinson's disease (Murata, 2004; Murata et al., 2007). In Japan, ZNS was approved for Parkinson's disease in 2009 by the Ministry of Health, Labor and Welfare. In this chapter, we review the dose-dependent effects of ZNS on neurotransmission and differences in the mechanisms underlying its antiepileptic and antiparkinsonian effects.

2. Antiepileptic mechanisms of ZNS

The major mechanism underlying the antiepileptic effects of ZNS (Rogawski & Porter, 1990) is inhibition of the voltage-gated Na^+ channel (Rock et al., 1989; Schauf, 1987). However, subsequent pharmacological studies have demonstrated that the target molecules of ZNS include T-type voltage-sensitive Ca^{2+} channel (Kito et al., 1996; Suzuki et al., 1992), Ca^{2+} induced Ca^{2+} releasing system (CICR) (Yamamura et al., 2009b; Yoshida et al., 2005), carbonic anhydrase (Yamamura et al., 2009a), redox (Tokumaru et al., 2000; Ueda et al., 2005; Ueda et al., 2003), neuronal depolarization-induced glutamate release (Okada et al., 1998; Yoshida et al., 2005), enhancement of release of inhibitory neurotransmitters, e.g., GABA (Yoshida et al., 2005), dopamine and serotonin (Murakami et al., 2001; Okada et al., 1999; Okada et al., 1992; Okada et al., 1995) and lack of affinity to $GABA_A$ receptor (Rock et al., 1989).

With regard to its antiparkinsonian action, ZNS enhances both the turnover and release of dopamine, and inhibits MAO-B activity and dopaminergic oxidative stress (Asanuma et al.,

2008; Komatsu et al., 2000; Leppik, 2004; Mori et al., 1998; Murata, 2004; Okada et al., 1992; Okada et al., 1995; Ueda et al., 2005). While the typical dose of ZNS is 300 to 600 mg/day for patients with epilepsy (Seino et al., 1988), a significant improvement in motor symptoms is reported in patients of Parkinson's disease treated with only 25 to 100 mg/day of ZNS (Murata, 2004; Murata et al., 2007).

Ion channel blockade
- Voltage-gated Na^+ channel
  - Enhancement of Na^+ channel inactivation
  - Inhibition of seizure-related repetitive neural firing
- Enhancement of N-type~stage
  - Inhibition of T-type Ca^{2+} channel
  - Inhibition of L-type Ca^{2+} channel
  - Inhibition of N-type and P-type Ca^{2+} channel during hyperexcitable stage
  - Enhancement of N-type and P-type Ca^{2+} channel during resting stage
- Ca^{2+} -induced Ca^{2+} releasing (CICR) channel
  - Enhancement of IP3R during resting stage without affecting RyR activity
  - Inhibition of IP3R and RyR during hyperexcitable stage

Neurotransmitter modulation
- Neuronal exocytosis
  - Enhancement of syntaxin/N-type Ca^{2+} channel during resting stage
  - Inhibition of synaptobrevin/P-type Ca^{2+} channel during hyperexcitable stage
- Glutamatergic system
  - Inhibition of glutamate release during hyperexcitable stage
  - Enhancement of glutamate transporter expression
- GABAergic system
  - No affinity for GABA receptors
  - Binding allosterically to GABA receptors
  - Downregulation of GABA transporter
- Monoaminergic system
  - Enhancement of dopamine and serotonin releases within therapeutic range
  - Inhibition of dopamine and serotonin releases at supratherapeutic range
  - Inhibition of MOA-B
  - Enhancement of monoamine synthesis (enhancement of turnover)

Other systems
- Carbonic anhydrase
  - Inhibition of cytosolic, mitochondrial and plasma membrane binding subtypes
  - Prevention of conversion excitatory features of $GABA_A$ receptor induced by epileptic hyperexcitability
- Redox system
  - Scavenging against free radical associated with cytosolic and plasma membrance in epileptogenic foci
  - Inhibition of DNA damage under oxidative stress
  - Suppression of lipid oxidation

Table 1. Possible antiepileptic mechanism of ZNS

2.1 Effects of ZNS on ion channels

Preclinical studies suggested that ZNS inhibits the propagation of epileptic hyperexcitability through neuronal membrane stabilization and prevention of synchronization of firing (Macdonald, 2002; Rock et al., 1989; Rogawski & Porter, 1990; Schauf, 1987). Ample evidence indicates that the modulation of activities of several types of ion channels is the major mechanism of the antiepileptic effect of ZNS (Macdonald, 2002; Rogawski & Porter, 1990; Seino & Leppik, 2007).

2.1.1 Effects of ZNS on voltage-gated Na^+ channel

The antiepileptic effects of ZNS on partial seizures are due to inhibition of voltage-gated Na^+ channels. In *in vitro* electrophysiological studies, ZNS reduced sustained repetitive firing by inhibiting voltage-gated Na^+ channels (Rock et al., 1989; Schauf, 1987). These inhibitory effects of ZNS probably increase the threshold of neuronal action potentials and lead a shift in the steady-state fast inactivation threshold of voltage-gated Na^+ channels (Macdonald, 2002; Rogawski & Porter, 1990; Seino & Leppik, 2007). The inhibitory effects of ZNS on Na^+ currents is probably induced by preferential binding to inactive voltage-gated Na^+ channels that produces use- and voltage-dependent blockade and slows the rate of recovery from inactivation (Macdonald, 2002)

2.1.2 Effects of ZNS on voltage-sensitive Ca^{2+} channel

The role of voltage-sensitive Ca^{2+} channel in epilepsy is entirely consistent with its ability to orchestrate numerous neuronal events thought to be altered in seizures such as neurotransmitter release, dendritic physiology, gene expression and notably epileptic seizure-induced neuronal apoptosis (Zhang et al., 2000). ZNS inhibits high-threshold voltage-sensitive Ca^{2+} channel (L-type Ca^{2+} channel)(Kito et al., 1996; Rossier et al., 1996). ZNS also inhibits low-threshold voltage-sensitive Ca^{2+} channel (T-type Ca^{2+} channel) in a concentration-dependent manner (Kito et al., 1996; Rossier et al., 1996; Suzuki et al., 1992). The T-type Ca^{2+} channel is activated by small depolarization of the neuronal plasma membrane; and the resulting Ca^{2+} influx generates low threshold spikes that can trigger a burst of action potentials mediated by Na^+ channels (Perez-Reyes, 2003). Therefore, antiepileptic actions of ZNS against childhood absence epilepsy and catastrophic childhood epilepsy are mediated through its inhibitory effects on T-type Ca^{2+} channel (Rogawski & Loscher, 2004a, b; White, 1999).

2.1.3 Effects of ZNS on CICR

The intraneuronal Ca^{2+} mobilization comprises both Ca^{2+} influx via voltage-sensitive Ca^{2+} channels and ligand-gated ion channels, as well as output from intracellular Ca^{2+} stores associated with the endoplasmic reticulum, namely the CICR, which is comprised of the ryanodine receptor (RyR) and inositol 1,4,5-trisphosphate receptor (IP3R) (Berridge, 1998). Several studies have indicated recently that functional abnormalities of CICR contribute to the rise in intraneuronal Ca^{2+} concentration associated with epileptic seizures (Matsumoto & Nagata, 1999; Matsumoto et al., 1996; Mori et al., 2005). Transient up-regulation of both c-Fos and Ryr-3 gene expression was observed in the hippocampus of the kainate-induced epilepsy model (Mori et al., 2005). Antagonists of both RyR and IP3R had no effect on the induction or persistence of epileptiform discharges, but both types of antagonists prevent seizure-induced neuronal death (Pal et al., 2001; Pelletier et al., 1999). During resting stage,

ZNS activates IP3R but has no effect on RyR (Yamamura et al., 2009c; Yoshida et al., 2005). Contrary to the resting stage, during neuronal hyperexcitability, ZNS inhibits the activities of both IP3R and RyR (Yamamura et al., 2009c; Yoshida et al., 2005). These actions of ZNS are similar to other antiepileptic drug, topiramate (Okada et al., 2005).

2.2 Effects of ZNS on other neuromodulating systems

2.2.1 Effects of ZNS on the redox system

Current research associates free radical damage with epilepsy (Komatsu et al 1995; Sudha et al 2001), and the use of antioxidants early in the treatment of seizure-related neuronal injury is an attractive strategy, since epileptic seizures cause neuronal cell damage through the production of free radicals (Komatsu et al., 2000; Sudha et al., 2001). ZNS protects neurons against free-radical damage by scavenging the hydroxyl and nitric oxide radicals and such action is dose-dependent (Leppik, 2004; Mori et al., 1998; Noda et al., 1999). Especially, ZNS provides scavenging effects against cytosolic and plasma membrane-targeting free radicals in epileptogenic foci (Komatsu et al., 2000; Tokumaru et al., 2000; Ueda et al., 2005; Ueda et al., 2003). The radical scavenging properties operate in not only the ZNS-related antiepileptic activity but also its neuroprotective action against hypoxic/ischemic brain damage (Hayakawa et al., 1994; Owen et al., 1997).

2.2.2 Effects of ZNS on carbonic anhydrase

It was initially thought that the inhibitory effects of ZNS on carbonic anhydrase do not contribute to the antiepileptic action of ZNS, since the IC_{50} value of ZNS is 188 times less potent than that of acetazolamide (Masuda & Karasawa, 1993). However, subsequent studies demonstrated that different affinities to carbonic anhydrase subtypes (Casini et al., 2003; Supuran, 2008). The Ki values for ZNS on cytosolic hCAII (35 nM), mitochondrial hCAV (20 nM) and plasma membrane binding hCAIX (5.1 nM) (Casini et al., 2003; Supuran, 2008) are lower than the therapeutic-relevant plasma concentrations of ZNS (Okada et al., 1999; Okada et al., 1995; Yamamura et al., 2009a). Activation of $GABA_A$ receptor opens its Cl^- channel, which is permeable to both HCO_3^- efflux and Cl^- influx (Staley et al., 1995). Under physiological conditions, the hyperpolarizing action of the Cl^- influx abolishes the depolarizing effect of HCO_3^- efflux (Staley et al., 1995). In contrast to physiological conditions, continuous neuronal hyperactivation, e.g., epileptic seizure, results in an increase in intraneuronal Cl^- concentration (Ge et al., 2006; Ge et al., 2007; Okada et al., 2003). A rise in Cl^- concentration in the synaptic active zone stimulates $GABA_A$ receptor to produce depolarizing action (Ge et al., 2006; Ge et al., 2007). Inhibition of carbonic anhydrase reduces intraneuronal HCO_3^- concentration with enhancement of Na^+-independent Cl^-/HCO_3^- exchange (Leniger et al., 2004). Thus, ZNS prevents the epileptic hyperexcitability-induced conversion of $GABA_A$ receptor activity from inhibitory to excitatory activity (Yamamura et al., 2009a).

2.3 Effects of ZNS on neurotransmitter system

The generation of epileptic seizures could be due to a relative imbalance between excitatory and inhibitory neurotransmission, resulting in increased neuronal excitability and abnormally frequent patterns of discharge (Hirose et al., 2000; Okada et al., 2002). Glutamate is one of the main excitatory neurotransmitters, and excessive release of glutamate seems to precipitate seizures in epileptic patients and in animal models of epilepsy (Hirose et al.,

2000; Okada et al., 2002). In contrast to glutamate, various other neurotransmitters, e.g., GABA, dopamine, serotonin and acetylcholine, are involve in the regulation of inhibitory transmission (Hirose et al., 2000; Okada et al., 2002; Okada et al., 2010).

2.3.1 Effects of ZNS on glutamatergic system

Both systemic administration of therapeutically-relevant dose and local perfusion of therapeutically-relevant concentration of ZNS reduced depolarization induced glutamate release in the hippocampus and frontal cortex (Okada et al., 1998; Yamamura et al., 2009a; Yamamura et al., 2009b; Yamamura et al., 2009c; Yoshida et al., 2005). It has been demonstrated that continuous stimulation induced by glutamate release has several components: (1) a Ca^{2+}-dependent initial rise, which is neuronal activity-independent, (2) this initial rise s followed by a series of Ca^{2+}-dependent phasic rises associated with neuronal activity, and (3) a small overflow of glutamate that persists in a Ca^{2+}-independent manner (Obrenovitch et al., 1993; Obrenovitch et al., 1996; Okada et al., 1998; Zilkha et al., 1995). Especially, the third component, which is Ca^{2+} independent and neuronal activity independent glutamate release, is probably spreading depression induced release (Okada et al., 1998). Therapeutically relevant concentrations of ZNS inhibit these three types of glutamate effects in the hippocampus (Okada et al., 1998).

2.3.2 Effects of ZNS on GABAergic system

ZNS has dual action against GABAergic transmission; enhancement of GABA release and protection against conversion $GABA_A$ receptor activity from inhibitory to excitatory action. ZNS tends to enhance the inhibitory function of $GABA_A$ receptor through interaction at allosteric or other binding sites (Mimaki et al., 1988) and GABAergic transmission via down-regulation of GABA transporter (Ueda et al., 2003). Inhibition of carbonic anhydrase reduces intraneuronal HCO_3^- concentration with enhancement of Na^+-independent Cl^-/HCO_3^- exchange (Leniger et al., 2004). Although there is no direct evidence that it activates $GABA_A$ receptor-associated neuronal events, ZNS enhances the Cl^- currents associated with $GABA_A$ receptor (Mimaki et al., 1988). These actions of ZNS are possibly modulated by inhibition of carbonic anhydrase activity similar to topiramate (Sills et al., 2000). Both systemic administration of therapeutically-relevant dose and local perfusion of therapeutically-relevant concentration of ZNS increased and decreased the basal and depolarization-induced releases of GABA in the hippocampus and frontal cortex, respectively (Okada et al., 1998; Yamamura et al., 2009a; Yamamura et al., 2009b; Yamamura et al., 2009c; Yoshida et al., 2005). Furthermore, the inhibitory interneurons release GABA (Hirose et al., 2000; Okada et al., 2002; Staley et al., 1995; Zhu et al., 2008).

2.3.3 Effects of ZNS on monoamine release

Systemic administration of ZNS affects monoamine release in the hippocampus, frontal cortex and striatum in a biphasic dose-dependent manner (Kawata et al., 1999; Murakami et al., 2001; Okada et al., 1999; Okada et al., 1992; Okada et al., 1995; Okada et al., 2002). At therapeutically-relevant dose, ZNS increases extracellular levels of monoamines, whereas ZNS at supra-therapeutic dose decreases monoamine release (Kawata et al., 1999; Murakami et al., 2001; Okada et al., 1999; Okada et al., 1992; Okada et al., 1995; Okada et al., 2002). Similar to its effect on the release of monoamines, both acute and chronic administration of therapeutically-relevant doses of ZNS enhance the turnover of dopamine and serotonin (i.e., monoamine synthesis) (Okada et al., 1999; Okada et al., 1992; Okada et al., 1995). In addition, ZNS inhibits monoamine oxidase activity. These stimulatory effects of ZNS on monoaminergic transmission, via enhancement of monoamine synthesis and release with inhibition of monoamine degradation, are observed after chronic administration (Okada et al., 1999; Okada et al., 1992; Okada et al., 1995).

3. Antiparkinsonian mechanisms of ZNS

In an open clinical trial of a combination of ZNS (50-200 mg/day) with antiparkinsonian drugs showed lessening of symptoms, wearing off of Parkinson's disease, and more than 30% improvement of total score of the Unified Parkinson's Disease Rating Score up to 3 years (Murata, 2004; Murata et al., 2001). The addition of ZNS to L-DOPA treatment in patients experiencing "wearing-off" fluctuations resulted in lessening of motor fluctuation and significant improvement of the duration, severity, and activities of daily living in "off " time and the score of motor examination. A more recent double blind controlled study from Japan demonstrated that the combination of lower than antiepileptically-relevant dose of ZNS (25-100 mg/day) and L-DOPA improved all cardinal symptoms of Parkinson's disease (Murata et al., 2007). Based on these clinical evidences, ZNS was released for use in Japan in March 2009 as a novel antiparkinsonian agent.

In a series of studies, we have reported a dose-dependent biphasic action for ZNS on striatal dopaminergic system, e.g., ZNS at 25–50 mg/kg (i.p.) increased whereas at 100 mg/kg (i.p.) it decreased striatal dopamine release. However, ZNS at lower than antiepileptically-relevant dose of ZNS failed to modulate striatal dopaminergic transmission (Murakami et al., 2001; Okada et al., 1999; Okada et al., 1992; Okada et al., 1995; Yamamura et al., 2009b). These results suggest possible differences in the mechanisms of the antiepileptic and antiparkinsonian actions of ZNS. In this regard, the mechanism of the antiparkinsonian action of ZNS remains poorly understood.

Ion channel blockade

- Inhibition of T-type voltage-sensitive Ca^{2+} channel
- Inhibition of dopamine-quinone formation
- Enhancement of glutathione synthesis
- Enhancement of transmission in indirect pathway

Table 2. Possible antiparkinsonian mechanism of ZNS

3.1 Inhibition of dopamine quinone formation

Under normal conditions, dopamine is stable in the synaptic vesicle; however, administration of L-DOPA to patients with Parkinson's disease damages the dopaminergic neuronal system (Sulzer et al., 2000). In patients with Parkinson's disease treated with L-DOPA, a large amount of dopamine remains in the cytosol away from the synaptic vesicle, since the damaged dopaminergic system has only a small dopamine pool for storage (Asanuma et al., 2008; Asanuma et al., 2003; Ogawa et al., 2005; Sulzer et al., 2000).

Despite the beneficial effects of L-DOPA, the toxicity of excess L-DOPA and dopamine has been well documented in many in vitro and in vivo animal studies using parkinsonian models (Asanuma et al., 2008; Asanuma et al., 2003; Ogawa et al., 2005; Sulzer et al., 2000).

Free excess dopamine is easily metabolized via type-B monoamine oxidase (MAO-B) or by auto-oxidation to produce cytotoxic reactive oxygen species (ROS), and then forms neuromelanin (Sulzer et al., 2000). In the oxidation of dopamine by MAO-B, dopamine is converted to DOPAC to generate general ROS hydrogen peroxide (Sulzer et al., 2000). Conversely, non-enzymatic and spontaneous auto-oxidation of L-DOPA and dopamine produces superoxide and reactive quinones, dopamine-quinone and DOPA-quinone, (Asanuma et al., 2003; Ogawa et al., 2005; Sulzer et al., 2000; Tse et al., 1976). The highly reactive dopamine-quinone or DOPA-quinone itself exerts predominant cytotoxicity in dopaminergic neurons and surrounding neurons, since these quinones are generated from free cytosolic dopamine away from the synaptic vesicle or from L-DOPA (Sulzer et al., 2000).

ZNS prevents dopamine-quinone formation induced by excess amount of cytosolic dopamine outside the synaptic vesicles (Asanuma et al., 2008).

3.2 Enhancement of glial glutathione synthesis

Glutathione acts as an antioxidant against ROS–induced neurodegeneration. Astrocytes, but not neurons, express cystine/glutamate exchange transporter, which takes up cystine, reduces it to cysteine, and consequently supplies cysteine, the substrate for glutathione synthesis, in neurons. Glutathione synthesis in neurons is dependent on the expression of the cystine/glutamate exchange transporter on astrocytes (Shih et al., 2006; Wang & Cynader, 2000). Other studies demonstrated that glutathione and its synthesis-related molecules provide protection for astrocytes against age-dependent nigrostriatal dopaminergic neuro-degeneration (Chinta et al., 2007; Solano et al., 2008). ZNS markedly increased glutathione levels by enhancing the astroglial cystine/glutamate exchange transporter and astroglial proliferation via S100β production or secretion. ZNS acts as a neuroprotectant against oxidative stress and progressive dopaminergic neurodegeneration (Asanuma et al., 2010).

3.3 Enhancement of transmission striato-pallidal indirect pathway

Parkinson's disease is characterized neuropathologically by a relative and selective loss of dopaminergic projection neurons within the substantia nigra pars compacta (SNc), and the formation of cytoplasmic inclusions within many surviving neurons (Gibb, 1991). The reduced population of dopaminergic neurons in SNc leads to the development of classical symptoms of Parkinson's disease through functional abnormalities in striatal output pathways, which are composed of direct and indirect pathways (Hauber, 1998). In the rat brain, the direct pathway is composed of striatal GABAergic neurons, which project to the substantia nigra pars reticulata (SNr), a region under dopamine D_1 receptor-mediated stimulatory regulation (Hauber, 1998). The indirect pathway comprises the striatal GABAergic neurons that project to the globus pallidus (GP) and are under dopamine D_2 receptor-mediated inhibitory regulation, the pallidal GABAergic neurons that project to the nucleus subthalamicus (STN) and the subthalamic glutamatergic neurons that project to GP and SNr (Hauber, 1998). Indeed, depletion of dopaminergic transmission produces over-inhibition of pallido-subthalamic GABAergic and disinhibition of subthalamonigral glutamatergic projections in the indirect pathway (DeLong, 1990; Hauber, 1998). Enkephalin is colocalized and acts as cotransmitter with GABA in striatal neurons that project to GP; however, enkephalin reduces the GABAergic inhibition in the indirect pathway via

inhibition of GABA release (Maneuf et al., 1994). Based on these effects, the δ opioid receptor and its endogenous agonist enkephalin have been proposed as a suitable target in the symptomatic therapy of Parkinson's disease (Hille et al., 2001; Maneuf et al., 1994).
Local administration of antiepileptic-relevant concentrations of ZNS in the striatum increases dopamine release, whereas the use of antiparkinsonian-relevant concentration of ZNS does not affect striatal dopamine release (Yamamura et al., 2009b). Local administration of both antiparkinsonian- and antiepileptic-relevant concentrations of ZNS in the striatum reduces the extracellular levels of GABA in STN and glutamate in SNr, but decreases extracellular levels of GABA in GP without affecting their level in SNr (Yamamura et al., 2009b). These concentration-dependent effects of ZNS on extracellular neurotransmitter levels are independent of dopamine and δ2 receptors; however, blockade of δ1 receptor inhibited the effects of ZNS (Yamamura et al., 2009b). Activation of δ1 receptor enhances the effects of ZNS on neurotransmitter level. Based on these results, we suggest that ZNS does not affect the direct pathway but inhibits the δ1 receptor-mediated indirect pathway.

4. Conclusion

It has been well established that ZNS is the first line antiepileptic drug in the treatment of partial, absence and generalized epilepsies. In addition, ZNS is a potentially useful agent in the treatment of Parkinson's disease. Its antiepileptic potential has been demonstrated in several clinical studies and meta-analysis studies; however, the antiparkinsonian potential has been demonstrated in only one randomized, placebo-controlled study.
The mechanisms of the antiepileptic action of ZNS have been investigated through various basic experiments, whereas the antiparkinsonian mechanisms remain to be clarified. Interestingly, the dose of ZNS used for the treatment of patients with Parkinson's disease is lower than its therapeutic range against epilepsy. To our knowledge, the pharmacological profile within the antiparkinsonian dose has demonstrated only an increase in glutathione synthesis and enhancement of transmission through the indirect pathway. Enhancement of the indirect pathway is probably involved in the improvement of symptoms of Parkinson's disease. In contrast, activation of glutathione synthesis prevents the progression of Parkinson's disease rather than improves symptoms. Therefore, ZNS likely improves long-term prognosis. More information is required to clarify the effects of ZNS on long-term prognosis of patients with Parkinson's disease (the long-term efficacy of ZNS). Based on clinical experience in the treatment of epilepsy for more than 20 years in Japan, ZNS is a relatively safe and well tolerated drug.

5. References

Asanuma, M., Miyazaki, I., Diaz-Corrales, F. J., Kimoto, N., Kikkawa, Y., Takeshima, M., Miyoshi, K. & Murata, M. (2010). Neuroprotective effects of zonisamide target astrocyte. *Ann Neurol* Vol. 67, pp. 239-249, ISSN 1531-8249

Asanuma, M., Miyazaki, I., Diaz-Corrales, F. J., Miyoshi, K., Ogawa, N. & Murata, M. (2008). Preventing effects of a novel anti-parkinsonian agent zonisamide on dopamine quinone formation. *Neurosci Res* Vol. 60, pp. 106-113, ISSN 0168-0102

Asanuma, M., Miyazaki, I. & Ogawa, N. (2003). Dopamine- or L-DOPA-induced neurotoxicity: the role of dopamine quinone formation and tyrosinase in a model of Parkinson's disease. *Neurotox Res* Vol. 5, pp. 165-176, ISSN 1029-8428

Bermejo, P. E. (2007). Zonisamide in patients with essential tremor and Parkinson's disease. *Mov Disord* Vol. 22, pp. 2137-2138, ISSN 0885-3185

Berridge, M. J. (1998). Neuronal calcium signaling. *Neuron* Vol. 21, pp. 13-26,

Brodie, M. J. (2004). Zonisamide clinical trials: European experience. *Seizure* Vol. 13 Suppl 1, pp. S66-72,

Casini, A., Abbate, F., Scozzafava, A. & Supuran, C. T. (2003). Carbonic anhydrase inhibitors: X-ray crystallographic structure of the adduct of human isozyme II with a bis-sulfonamide-two heads are better than one? *Bioorg Med Chem Lett* Vol. 13, pp. 2759-2763, ISSN 0960-894X

Chinta, S. J., Kumar, M. J., Hsu, M., Rajagopalan, S., Kaur, D., Rane, A., Nicholls, D. G., Choi, J. & Andersen, J. K. (2007). Inducible alterations of glutathione levels in adult dopaminergic midbrain neurons result in nigrostriatal degeneration. *J Neurosci* Vol. 27, pp. 13997-14006, ISSN 1529-2401

DeLong, M. R. (1990). Primate models of movement disorders of basal ganglia origin. *Trends Neurosci* Vol. 13, pp. 281-285, ISSN 0166-2236

Ge, S., Goh, E. L., Sailor, K. A., Kitabatake, Y., Ming, G. L. & Song, H. (2006). GABA regulates synaptic integration of newly generated neurons in the adult brain. *Nature* Vol. 439, pp. 589-593, ISSN 1476-4687

Ge, S., Pradhan, D. A., Ming, G. L. & Song, H. (2007). GABA sets the tempo for activity-dependent adult neurogenesis. *Trends Neurosci* Vol. 30, pp. 1-8, ISSN 0166-2236

Ghaemi, S. N., Shirzadi, A. A., Klugman, J., Berv, D. A., Pardo, T. B. & Filkowski, M. M. (2008). Is adjunctive open-label zonisamide effective for bipolar disorder? *J Affect Disord* Vol. 105, pp. 311-314, ISSN 0165-0327

Ghaemi, S. N., Zablotsky, B., Filkowski, M. M., Dunn, R. T., Pardo, T. B., Isenstein, E. & Baldassano, C. F. (2006). An open prospective study of zonisamide in acute bipolar depression. *J Clin Psychopharmacol* Vol. 26, pp. 385-388, ISSN 0271-0749

Gibb, W. R. (1991). Neuropathology of the substantia nigra. *Eur Neurol* Vol. 31 Suppl 1, pp. 48-59, ISSN 0014-3022

Hauber, W. (1998). Involvement of basal ganglia transmitter systems in movement initiation. *Prog Neurobiol* Vol. 56, pp. 507-540, ISSN 0301-0082

Hayakawa, T., Higuchi, Y., Nigami, H. & Hattori, H. (1994). Zonisamide reduces hypoxic-ischemic brain damage in neonatal rats irrespective of its anticonvulsive effect. *Eur J Pharmacol* Vol. 257, pp. 131-136, ISSN 0014-2999

Hille, C. J., Fox, S. H., Maneuf, Y. P., Crossman, A. R. & Brotchie, J. M. (2001). Antiparkinsonian action of a delta opioid agonist in rodent and primate models of Parkinson's disease. *Exp Neurol* Vol. 172, pp. 189-198, ISSN 0014-4886

Hirose, S., Okada, M., Kaneko, S. & Mitsudome, A. (2000). Are some idiopathic epilepsies disorders of ion channels?: A working hypothesis. *Epilepsy Res* Vol. 41, pp. 191-204, ISSN 0920-1211

Kanba, S., Yagi, G., Kamijima, K., Suzuki, T., Tajima, O., Otaki, J., Arata, E., Koshikawa, H., Nibuya, M., Kinoshita, N. & et al. (1994). The first open study of zonisamide, a novel anticonvulsant, shows efficacy in mania. *Prog Neuropsychopharmacol Biol Psychiatry* Vol. 18, pp. 707-715,

Karceski, S., Morrell, M. J. & Carpenter, D. (2005). Treatment of epilepsy in adults: expert opinion, 2005. *Epilepsy Behav* Vol. 7 Suppl 1, pp. S1-64; quiz S65-67, ISSN 1525-5050

Kawata, Y., Okada, M., Murakami, T., Mizuno, K., Wada, K., Kondo, T. & Kaneko, S. (1999). Effects of zonisamide on K+ and Ca2+ evoked release of monoamine as well as K+ evoked intracellular Ca2+ mobilization in rat hippocampus. *Epilepsy Res* Vol. 35, pp. 173-182, ISSN 0920-1211

Kito, M., Maehara, M. & Watanabe, K. (1996). Mechanisms of T-type calcium channel blockade by zonisamide. *Seizure* Vol. 5, pp. 115-119, ISSN 1059-1311

Komatsu, M., Hiramatsu, M. & Willmore, L. J. (2000). Zonisamide reduces the increase in 8-hydroxy-2'-deoxyguanosine levels formed during iron-induced epileptogenesis in the brains of rats. *Epilepsia* Vol. 41, pp. 1091-1094, ISSN 0013-9580

Leniger, T., Thone, J. & Wiemann, M. (2004). Topiramate modulates pH of hippocampal CA3 neurons by combined effects on carbonic anhydrase and Cl-/HCO3-exchange. *Br J Pharmacol* Vol. 142, pp. 831-842, ISSN 0007-1188

Leppik, I. E. (2004). Zonisamide: chemistry, mechanism of action, and pharmacokinetics. *Seizure* Vol. 13 Suppl 1, pp. S5-9; discussion S10, ISSN 1059-1311

Macdonald, R., 2002. Zonisamide, Mechanisms of action. In: Mattson RH, M. B., Perucca E, (Ed), Antiepileptic drugs 5th edn. Lippincott Williams & Wilkins, Philadelphia, pp. 867-872.

Maneuf, Y. P., Mitchell, I. J., Crossman, A. R. & Brotchie, J. M. (1994). On the role of enkephalin cotransmission in the GABAergic striatal efferents to the globus pallidus. *Exp Neurol* Vol. 125, pp. 65-71, ISSN 0014-4886

Masuda, Y. & Karasawa, T. (1993). Inhibitory effect of zonisamide on human carbonic anhydrase in vitro. *Arzneimittelforschung* Vol. 43, pp. 416-418, ISSN 0004-4172

Matsumoto, M. & Nagata, E. (1999). Type 1 inositol 1,4,5-trisphosphate receptor knock-out mice: their phenotypes and their meaning in neuroscience and clinical practice. *J Mol Med* Vol. 77, pp. 406-411,

Matsumoto, M., Nakagawa, T., Inoue, T., Nagata, E., Tanaka, K., Takano, H., Minowa, O., Kuno, J., Sakakibara, S., Yamada, M., Yoneshima, H., Miyawaki, A., Fukuuchi, Y., Furuichi, T., Okano, H., Mikoshiba, K. & Noda, T. (1996). Ataxia and epileptic seizures in mice lacking type 1 inositol 1,4,5-trisphosphate receptor. *Nature* Vol. 379, pp. 168-171,

McElroy, S. L., Suppes, T., Keck, P. E., Jr., Black, D., Frye, M. A., Altshuler, L. L., Nolen, W. A., Kupka, R. W., Leverich, G. S., Walden, J., Grunze, H. & Post, R. M. (2005). Open-label adjunctive zonisamide in the treatment of bipolar disorders: a prospective trial. *J Clin Psychiatry* Vol. 66, pp. 617-624,

Mimaki, T., Suzuki, Y., Tagawa, T., Tanaka, J., Itoh, N. & Yabuuchi, H. (1988). [3H]zonisamide binding in rat brain. *Jpn J Psychiatry Neurol* Vol. 42, pp. 640-642, ISSN 0912-2036

Mori, A., Noda, Y. & Packer, L. (1998). The anticonvulsant zonisamide scavenges free radicals. *Epilepsy Res* Vol. 30, pp. 153-158, ISSN 0920-1211

Mori, F., Okada, M., Tomiyama, M., Kaneko, S. & Wakabayashi, K. (2005). Effects of ryanodine receptor activation on neurotransmitter release and neuronal cell death following kainic acid-induced status epilepticus. *Epilepsy Res* Vol. 65, pp. 59-70. ISSN 0920-1211

Murakami, T., Okada, M., Kawata, Y., Zhu, G., Kamata, A. & Kaneko, S. (2001). Determination of effects of antiepileptic drugs on SNAREs-mediated hippocampal monoamine release using in vivo microdialysis. *Br J Pharmacol* Vol. 134, pp. 507-520, ISSN 0007-1188

Murata, M. (2004). Novel therapeutic effects of the anti-convulsant, zonisamide, on Parkinson's disease. *Curr Pharm Des* Vol. 10, pp. 687-693,

Murata, M., Hasegawa, K. & Kanazawa, I. (2007). Zonisamide improves motor function in Parkinson disease: a randomized, double-blind study. *Neurology* Vol. 68, pp. 45-50,

Murata, M., Horiuchi, E. & Kanazawa, I. (2001). Zonisamide has beneficial effects on Parkinson's disease patients. *Neurosci Res* Vol. 41, pp. 397-399,

Noda, Y., Mori, A. & Packer, L. (1999). Zonisamide inhibits nitric oxide synthase activity induced by N-methyl-D-aspartate and buthionine sulfoximine in the rat hippocampus. *Res Commun Mol Pathol Pharmacol* Vol. 105, pp. 23-33, ISSN 1078-0297

Obrenovitch, T. P., Richards, D. A., Sarna, G. S. & Symon, L. (1993). Combined intracerebral microdialysis and electrophysiological recording: methodology and applications. *J Neurosci Methods* Vol. 47, pp. 139-145, ISSN 0165-0270

Obrenovitch, T. P., Urenjak, J. & Zilkha, E. (1996). Evidence disputing the link between seizure activity and high extracellular glutamate. *J Neurochem* Vol. 66, pp. 2446-2454, ISSN 0022-3042

Ogawa, N., Asanuma, M., Miyazaki, I., Diaz-Corrales, F. J. & Miyoshi, K. (2005). L-DOPA treatment from the viewpoint of neuroprotection. Possible mechanism of specific and progressive dopaminergic neuronal death in Parkinson's disease. *J Neurol* Vol. 252 Suppl 4, pp. IV23-IV31, ISSN 0340-5354

Okada, M., Hirano, T., Kawata, Y., Murakami, T., Wada, K., Mizuno, K., Kondo, T. & Kaneko, S. (1999). Biphasic effects of zonisamide on serotonergic system in rat hippocampus. *Epilepsy Res* Vol. 34, pp. 187-197,

Okada, M., Kaneko, S., Hirano, T., Ishida, M., Kondo, T., Otani, K. & Fukushima, Y. (1992). Effects of zonisamide on extracellular levels of monoamine and its metabolite, and on Ca2+ dependent dopamine release. *Epilepsy Res* Vol. 13, pp. 113-119, ISSN 0920-1211

Okada, M., Kaneko, S., Hirano, T., Mizuno, K., Kondo, T., Otani, K. & Fukushima, Y. (1995). Effects of zonisamide on dopaminergic system. *Epilepsy Res* Vol. 22, pp. 193-205,

Okada, M., Kawata, Y., Mizuno, K., Wada, K., Kondo, T. & Kaneko, S. (1998). Interaction between Ca^{2+}, K^{+}, carbamazepine and zonisamide on hippocampal extracellular glutamate monitored with a microdialysis electrode. *Br J Pharmacol* Vol. 124, pp. ISSN 1277-1285

Okada, M., Yoshida, S., Zhu, G., Hirose, S. & Kaneko, S. (2005). Biphasic actions of topiramate on monoamine exocytosis associated with both soluble N-ethylmaleimide-sensitive factor attachment protein receptors and Ca(2+)-induced Ca(2+)-releasing systems. *Neuroscience* Vol. 134, pp. 233-246, ISSN 0306-4522

Okada, M., Zhu, G., Hirose, S., Ito, K. I., Murakami, T., Wakui, M. & Kaneko, S. (2003). Age-dependent modulation of hippocampal excitability by KCNQ-channels. *Epilepsy Res* Vol. 53, pp. 81-94, ISSN 0920-1211

Okada, M., Zhu, G., Yoshida, S., Kanai, K., Hirose, S. & Kaneko, S. (2002). Exocytosis mechanism as a new targeting site for mechanisms of action of antiepileptic drugs. *Life Sci* Vol. 72, pp. 465-473, ISSN 0024-3205

Okada, M., Zhu, G., Yoshida, S. & Kaneko, S. (2010). Validation criteria for genetic animal models of epilepsy. *Epilepsy & Seizure* Vol. 3, pp. 109-120,

Owen, A. J., Ijaz, S., Miyashita, H., Wishart, T., Howlett, W. & Shuaib, A. (1997). Zonisamide as a neuroprotective agent in an adult gerbil model of global forebrain ischemia: a histological, in vivo microdialysis and behavioral study. *Brain Res* Vol. 770, pp. 115-122, ISSN 0006-8993

Pal, S., Sun, D., Limbrick, D., Rafiq, A. & DeLorenzo, R. J. (2001). Epileptogenesis induces long-term alterations in intracellular calcium release and sequestration mechanisms in the hippocampal neuronal culture model of epilepsy. *Cell Calcium* Vol. 30, pp. 285-296, ISSN 0143-4160

Pelletier, M. R., Wadia, J. S., Mills, L. R. & Carlen, P. L. (1999). Seizure-induced cell death produced by repeated tetanic stimulation in vitro: possible role of endoplasmic reticulum calcium stores. *J Neurophysiol* Vol. 81, pp. 3054-3064, ISSN 0022-3077

Perez-Reyes, E. (2003). Molecular physiology of low-voltage-activated t-type calcium channels. *Physiol Rev* Vol. 83, pp. 117-161, ISSN 0031-9333

Rock, D. M., Macdonald, R. L. & Taylor, C. P. (1989). Blockade of sustained repetitive action potentials in cultured spinal cord neurons by zonisamide (AD 810, CI 912), a novel anticonvulsant. *Epilepsy Res* Vol. 3, pp. 138-143, ISSN 0920-1211

Rogawski, M. A. & Loscher, W. (2004a). The neurobiology of antiepileptic drugs. *Nat Rev Neurosci* Vol. 5, pp. 553-564, ISSN 1471-003X

Rogawski, M. A. & Loscher, W. (2004b). The neurobiology of antiepileptic drugs for the treatment of nonepileptic conditions. *Nat Med* Vol. 10, pp. 685-692, ISSN 1078-8956

Rogawski, M. A. & Porter, R. J. (1990). Antiepileptic drugs: pharmacological mechanisms and clinical efficacy with consideration of promising developmental stage compounds. *Pharmacol Rev* Vol. 42, pp. 223-286, ISSN 0031-6997

Rossier, M. F., Burnay, M. M., Vallotton, M. B. & Capponi, A. M. (1996). Distinct functions of T- and L-type calcium channels during activation of bovine adrenal glomerulosa cells. *Endocrinology* Vol. 137, pp. 4817-4826, ISSN 0013-7227

Schauf, C. L. (1987). Zonisamide enhances slow sodium inactivation in Myxicola. *Brain Res* Vol. 413, pp. 185-188, ISSN 0006-8993

Seino, M. (2004). Review of zonisamide development in Japan. *Seizure* Vol. 13 Suppl 1, pp. S2-4,

Seino, M. & Leppik, I., 2007. Zonisamide. In: Engel, J., Jr. and Pedley, TA., , (Ed), Epilepsy: a comprehensive text book Lippincott Williams & Wilkins, Philadelphia, pp. 1695-1701.

Seino, M., Ohkuma, T. & MIyasaka, M. (1988). Efficacy evaluation of AD-810 (zonisamide), results of a duble blind comparison with carbamazepine (CBZ). *J Clin Exp Med* Vol. 44, pp.

Shih, A. Y., Erb, H., Sun, X., Toda, S., Kalivas, P. W. & Murphy, T. H. (2006). Cystine/glutamate exchange modulates glutathione supply for neuroprotection from oxidative stress and cell proliferation. *J Neurosci* Vol. 26, pp. ISSN 10514-10523,

Sills, G. J., Leach, J. P., Kilpatrick, W. S., Fraser, C. M., Thompson, G. G. & Brodie, M. J. (2000). Concentration-effect studies with topiramate on selected enzymes and intermediates of the GABA shunt. *Epilepsia* Vol. 41 Suppl 1, pp. S30-34, ISSN 0013-9580

Solano, R. M., Casarejos, M. J., Menendez-Cuervo, J., Rodriguez-Navarro, J. A., Garcia de Yebenes, J. & Mena, M. A. (2008). Glial dysfunction in parkin null mice: effects of aging. *J Neurosci* Vol. 28, pp. 598-611, ISSN 1529-2401

Staley, K. J., Soldo, B. L. & Proctor, W. R. (1995). Ionic mechanisms of neuronal excitation by inhibitory GABAA receptors. *Science* Vol. 269, pp. 977-981, ISSN 0036-8075

Sudha, K., Rao, A. V. & Rao, A. (2001). Oxidative stress and antioxidants in epilepsy. *Clin Chim Acta* Vol. 303, pp. 19-24, ISSN 0009-8981

Sulzer, D., Bogulavsky, J., Larsen, K. E., Behr, G., Karatekin, E., Kleinman, M. H., Turro, N., Krantz, D., Edwards, R. H., Greene, L. A. & Zecca, L. (2000). Neuromelanin biosynthesis is driven by excess cytosolic catecholamines not accumulated by synaptic vesicles. *Proc Natl Acad Sci U S A* Vol. 97, pp. 11869-11874, ISSN 0027-8424

Supuran, C. T. (2008). Carbonic anhydrases: novel therapeutic applications for inhibitors and activators. *Nat Rev Drug Discov* Vol. 7, pp. 168-181, ISSN 1474-1784

Suzuki, S., Kawakami, K., Nishimura, S., Watanabe, Y., Yagi, K., Seino, M. & Miyamoto, K. (1992). Zonisamide blocks T-type calcium channel in cultured neurons of rat cerebral cortex. *Epilepsy Res* Vol. 12, pp. 21-27, ISSN 0920-1211

Tokumaru, J., Ueda, Y., Yokoyama, H., Nakajima, A., Doi, T., Mitsuyama, Y., Ohya-Nishiguchi, H. & Kamada, H. (2000). In vivo evaluation of hippocampal anti-oxidant ability of zonisamide in rats. *Neurochem Res* Vol. 25, pp. 1107-1111, ISSN 0364-3190

Tse, D. C., McCreery, R. L. & Adams, R. N. (1976). Potential oxidative pathways of brain catecholamines. *J Med Chem* Vol. 19, pp. 37-40, ISSN 0022-2623

Ueda, Y., Doi, T., Tokumaru, J., Nakajima, A. & Nagatomo, K. (2005). In vivo evaluation of the effect of zonisamide on the hippocampal redox state during kainic acid-induced seizure status in rats. *Neurochem Res* Vol. 30, pp. 1117-1121, ISSN 0364-3190

Ueda, Y., Doi, T., Tokumaru, J. & Willmore, L. J. (2003). Effect of zonisamide on molecular regulation of glutamate and GABA transporter proteins during epileptogenesis in rats with hippocampal seizures. *Brain Res Mol Brain Res* Vol. 116, pp. 1-6, ISSN 0169-328X

Wang, X. F. & Cynader, M. S. (2000). Astrocytes provide cysteine to neurons by releasing glutathione. *J Neurochem* Vol. 74, pp. 1434-1442, ISSN 0022-3042

White, H. S. (1999). Comparative anticonvulsant and mechanistic profile of the established and newer antiepileptic drugs. *Epilepsia* Vol. 40 Suppl 5, pp. S2-10, ISSN 0013-9580

Willmore, L. J. (2004). Zonisamide overview of the United States experience. *Seizure* Vol. 13 Suppl 1, pp. S57-58,

Yamamura, S., Hamaguchi, T., Ohoyama, K., Sugiura, Y., Suzuki, D., Kanehara, S., Nakagawa, M., Motomura, E., Matsumoto, T., Tanii, H., Shiroyama, T. & Okada, M. (2009a). Topiramate and zonisamide prevent paradoxical intoxication induced by carbamazepine and phenytoin. *Epilepsy Res* Vol. 84, pp. 172-186, ISSN 1872-6844

Yamamura, S., Ohoyama, K., Nagase, H. & Okada, M. (2009b). Zonisamide enhances delta receptor-associated neurotransmitter release in striato-pallidal pathway. *Neuropharmacology* Vol. 57, pp. 322-331, ISSN 1873-7064

Yamamura, S., Saito, H., Suzuki, N., Kashimoto, S., Hamaguchi, T., Ohoyama, K., Suzuki, D., Kanehara, S., Nakagawa, M., Shiroyama, T. & Okada, M. (2009c). Effects of zonisamide on neurotransmitter release associated with inositol triphosphate receptors. *Neurosci Lett* Vol. 454, pp. 91-96, ISSN 1872-7972

Yoshida, S., Okada, M., Zhu, G. & Kaneko, S. (2005). Effects of zonisamide on neurotransmitter exocytosis associated with ryanodine receptors. *Epilepsy Res* Vol. 67, pp. 153-162, ISSN 0920-1211

Zhang, X., Velumian, A. A., Jones, O. T. & Carlen, P. L. (2000). Modulation of high-voltage-activated calcium channels in dentate granule cells by topiramate. *Epilepsia* Vol. 41 Suppl 1, pp. S52-60, ISSN 0013-9580

Zhu, G., Okada, M., Yoshida, S., Ueno, S., Mori, F., Takahara, T., Saito, R., Miura, Y., Kishi, A., Tomiyama, M., Sato, A., Kojima, T., Fukuma, G., Wakabayashi, K., Hase, K., Ohno, H., Kijima, H., Takano, Y., Mitsudome, A., Kaneko, S. & Hirose, S. (2008). Rats harboring S284L Chrna4 mutation show attenuation of synaptic and extrasynaptic GABAergic transmission and exhibit the nocturnal frontal lobe epilepsy phenotype. *J Neurosci* Vol. 28, pp. 12465-12476, ISSN 1529-2401

Zilkha, E., Obrenovitch, T. P., Koshy, A., Kusakabe, H. & Bennetto, H. P. (1995). Extracellular glutamate: on-line monitoring using microdialysis coupled to enzyme-amperometric analysis. *J Neurosci Methods* Vol. 60, pp. 1-9, ISSN 0165-0270

3

Role of Mitochondria in Epilepsy

Massoud Houshmand

National Institute for Genetic Engineering and Biotechnology, Tehran, Iran

1. Introduction

The dramatic clinical presentation of many seizure disorders has been recognized for millennia. Many prominent individuals have been affected including Julius Caesar, James Madison, Peter Tchaikovsky, Alfred Nobel and Leo Tolstoy. Distinguishing types of seizures has helped direct treatment, clarify prognosis and, more recently, provide insight into basic pathophysiology. Clearly, the generic "seizure" involves neuronal dysfunction. Often, there are no physical changes in brain cells. Nutritional and toxic aspects of seizures have been studied in past decades. Perhaps more valuable in terms of cellular biology have been insights gained from examination of well-defined seizure types. Of particular interest has been a group of neuromuscular disorders genetically linked to the mitochondrial genome.

2. Mitochondrial genetic

Mitochondria are the powerhouses of our cells. They are responsible for heat production and generating energy as adenosine triphosphate (ATP), therefore mitochondria play a major role in initiating the process of apoptosis. Mitochondria produce more than 90% of our cellular energy by oxidative phosphorylation (OXPHOS) (Wallace D.C, 1999 and 2005, Gupta, 2001, Spees, J et al 2006) (DiMauro, S., Schon, E. A. 2003). Energy production is the result of two closely coordinated metabolic processes including the tricarboxylic acid (TCA) cycle, also known as the Krebs or citric acid cycle, and the electron transport chain (ETC). The TCA cycle converts carbohydrates and fats into some ATP, but its major job is the capture of electrons by the coenzymes NADH and FADH which shuttle this energy to the ETC. The synthesis of ATP occurs through the respiratory which is located at the inner mitochondrial membrane and consists of five protein complexes (Complexes I–V). Most of the oxygen that is consumed that reduced to water through four consecutive one-electron reductions. (Brookes, P et al. 2004). Current theory holds that mitochondria are the descendants of aerobic bacteria that colonized an ancient prokaryote between 1 and 3 billion years ago (Vellai T et al. 1998 and Roger AJ et al. 1996).
A single somatic cell can contain from of 200 to 2000 mitochondria (Veltri K et al 1990 and Gray M.W, et al 1989), while human germ cells such as spermatozoa contain a fixed number of 16 mitochondria and oocytes have up to 100000 (Szewczyk A et al 2002). The largest numbers of mitochondria are found in the most metabolically active cells, such as skeletal, cardiac muscle, the liver and brain. Mitochondria are found in every human cell except mature erythrocytes (Cohen, B. H., and Gold, D. R. 2001).

Mitochondria are controlled by both nuclear and mitochondrial genomes therefore, there are several very unique features of the mitochondrial genome. Mitochondrial DNA comprises 0.1–2% of the total DNA in most mammalian cells. MtDNA consists of a 16.5 kb doublestranded circular DNA molecule that is maternally inherited (Anderson et al. 1981). MtDNA has 2 strands: a guanine-rich heavy strand (or outer strand) and cytosine-rich light strand (or inner strand). The comprision of ETC 13 polypeptide genes can be classified as fallow:

1. MtDNA also encodes the 12S and 16S rRNA genes, and the 22 tRNA genes, which are required for mitochondrial protein synthesis. MtDNA encodes 7 subunits (ND1, 2, 3, 4, 4L, 5, and 6) of the 46 subunits constituting complex I, one of 11 subunits of complex III, 3 of 13 subunits of complex IV, and 2 of 17 subunits of complex V (Reddy PH and Beal MF, 2005). The rest of the polypeptides of the ETC complexes, including all the subunits of Complex II (succinate dehydrogenase), as well as approximately 1500 other proteins which function in mitochondria are encoded by nuclear genes, synthesized in the cytosol and imported into mitochondria through various protein import systems.
2. Genetic information is not distributed equally on the two mtDNA strands. The two mtDNA strands can be separated by denaturing cesium chloride gradient centrifugation (Kasamatsu H, and Vinograd J, 1974). Most of the information is encoded in the heavy (purine-rich) strand. The light (pyrimidine-rich) strand contains genetic information for only one polypeptide and eight tRNAs.
3. Mitochondrial genes have no introns and intergenic sequences are absent or limited to a few bases. Some genes overlap and in some instances, termination codons are not encoded (Ojala D, et al., 1981).
4. Human mtDNA is exclusively inherited through the maternal lineage. Mitochondria from spermatozoa penetrate to the ovum but they are selectively marked with ubiquitin and apparently removed (Sutovsky P et al.1999). It has been recently found that even before the elimination of the spermatozoa mitochondria, the mtDNA is degraded (Nishimura Y. et al. 2006).Spermatozoa are germinal cells but the behavior of their mitochondria is similar to that of somatic cells. They are very active (E. Ruiz-Pesini et al 2007)and produce many mutagenic reactive oxygen species (ROS). Thus, by removing the paternal mtDNA, the possibility of transmitting mtDNA mutations decreases enormously. In fact, the only known human paternal contribution to the next generation is associated with a pathologic mutation in the mtDNA (M. Schwartz et al 2002).
5. Mitochondria do not have histones. However, mammalian mtDNA is organized in nucleoids, which can be seen under the microscope as punctuate structures containing mtDNA and proteins which localize to the matrix surface of the mitochondrial inner membrane. Another important piece of information about mtDNA is whether this genome is totally dependent upon nuclear-encoded proteins for its maintenance and transcription. Regarding replication, mtDNA replicates throughout the lifespan of an organism in both proliferating and post-mitotic cells in order to maintain a constant supply of genetic material so that mitochondria can undergo continuous turnover.
6. Mammalian mitochondria have multi-copies of own genome (approximately 103 to 104 copies/cell). Mitochondria which is replicated and expressed within mitochondria (Clayton, 1982, 1984).
7. While the ovum has about 100,000 copies of mtDNA, during oogenesis, the number of mtDNA molecules that will populate the next generation is very small, with estimates ranging as low as one to a few mtDNA genomes (known as the "bottleneck") (Wallace

DC, et al 2001and Howell N, et al 2000). Thus, a heteroplasmic mother frequently will have children with widely different average levels of mutant heteroplasmy.

8. Unlike nuclear genes in which there are usually two copies per cell, mtDNA is at high copy number with hundreds to tens of thousands of copies per cell (Smeitink J, et al 2001). Thus, while in nuclear genetics there are homozygotes (100% mutant) and heterozygotes (50% mutant) within mtDNA, mutant proportions can vary anywhere between 0% and 100% across the spectrum (e.g., 0.42% or 78.3% mutant). When two (and very rarely more) mtDNA sequences coexist in the same mitochondrion, cell, tissue or individual, the term "heteroplasmy" is applied. In clinical diagnostics, one usually discusses heteroplasmy as consisting of a "wild-type" (normal) mtDNA sequence and a "mutant" (disease-associated) mtDNA sequence, although this is not always the case as benign polymorphisms can also be heteroplasmic, in other words, both mtDNA sequences may be unrelated to disease (Tzen CY, et al 2001).
9. A critical number of mutated mtDNAs must be present before tissue dysfunction and clinical signs become apparent, so-called threshold effect. Tissues with high requirements for oxidative energy metabolism, such as muscle, heart, brain, and neurosensory organs have relatively low thresholds and are particularly vulnerable to mtDNA mutations.

3. Mitochondrial disorders

Hereditary mitochondrial disorders are caused by mutations in the mtDNA, or nuclear DNA (nDNA), resulting in impaired respiratory chain activity or oxidative phosphorylation. Phenotypically, mitochondrial disorders present as single or multi system diseases, with onset between birth and senescence (Zeviani M, Di DonatoS 2004). Mitochondrial disorders usually have a progressive course which is why single organ affection turns into multi-system affection during the disease course. Mitochondrial disorders manifest in tissues/organs with high-energy demand (Montirosso R, et al.2002) and are aggravated by fever, infection, stress, or certain drugs (Longo N. 2003). Systems/organs most frequently clinically or sub-clinically affected in mitochondrial disorders are the peripheral nervous system, the central nervous system (CNS), endocrine glands, heart, ears, eyes, gastrointestinal tract, liver, kidneys, bone marrow, and dermis (Finsterer J. 2004).Various combinations of organ affection constitute mitochondrial syndromes for which well-known acronyms have been adopted.

The second most frequently affected system is the CNS (Finsterer J et al 2001). Similar to other organs, the CNS may be affected alone or together with one or several other tissues. Most frequently the CNS is affected together with the skeletal muscles for which the term _encephalomyopathy_ was coined (Riggs JE, et al 1984, Leonard JV, Schapira AHV 2000).

The frequency of mtDNA diseases is high. It has been estimated that one out of approximately 8000 individuals harbors a pathogenic mtDNA mutation (Chinnery P.F. et al 2000). Mitochondrial diseases are mostly caused by defects in the enzymes involved in respiration and OXPHOS (Wallace D.C, 1999 and 2005, Gupta, 2001, Spees, J et al 2006, DiMauro, S., Schon, E. A 2003). They may arise from mutations in nuclear DNA or mtDNA. It has been documented that some mitochondrial diseases are caused by specific mutations in nuclear genes, which are involved in the replication and maintenance of mtDNA and respiratory chain function of mitochondria. These diseases may be resulted from defects in the citric acid cycle, β-oxidation of fatty acids, the urea cycle, and the respiration and OXPHOS system, respectively.

A striking feature of mtDNA disorders is their clinical heterogeneity, ranging from single-organ involvement to severe multisystem disease. The same mutation or different mutations in the same mtDNA gene may present with very different clinical manifestations while the same clinical phenotype may be caused by different mutations.

This variability in clinical manifestation may be due to several factors, including the ratio of wild-type to mutant mtDNA, varying thresholds of biochemical expression for both the mutation and the tissue involved, and the modulating effect of nuclear and other mitochondrial genes. Since 1988, more than 100 distinct mtDNA point mutations have been identified in patients with diverse clinical phenotypes (Schon EA, et al 2002. and Servidei S, 2002).

Organ system	**Possible symptom or disease**
Muscles	Hypotonia, weakness, cramping, muscle pain, ptosis, opthalmoplagia
Brain	Developmental delay, mental retardation, autism, dementia, seizures, neuropsychiatric disturbances, atypical cerebral palsy, atypical migraines, autism, and stroke like events
Nerves	Neuropathic pain and weakness, acute and chronic inflammatory demyelinating polyneuropathy, absent deep tendon reflexes, neuropathic gastrointestinal problem, fainting, absent or excessive sweating aberrant temperature regulation
Kidneys	Proximal renal tubular dysfunction: possible loss of protein, magnesium, phosphorus, calcium, and other electrolytes
Heart	Cardiac conduction defects, cardiomyopathy
Liver	Hypoglycemia, gluconeogenic defects, nonalcoholic liver failure
Eyes	Optic neuropathy and retinitis pigmentosa
Ears	Sensorineural hearing loss, aminoglycoside sensitivity
Pancreas	Diabetes and exocrine pancreatic failure
Systemic	Failure to gain weight, short stature, fatigue, respiratory problems including intermittent air hunger

Table 1. Signs, symptoms and diseases associated with mitochondrial dysfunction

Myopathies

1. Chronic progressive external ophthalmoplegia (CPEO), with or without retinitis pigmentosa or limb weakness and fatigue, is the commonest clinical manifestation of an OXPHOS mtDNA defect. The age of onset is usually during the second or third decades but late-onset mitochondrial myopathy is well recognized. The clinical course is usually benign in that additional tissue or organ failure rarely develops and the risk of serious disability is very low.
2. Kearns-Sayre syndrome (KSS) is a subtype of CPEO with onset before age 20 and one of the following: cardiac conduction defects, cerebellar ataxia or CSF protein greater than 100 mg/dl. Some patients have additional manifestations, including dementia or endocrinopathies. These patients may develop additional features such as deafness, diabetes, endocrine dysfunction, and behavioural disorders. The prognosis is much worse than that for isolated CPEO, and few patients survive beyond the age of 30. Isolated limb myopathy is a frequent manifestation of mtDNA disorders, taking the

form of a proximal limb weakness with fatigue. Deterioration is usual but it is slow and the patient is unlikely to need a wheelchair. This spectrum of phenotypes is often caused by a single large mtDNA deletion, especially the 5-kb "common deletion", but additional possibilities include deletion/duplications and mtDNA point mutations including A3243G (Wallace DC, et al 2001).

Leber's hereditary optic neuropathy (LHON)

1. LHON is the commonest cause of blindness in healthy young men. It is maternally inherited and manifests in late adolescence or early adulthood as bilateral sequential visual failure. 90% of patients are affected by age 40 and virtually all by age 50. Although the disease is usually confined to the optic nerve some patients also have cardiac conduction defects or encephalopathic features, particularly dystonia. The preponderance of males (about 80%) among LHON patients and the high proportion of symptomless carriers have prompted the suggestion that factors other than mtDNA mutations contribute to pathogenesis. LHON is usually caused by homoplasmic mtDNA mutations (100% mutant); the most common are G11778A, G3460A and T14484C (Wallace DC, et al 2001). Penetrance is low, and males are three to four times more likely to become blind than females.

Encephalomyopathies

Any combination of encephalopathic features (dementia/mental retardation, ataxia, seizures, myoclonus, deafness, dystonia) may occur alone, in combination, or in association with myopathy. However, certain syndromes have emerged that remain a useful means for classification even though the syndromes may overlap considerably.

1. **Mitochondrial encephalopathy, lactic acidosis and stroke-like episodes (MELAS)** is probably the commonest of the mitochondrial encephalomyopathies. This syndrome is characterized by stroke-like episodes, often reversible, with onset generally between age 5–15 years but can be anywhere between infancy and adulthood. Most cases are caused by heteroplasmy for the A3243G mutation; however, T3271C, other heteroplasmic mtDNA point mutations, large rearrangements and presumed nuclear defects (with normal mtDNA) can cause the MELAS phenotype. Ragged-red fibers and abnormal electron transport chain activities are frequently absent, particularly in younger children. Although the A3243G mutation is usually thought of as being causal for MELAS, the mutation is more often associated with maternally inherited diabetes, deafness, cognitive impairment, short stature and/or migraine, as well as a wide variety of other disease manifestations (Wallace DC, et al 200; Shah NS, et al 2002; Harrison TJ, et al 1997; and Majamaa K, et al 1998).
2. **Leigh syndrome**_Also called subacute necrotizing encephalopathy, this disorder is characterized by cranial nerve abnormalities, respiratory dysfunction and ataxia with hyperintense signals on T2-weighed images in the basal ganglia, cerebellum or brain stem. Age of onset is from infancy to early childhood. As in many other mitochondrial disorders, Leigh disease is usually but not always progressive and lethal, and progression often occurs associated with infection. There is significant genetic heterogeneity, including mutations on both genomes. Very high mutant loads of the T8993G/C mtDNA mutation (usually > 95%) are one common cause of Leigh syndrome. The most common nuclear DNA related causes of Leigh disease are complex I deficiency (including NDUFV1 mutations), complex IV deficiency (including SURF1 mutations), and PDHC deficiency (Wallace DC, et al 2001).

3. **Myoclonic epilepsy and ragged-red fiber disease (MERRF)** this syndrome consists of progressive epilepsy and dementia, with onset in late childhood or adulthood. Most cases have heteroplasmy for A8344G, a point mutation in the tRNA lysine gene. Some patients have multiple symmetrical lipomatosis, which are large subcutaneous fat masses, usually located around the neck (Shoffner JM. 2001). Ragged-red fibers refer to subsacrolemmal collections of mitochondria that stain red on modified Gomori trichrome stain. They are present in many patients with different presentations of mitochondrial disease but are not common in affected children. Myoclonus may occur in association with generalized seizures. The prognosis is variable but a useful pointer is the mutant load in the blood.

Syndrome	Symptom
Kearn-Sayre Syndrome (KSS)	External ophtalmoplegia, cardiac conduction defects, and sensorineural hearing loss
Leber hereditary optic neuropathy (LHON)	Visual loss in young adulthood
Mitochondrial encephalomyopathy, lactic acidosis, and stroke-like syndrome (MELAS)	Varying degrees of cognitive impairment and dementia, lactic acidosis, strokes, and transient ischemic attacks
Myoclonic epilepsy and ragged-red fibers (MEERF)	Progressive myoclonic epilepsy, clumps of diseased mitochondria accumulate in the subsarcolemmal of the muscle fibers
Leigh syndrome subacute sclerosis encephalopathy	Seizures, altered states of consciousness, dementia, ventilator failure
Neuropathy, ataxia, retinitis, pigmentosa, and ptosis (NARP)	Dementia, in addition to the symptoms described in the acronym
Myoneurogenic gastrointestinal encephalopathy (MINGIE)	Gastrointestinal pseudo-obstruction, neuropathy

Table 2. Inherited conditions in which mitochondrial dysfunction has been implicated

Mitochondrial Investigation

1. *Biochemistry:*_Blood lactate concentrations and lactate: pyruvate ratios may be increased at rest and rise significantly above those for matched controls after exercise. In patients with encephalopathy, particularly in infants, CSF lactate may be raised. Creatine kinase levels are either normal or only mildly increased. Biochemical analysis of isolated mitochondria or muscle tissue by enzyme studies, polarography, or spectroscopy may identify the site(s) of the defect within the respiratory chain and this can help to direct molecular genetic analysis.
2. *Electrophysiology:*_The electromyogram is normal or only mildly myopathic while nerve conduction studies may demonstrate a peripheral (predominantly axonal) neuropathy.
3. *Imaging:*_Cranial computed tomography demonstrates cerebral and cerebellar atrophy in many encephalopathic patients; basal ganglia calcification may be seen in MELAS. Magnetic resonance imaging in MELAS-associated stroke reveals increased T2 weighted signals in the grey and white matter, typically of the occipital or parieto-occipital areas. Symmetrical changes in the basal ganglia and brainstem are frequently observed in those with Leigh syndrome.
4. *Histology:*_Muscle biopsy is diagnostic, although occasional patients, with mitochondrial myopathy due to mtDNA mutations and those with LHON may have normal biopsies.

Histochemical analysis typically reveals ragged red fibers on Gomoritrichrome staining and these fibers stain strongly for succinate dehydrogenase (SDH, complex II). These fibers often stain negatively for COX (complex IV) in CPEO, KSS, or MERRF but positively in MELAS. Maternally inherited Leigh syndrome patients or others presenting in infancy may have no ragged red fibers and demonstrate COX-negative fibers only.

5. *Molecular genetics:*_Whilst muscle biopsy may prove diagnostic clinically, molecular genetic analysis is necessary for genetic counseling. MtDNA rearrangements are not usually found in blood whilst point mutations are; both types are seen in muscle. Thus a negative result for mutation analysis of mtDNA in blood does not exclude mitochondrial OXPHOS disease. Single mtDNA deletion is the commonest mutation identified in patients presenting in adolescence or adulthood. These mutations are seen most frequently in CPEO with or without myopathy and in KSS although they may occasionally be identified in patients with other phenotypes, including MELAS. mtDNA duplications often accompany deletions and may represent an intermediate stage from the wild-type molecule to deletion although their pathogenicity is uncertain. mtDNA tRNA mutations are probably the commonest of the single base change abnormalities. A3243G (A->G transition at bp 3243) in the tRNALeu(UUR) gene is most frequently found in MELAS and G8344A in tRNALys in MERRF. Many other tRNA mutations have been associated with other clinical phenotypes. Again, there is no strict relation between phenotype and genotype. The primary mutations associated with LHON (G11778A, G3460A, T14484C) are in complex I genes ND4, ND1, and ND6, respectively. G11778A is by far the commonest mutation and is found in over 50% of LHON families in the UK. A variety of secondary mutations may cause LHON if present in combination but only the primary ones seem capable of causing LHON on their own. The mutations are distributed in all tissues and are present in blood in high load, often being homoplasmic.

However, a systematic search for new mtDNA mutations is usually undertaken only in highly selected patients, when there is a strong indication that symptoms are attributable to a mitochondrial defect and the trait is transmitted maternally (Houshmand et al 1994)

Phenotype	Mutation	Gene
LHON	3460 G->A	MT-ND1
	11778 G->A	MT-ND4
	14484 T->C	MT-ND6
Leigh, NARP	8993 T->G	MT-ATP 6
MELAS, Diabetes	3243 A->G	MT- TL1
MERRF	8344 A->G	MT-TK
Non syndromic deafness	1555 A->G	MT-RNR1

Table 3. Mitochondrial DNA Mutations frequently associated to specific phenotype MITOMAP: A Human Mitochondrial Genome Database. http://www.mitomap.org

4. Mitochondrial epilepsy

The genetic forms of progressive myoclonus epilepsies (PMEs) are a clinically variable and causally rare heterogenous group, mostly autosomal recessive disorders. The exceptions to autosomal recessive mode of inheritance are autosomal dominant dentatorubral-pallidoluysian atrophy and MERRF.

Model	Samples	Experimental findings	Reference
kainic acid, -treated rats	Hippocampal slices	Increased basal energy turnover with glucose as substrate Higher uncoupled rate of respiration	Kunz et al.(1999
Temporal lobe epilepsy (human)	Hippocampal specimens	Mitochondrial Complex I deficiency and ultrastructural abnormalities of mitochondria in the epileptic focus	Kunz et al.(2000
Perforant path stimulation model of rats	Whole brain tissues	Reduction of brain aconitase and <-ketoglutarate dehydro genase activities Decrease in reduced glutathione levels	Cock et al.(2002
Pilocarpine-treated rats	Hippocampal tissues and slices	Decline of the activities of Complexes I and IV and lower mitochondrial membrane potential in CA1 and CA3 sub fields Decrease in mitochondrial DNA copy number in CA3	Kudin et al.(2002
Perforant path stimulation model of rats	Hippocampal tissues	Reductions in glutathione, <-ketoglutarate dehydrogenase, aconitase, citrate synthase, and Complex I activities	Gibbs et al.(2006
Pilocarpine-treated rats	Hippocampal tissues	Depression of mitochondrial- and nuclear-encoded COX activity and COX III expression Mitochondrial ultrastructural damage	Gao et al.(2007
Intracerebroventricular infusion of homocysteic acid in rats	Cerebral cortex	Mitochondrial Complex I inhibition	Folbergrová et al.(2007
Microinjection of KA into the hippocampus of rats	Hippocampal tissues	Dysfunction of Complex I in the mitochondrial electron transport chain and mitochondrial ultrastructural injury	Chuang et al.(2004

Table 4. Evidences of mitochondrial dysfunction following epileptic seizures from animal and human studies

Only a few mtDNA pathologic point mutations account for the majority of cases. An interesting common feature of these mutations is that they are usually associated with very well-defined phenotypes, although some particular mtDNA mutations are associated with very different phenotypes.

Epilepsy is also a frequent CNS manifestation of mitochondrial disorders (Abu-Amero KK, et al/2005; Patel MN, 2002; Tsuji M, et al. 2003). Epilepsy may start at infancy as infantile spasms (Blanco-Barca O. et al. 2004; Desguerre I, et al. 2003; Shah NS, et al. 2002), West syndrome (Tsuji M, et al. Blanco-Barca O. et al. 2004), myoclonic jerks (Van Goethem G, et al. 2003; Arenas J, et al. 1999; Casali C, et al. 1999), astatic seizures (Toyono M, et al. 2001), or juvenile myoclonic epilepsy (Minassian BA, et al.1995). In adultpatients myoclonic jerks or focal or generalized epilepsy may occur (Arenas J, et al. 1999;, Mitani M, et al. 2000). In single cases epilepsy a partial is continua have been reported (Balestri P, Grosso S. 2000). Epilepsy is particularly prevalent inpatients with MELAS, MERRF, LS, or NARP. Epidemiological studies have shown that epilepsy patients are more likely to have affected mothers than fathers.

It is a well-known fact that epileptic seizures can be presenting signs of mitochondrial dysfunction in the central nervous system. Thus, generalized seizures have been observed in several forms of myoclonus epilepsy associated with mutations in the mitochondrial DNA polymerase γ (POLG) (Naviaux and Nguyen 2004; Zsurka et al. 2008), mitochondrial tRNALys (MT-TK) (Shoffner et al. 1990; Zeviani et al. 1993) and tRNAPhe (MT-TF) (Zsurka et al.2010) genes. Partial seizures are frequently noticed in mitochondrial encephalopathies, including the MELAS syndrome, associated with mutations in the mitochondrial tRNALeu gene (MT-TL1) (Goto et al. 1990). More recently, evidence for a more general involvement of mitochondria also in sporadic forms of epilepsy has been accumulated (Kann et al. 2005; Kunz et al. 2000; Kunz 2002). This might be related to the fact that mitochondria are intimately involved in pathways leading to neuronal cell death (Krajewski et al. 1999; Blümcke et al. 1999) as seen in experimental and human epilepsy. On the other hand, more recent data substantiate the evidence, that mitochondrial dysfunction might play a direct pathogenic role in the process of epileptogenesis and seizure generation in certain types of epilepsy.

Syndrome	PSY	NPD	SLE	MIG	EPI	EPS	SPS	ATX	HYP	HRM	DRT	DPG	NYS
MELAS	+	+	+	+	+	-	-	+	-	+	-	-	-
MERRF	+	+	+	-	+	-	+	+	-	+	+	-	-
LS	+	+	-	+	+	+	+	+	+	-	-	-	+
LHON	+	-	-	-	-	+	-	-	-	-	-	-	-
KSS	+	+	+	-	-	-	-	+	-	+	-	+	-
NARP	+	+	-	-	+	-	-	+	-	-	-	-	-

CNS, central nervous system; PSY, psychiatric abnormalities; NPD, neuropsychological deficits; SLE, stroke-like-episodes; MIG, migraine; EPI, epilepsy; EPS, extrapyramidal manifestations; SPS, spasticity, hyperreflexia; ATX, ataxia; HYP, muscle hypotonia; HRM, hypopituitarism; DRT, dysarthria; DPG, dysphagia; NYS, nystagmus; MELAS, mitochondrial encephalomyopathy, lactic acidosis, stroke-like episodes; MERFF, myoclonic epilepsy and ragged red fibers; LS, Leigh syndrome, maternally inherited Leigh syndrome; LHON, Leber's hereditary optic neuropathy; KSS, Kearns-Sayre syndrome; NARP, neurogenic muscle, weakness, ataxia, and retinitis pigmentosa;

Table 5. CNS manifestations of syndromic mitochondrial disease

The clinical syndrome was first recognized by Fukuhara et al.(1980), when he described the "canonical" signs of 1) myoclonus, 2) generalized tonic clonic and absence seizures, 3) ataxia, and 4) ragged red fibres in the muscle biopsy. MERRF usually starts in childhood but it is not uncommon in adults. Deafness in PME should make one consider MERRF, especially if dementia, dysarthria short stature, optic atrophy, neuropathy, lactic acidosis, hypoventilation, and migraine are present. Inheritance is consistent with mitochondrial (maternal) transmission. Muscle biopsy demonstrates subsarcolemmal aggregates of mitochondria, the so-called ragged-red Fibres. Giant visual evoked potentials are recorded in all cases. Shoffner et al. (1990) were the first to demonstrate the typical A-to-G substitution at nucleotide 8344 in the mitochondrial DNA, which affects the pseudouridine loop of the mitochondrial tRNALys. The A8344G mutation is present in 90% of patients with MERRF. Two other mutations (T8356C and G8363A) in the tRNAlys gene have also been associated with MERRF. How these mutations produce the disease phenotype is unclear, although it is suspected to be a defect of oxidative energy production.

Syndrome	tRNA	Protein	Single Deletion	Multiple Deletion	Duplication	nDNA
MELAS	+	+	+	+	-	-
MERRF	+	-	-	+	-	+
LS	+	+	-	-	-	+
LHON	-	+	-	-	-	-
KSS	-	-	+	+	+	-
NARP	-	+	-	-	-	-

MELAS, mitochondrial encephalomyopathy, lactic acidosis, stroke-like episodes; MERFF, myoclonic epilepsy and ragged red fibers; LS, Leigh syndrome, maternally inherited Leigh syndrome; LHON, Leber's hereditary optic neuropathy; KSS, Kearns-Sayre syndrome; NARP, neurogenic muscle, weakness, ataxia, and retinitis pigmentosa;

Table 6. Genetic heterogeneity of mitochondrial disease with CNS involvements

MERRF syndrome is a devastating neuromuscular disorder characterized by myoclonic epilepsy, general weakness, muscle wasting, cerebellar ataxia, deafness, and dementia transmitted through maternal lineages (Shoffner JM et al 1990). Additional manifestations such as short stature, optic atrophy, peripheral neuropathy, cardiomyopathy, myoglobinuria, and renal tubular dysfunction have also been documented (Eroll et al 2009) Common clinical manifestations include myopathy, neuropathy, hearing loss, dementia, short stature, and optic atrophy. Less commonly, cardiomyopathy, pigmentary retinopathy, pyramidal signs, ophthalmoparesis, multiple lipomas, and diabetes mellitus can occur. (Chinnery PF et al. 1997)There is an overlap with the syndrome of MELAS, but MERRF usually has a longer course and is associated with milder behavioural and cognitive deficits. (DiMauro S et al. 2002)

In patients with MERRF, the EEG shows generalised spike-and-wave discharges at 2–5 Hz, with background slowing that progress as the disease advances. Focal epileptiform discharges can also be seen.(So N. et al. 1989) Muscle biopsy shows ragged red fibres in over 90% of patients.(Hirano M et al 1996) Biochemical studies of respiratory-chain enzymes in muscle extracts usually show decreased activity.(Boulet L et al. 1992) Besides, lactate and pyruvate are commonly elevated in serum at rest and increased excessively after moderate physical activities (Ozawa M et al 1995). Brain MRI may show brain atrophy and basal ganglia calcifications. (DiMauro S et al. 2002) Grey-matter signal changes on T2-weighted images are sometimes seen, with deep cerebral nuclei being more involved than the cerebral cortex. When signal changes are seen in the white matter, the peripheral white matter is the earliest to beinvolved. (BarkovichAJ et al 1993). When myoclonus and myoclonic seizures are combined with deafness, ataxia, and neuromyopathy, MERRF should be considered.

Syndrome type	Age at onset Year	Seizures at onset	Visual	Cerebellar	Pyramidal tract	Extrapyramidal tract	Dementia	Neuropathology	Death
Mitochondrial encephalomyopathy with ragged-red fibers or MERRF	3±65	Photosensitive generalized or partial seizures with lactic acidosis and neuromyopathy, short stature, and migraine, deafness	Rare optic atrophy	Can occur	Dysarthria ataxia	No	Slowly progressive	Ragged-red fibers on muscle biopsy; abnormality in mito chondrial respiratory chain consisting of a heteroplasmic A16 mutation in position 8.344; treatment with coenzyme Q	3±30 years from onset

Table 7. Spectrum of MERRF Syndrome

Debilitating if not fatal, these epileptic encephalopathies are characterized by the triad of myoclonus, epilepsy, and progressive neurologic deterioration. Myoclonus or myoclonias consist of stimulus sensitive, segmental or par cellar, arrhythmic, and asynchronous lightning like muscular jerks that affect any muscle group in the body. Epilepsy is also stimulus sensitive and consists of generalized tonic± clonic or clonic±tonic±clonic seizures (grand mal) and absences. Neurologic deterioration consists of mental decline leading to dementia, cerebellar ataxia, and various progressive neurologic manifestations, depending on the cause.

5. Genetics and diagnosis

The most common molecular defect is an adenosine to guanine substitution at nucleotide pair 8344 (8344A→G) in the tRNALys gene of mitochondrial DNA. (Shoffner JM et al 1990) Although few less frequent point mutations of mtDNA were also found in MERRF patients (Virgilio R et al 2009, and Blakely EL et al 2009). Besides, molecular genetic studies of several MERRF pedigrees and biochemical studies of skin fibroblasts showed a positive correlation between the A8344G mutation in the tRNALys gene of mtDNA and the reduction in the activities of respiratory enzyme Complexes I and IV (James AM et al. 1996 and 1999).

Another rare identified molecular cause of MERRF is a tyrosine to cytosine substitution (8356T→C) in the same gene, (Silvestri G et al. 1992) and another is a guanine to adenosine substitution (8363G→A). (Santorelli FM et. Al 1996) However, in some individuals, a mutation has not been identified. Clinical clues to the presence of MERRF include deafness, optic atrophy, myopathy, lipomas, intrafamilial variation in age of onset, and maternal transmission. Ragged red fibres and mutations in germline DNA (eg, peripheral blood) can be used to confirm the diagnosis. (Hammans SR et al. 1991)

Defects in mitochondrial respiratory enzyme Complexes I and IV accompanied with RRF are the most prominent biochemical defects in the muscle of MERRF patients (Antonická H et al 1999)

Phenotype	Mitochondrial gene	Mutations	References
MELAS	tRNALeu(UUR)	A3243G, T3271C,A3252G, C3256T,A3260G, T3291C	(Goto et al., 1990, 1991,1994; Morten et al., 1993;Nishino et al., 1996;Sato et al., 1994)
	tRNAPhe	G583A	(Hanna et al., 1998)
	tRNAVal	G1642A	(Taylor et al., 1996)
	tRNAGln	G4332A	(Bataillard et al., 2001)
	tRNACys	A5814G	(Manfredi et al., 1995)
	tRNALys	A8296G,T8316C, T8356C	(Campos et al., 2000; Sakuta and Nonaka, 1989; Zeviani et al., 1993)
	COX III	T9957C	(Manfredi et al., 1996)
	ND5	G13513A	(Santorelli et al., 1997)
	ND6	G14453A	(Ravn et al., 2001)
	Cyt b	del 14787-90	(De Coo et al., 1999)
MERRF	tRNALys	A8344G, T8356C	(Shoffner et al., 1990; Zeviani et al., 1993)
	tRNAPhe	G611A	(Mancuso et al., 2004
Atypical MERRF	tRNALeu(UUR)	G3255A	(Nishigaki et al., 2003)
	tRNASer(UCN	7472 Ins C	(Pulkes et al., 2005)
	tRNAAsp	A7543G	(Shtilbans et al., 1999)
	tRNALys	G8342A	(Tiranti et al., 1999)
	tRNAHis	G12147A	(Taylor et al., 2001)
	ND3	T10191C	(Taylor et al., 2004
	ND5	G13042A	(Naini et al., 2005)
Seizures, PEO, diabetes, and deafness	tRNALeu(UUR)	A3256G	(Moraes et al., 1993)
Cardiomyopathy, deafness, and seizures	tRNAIle	A4269G, C4320T	(Taniike et al., 1992; Santorelli et al., 1997)
ME with recurrent episodes of epilepsia partialis continua	tRNASer(UCN	T7512C	(Jaksch et al., 1998; Schuelke et al., 1998)
	COX I	C6489A	(Varlamov et al., 2002)
Leigh syndrome	ATP6	T8993G,T8993C	(Canafoglia et al., 2001; De Vries et al., 1993)
	tRNALys	G8363A	(Shtilbans et al., 2000)
LHON	ND1	G3460A	(Brown et al., 2001)
	ND2	C4640A	(Brown et al., 2001)

ME — mitochondrial encephalopathy; MERRF — myoclonus epilepsy with 'ragged redfibers'; MELAS — mitochondrial encephalopathy with lactic acidosis and stroke-likeepisodes; PEO — progressive external ophthalmoplegia; LHON — Leber's hereditaryoptical neuropathy; RC — respiratory chain.

Table 8. Epileptic phenotypes in mitochondrial gene-related mitochondrial disorders.

Type of defect	Biochemical defect	Clinical phenotype	Defective gene
Genes altering the stability of mitochondrial DNA	mtDNA depletion	Alpers syndrome	POLG
	mtDNA depletion	Infantile encephalopathy and hepatopathy	DGUOK
	mtDNA depletion	Infantile encephalomyopathy	SUCLG1
	multiple mtDNA deletions	MNIGIE	TYMP
Genes encoding structural components of OXPHOS complexes	complex I deficiency	Leigh syndrome or encephalomyopathy	NDUFS1, NDUFS2, NDUFS3, NDUFS4, NDUFS6, NDUFS7, NDUFS8, NDUFV1, NDUFV2
	complex II deficiency	Leigh syndrome	SDHA, SDHB, SDHC, SDHD
Genes encoding assembly factors of OXPHOS complexes	complex I deficiency	Encephalopathy	NDUFA12
	complex III deficiency	Encephalopathy, tubulopathy and hepatopathy	BCS1L
	complex IV deficiency	Leigh syndrome	SURF1
	complex IV deficiency	Infantile cardioencephalo-pathy	SCO2
	complex IV deficiency	Infantile encephalo-pathy	SCO1, COX10
Genes encoding factors involved in the biogenesis of mitochondria, including OXPHOS	Transporter of carrier proteins	X-linked deafness-dystonia syndrome	DDP1
	Iron exporter	X-linked ataxia/sideroblastic anemia syndrome	ABC7
	Iron storage protein	Friedreich's ataxia	FRDA (Frataxin)
	Metalloprotease, involved in protein turnover	Hereditary spastic paraplegia	SPG7 (Paraplegin)
	Dynamin-related protein, possibly involved in mitochondrial fission and fusion	Autosomal dominant optic atrophy	OPA1

Table 9. Epilepsy phenotypes in patients with nuclear gene-related mitochondrial disorders Table modified according to M. Hirano et al. (2008).

Gene	Protein function	Phenotype
Genes encoding structural components of OXPHOS complexes		
NDUFS1	Complex I	Leigh syndrome
NDUFS2	Complex I	Cardio-encephalomyopathy
NDUFS4	Complex I	Atypical Leigh syndrome
NDUFS7	Complex I	Leigh syndrome
NDUFS8	Complex I	Leigh syndrome
NDUFV1	Complex I	Leukodystrophy, myoclonus, Leigh syndrome
SDHA	Complex II	Leigh syndrome
SDHB	Complex II	Phaeochromocytoma, cervical paraganglioma
SDHC, SDHD	Complex II	Hereditary paraganglioma
Synthesis of CoQ_{10}	Complex I, II, III	Ataxia, myopathy, seizures
Genes encoding assembly factors of OXPHOS complexes		
SURF1	COX assembler	Leigh syndrome
SCO1	COX assembler	Ketacidotic coma, hepatopathy
SCO2	COX assembler	Infantile cardiomyopathy
COX10	COX assembler	Tubulopathy, leucodystrophy
COX15	COX assembler	Hypertrophic cardiomyopathy
LRPPRC	Putative mtDNA transcript processing factor	Leigh syndrome (French-Canadian)
BCS1L	Complex III assembler	Tubulopathy, encephalopathy, liver failure GRACILE syndrome
Genes altering the stability of mitochondrial DNA		
ANT1	Nucleotide pool	adCPEO
C10 ORF2 (Twinkle)	Nucleotide pool	adCPEO
POLG1	mtDNA replication	adCPEO, arCPEO
TP	Nucleotide pool	MNGIE
DGUOK	Nucleotide pool	MDS, hepato-cerebral form
TK2	Nucleotide pool	MDS, myopathic form
DNC	Nucleotide pool	Congenital microcephaly of Amish
Genes encoding factors involved in the biogenesis of mitochondria, including OXPHOS		
DDP1	Transporter of carrier proteins	X-linked deafness-dystonia syndrome
ABC7	Iron exporter	X-linked ataxia/sideroblastic anemia syndrome
FRDA (Frataxin)	Iron storage protein	Friedreich's ataxia
SPG7 (Paraplegin)	Metalloprotease, involved in protein turnover	Hereditary spastic paraplegia
OPA1	Dynamin-related protein, possibly involved in mitochondrial fission and fusion	Autosomal dominant optic atrophy
TAZ (Tafazzin)	Homologous to phospholipid acyltransferases, abnormality of cardiolipin metabolism	Barth syndrome

GRACILE, Growth Retardation, Aminoaciduria, Cholestasis, Iron overload, Lactacidosis, Early death
AdCPEO, autosomal dominant Chronic External Opthalmoplegia
ArCPEO, autosomal recessive Chronic External Ophthalmoplegia
MNGIE, Mitochondrial Neuro-Gastro-Intestinal Encephalomyopathy
MDS, Mitochondrial DNA Depletion Syndrome

Table 10. Clinical-genetic classification of mitochondrisl disorders.

Mitochondrial dysfunction not only decreases the production of ATP but also increases the reactive oxygen species (ROS) generation through the electron leak from the respiratory chain in mitochondria (James AM et al. 1996 and 1999). Consequently, enhanced oxidative stress and oxidative damage have been often observed in the affected tissues of MERRF patients (Bacman SR et al. 2003). Normally, the expression and activity levels of antioxidant enzymes are induced to change so prevent cells from ROS-induced oxidative damage. Long-term exposure to ROS of the affected cells in MERRF patients may initiate and expedite a vicious cycle to result in further increase of ROS production and enhanced oxidative damage to DNA, RNA, lipids, and proteins in mitochondria (Liu CY et al 2009).

Nuclear disease genes associated with mitochondrial disease can be provisionally classified into four groups: (1) genes encoding structural components of OXPHOS complexes; (2) genes encoding assembly factors of OXPHOS complexes; (3) genes altering the stability of mitochondrial DNA; (4) genes encoding factors involved in the biogenesis of mitochondria, including OXPHOS.

A8296G mutation was found in MT-TK and Ahadi et al (2008) suggest that this mutation is a rare polymorphism or may be a pathogenic mutation in combination with other mutations outside of the *MT-TK* gene.

6. Therapy

Mitochondrial dysfunction has been identified as a potential cause of epileptic seizure and therapy-resistant forms of sere epilepsy. Experimental and human studies have suggested that excessive free radical generation and a deficient antioxidant system are directly or indirectly implicated as taking part in the pathogenesis of epilepsy, resulting in seizure recurrence and resistance to treatment with antiepileptic drugs.

Antiepileptic drugs alter the neuronal oxidative status and increase membrane lipid peroxidation, leading to the increase risk of seizure recurrence. Epileptic patients and experimental animals with the antioxidant supplementations, such as vitamin E, melatonin and resveratrol, improve the oxidative damage in mitochondrial dysfunction. Hence, the antioxidant supply is beneficial for the prevention of mitochondrial dysfunction and recurrence of epilepsy. In addition, the detection of brain oxidative status is important for predicting the prognosis of patients with medication or surgery.

In MERRF patients with secondary cytochrome-c oxidase deficiency intravenous administration of copper has been reported to be beneficial (Ohinata J, et al 2002). Seizures in mitochondrial diseases can be effectively treated with conventional antiepileptic drugs. If possible, however, valproate should be avoided because of its mitochondrial and liver toxicity and its hematological side effects. In addition, carbamazepine or oxcarbamazepine should be avoided because of its liver toxicity and its hematologic side effects, particularly in mitochondrial diseases patients who frequently also manifest with anemia, leucopenia, or thrombocytopenia. Furthermore, carbamazepine and oxcarbamazepine may cause or worsen hyponatriemia, and thus increase the risk of triggering further seizures. According to personal observations, topiramate may worsen wasting in mitochondrial diseases patients with myopathy. The most well tolerated antiepileptic drugs appear to be lamotrigine, gabapentin, lorazepam, and levetirazetam. For acute seizure control intravenous valproate is sometimes inevitable. Other options for intravenous antiepileptic acute therapy are lorazepam or phenytoin. In single cases with resistance to antiepileptic drugs succinate (6 g/day) may reduce seizure frequency. Uncinatus crises in MELAS can be effectively resolved with lorazempam.

7. References

Abu-Amero KK, Bosley TM, Bohlega S, Hansen E. Mitochondrial T9957C mutation in association with NAION and seizures but not MELAS. Ophthalmic Genet 2005;26:31–6.

Ahadi A. M, Sadeghizadeh M, Houshmand M, Gharagoozli K, Banoei M. M, ShafaShariatPanahai M. An A8296G mutation in the MT-TK gene of a patient with epilepsy - a disease-causing mutation or rare polymorphism?Neurologia i NeurochirurgiaPolska 2008; 42, 3

Antonická H, Floryk D, Klement P, Stratilová L, Hermanská J, Houstková H, Kalous M, Drahota Z, Zeman J, Houstek J (1999) Defective kinetics of cytochrome c oxidase and alteration of mitochondrial membrane potential in fibroblasts and cytoplasmic hybrid cells with the mutation for myoclonus epilepsy with ragged0red fibres (MERRF) at position 8344 nt. Biochem J 3:537–544

Arenas J, Campos Y, Bornstein B et al. A double mutation (A8296G and G8363A) in the mitochondrial DNA tRNA(Lys) gene associated with myoclonus epilepsy with ragged- red fibers. Neurology 1999;52:377–82.,

Bacman SR, Atencio DP, Moraes CT (2003) Decreased mitochondrial tRNALys steady-state levels and aminoacylation are associated with the pathogenic G8313A mitochondrial DNA mutation. Biochem J 15:131–136

Balestri P, Grosso S. Endocrine disorders in two sisters affected by MELAS syndrome. J Child Neurol 2000;15:755–8.

Barkovich AJ, Good WV, Koch TK, Berg BO. Mitochondrial disorders: analysis of their clinical and imaging characteristics. *Am J Neuroradiol*1993; 14: 1119–37.

Bataillard, M., Chatzoglou, E., Rumbach, L., Sternberg, D., Tournade, A., Lafort, P., Jardel,C., Maisonobe, T., Lombes, A., 2001. Atypical MELAS syndrome associated with anew mitochondrial tRNA glutamine point mutation. Neurology 56, 405–407.

Berkovic SF, Carpenter S, Evans A, et al. Myoclonus epilepsy and ragged-red fibers (MERRF). A clinical, pathological, biochemical, magnetic resonance spectroscopic and positron emission tomographic study. *Brain* 1989; 112: 1231–60.

Blakely EL, Trip SA, Swalwell H, He L, Wren DR, Rich P, Turnbull DM, Omer SE, Taylor RW (2009) A new mitochondrial transfer RNAPro gene mutation associated with myoclonic epilepsy with ragged-red fibers and other neurological features. Arch Neurol 66:399–402

Blanco-Barca O, Pintos-Martinez E, Alonso-Martin A et al. Mitochondrial encephalomyopathies and West'ssyndrome: a frequently underdiagnosed association. Rev Neurol 2004;39:618–23.

Blümcke I, Zuschratter W, Schewe JC, Suter B, Lie AA, Riederer BM, Meier B, Schramm J, Elger CE, Wiestler OD (1999) J Comp Neurol 414:437–453

Boulet L, Karpati G, Shoubridge EA. Distribution and threshold expression of the tRNALys mutation in skeletal muscle of patients with myoclonic epilepsy and ragged-red fibers (MERRF). *Am J Hum Genet* 1992; 51: 1187–200

Brookes, P. S., Yoon, Y., Robotham, J. L., Anders, M. W., Sheu, S. S., Calcium, ATP, and ROS: A mitochondrial love hate triangle. Am. J. Physiol. Cell Physiol. 2004, 287, C817–833.

Brown, M.D., Zhadanov, S., Allen, J.C., Hosseini, S., Newman, N.J., Atamonov, V.V.,Mikhailovskaya, I.E., Sukernik, R.I.,Wallace, D.C., 2001. Novel mtDNA mutations andoxidative phosphorylation dysfunction in Russian LHON families. Hum. Genet. 109,33–39.

Campos, Y., Lorenzo, G., Martin, M.A., Torregrosa, A., delHoyo, P., Rubio, J.C., Garcia,A., Arenas, J., 2000. A mitochondrial tRNA(Lys) gene mutation (T8316C) in apatient with mitochondrial myopathy, lactic acidosis, and stroke-like episodes.Neuromuscul.Disord. 10, 493–496.

Canafoglia, L., Franceschetti, S., Antozzi, C., Carrara, F., Farina, L., Granata, T., Lamantea,E., Savoiardo, M., Uziel, G., Villani, F., Zeviani, M., Avanzini, G., 2001. Epilepticphenotypes associated with mitochondrial disorders. Neurology 56, 1340–1346.

Casali C, Fabrizi GM, Santorelli FM et al. Mitochondrial G8363A mutation presenting as cerebellar ataxia andlipomas in an Italian family. Neurology 1999;52:1103–4.

Chinnery PF, Howell N, Lightowlers RN, Turnbull DM. Molecular pathology of MELAS and MERRF.The relationship between mutation load and clinical phenotypes.*Brain* 1997;120: 1713–21.

Chinnery P.F., M.A. Johnson, T.M.Wardell, R. SinghKler, C. Hayes, D.T. Brown, R.W. Taylor, L.A. Bindoff, D.M. Turnbull, The epidemiology of pathogenic mitochondrial DNA mutations, Ann. Neurol. 48 (2000) 188–193.

Chuang YC, Chang AYW, Lin JW, et al. Mitochondrial dysfunction and ultrastructural damage in the hippocampus during kainic acid-induced status epilepticus in the rat. Epilepsia 2004;45:1202-9.

Clayton DA. Replication of animal mitochondrial DNA. Cell 1982;28:693–705.

Clayton DA. Transcription of the mammalian mitochondrial genome. Annu Rev Biochem 1984;53:573–94.

Cock HR, Tong X, Hargreaves IP, et al. Mitochondrial dysfunction associated with neuronal death following status epilepticus in rat. Epilepsy Res 2002;48:157-68.

Cohen, B. H., Gold, D. R., Mitochondrial cytopathy in adults: What we know so far. Cleve.Clin. J. Med. 2001, 68, 625 - 626, 629–642.

De Coo, I.F., Renier, W.O., Ruitenbeek, W., TerLaak, H.J., Bakker, M., Schägger, H.,Van Oost, B.A., Smeets, H.J., 1999. A 4-base pair deletion in the mitochondrialcytochrome b gene associated with parkinsonism/MELAS overlap syndrome. Ann.Neurol. 45, 130–133.

Desguerre I, Pinton F, Nabbout R et al. Infantile spasms with basal ganglia MRI hypersignal may reveal mitochondrialdisorder due to T8993G mtDNA mutation. Neuropediatrics 2003;34:265–9.

De Vries, D.D., van Engelen, B.G., Gabrels, F.J., Ruitenbeek, W., van Oost, B.A., 1993. Asecond missense mutation in the mitochondrial ATPase 6 gene in Leigh's syndrome.Ann. Neurol. 34, 410–412.

DiMauro S, Hirano M, Kaufmann P, et al. Clinical features and genetics of myoclonic epilepsy with ragged-red fibers. *AdvNeurol*2002; 89: 217–29.

DiMauro, S., Schon, E. A., Mitochondrial respiratory-chain diseases.N. Engl. J. Med. 2003, 348, 2656 -2668.

Erol I, Alehan F, Horvath R, Schneiderat P, Talim B (2009) Demyelinating disease of central and peripheral nervous systems associated with a A8344G mutation in tRNALys. NeuromusculDisord 19:275–278

Finsterer J. Mitochondriopathies. Eur J Neurol 2004;11:163–86.

Finsterer J, Jarius C, Eichberger H. Phenotype variability in 130 adult patients with respiratory chain disorder. J Inherit Metab Dis 2001;24:560–76.

Folbergrová J, Je˘sina P, Drahota Z, et al. Mitochondrial complex I inhibition in cerebral cortex of immature rats following homocysteic acid-induced seizures. Exp Neurol 2007;204:597-609.

Fukuhara N, Tokiguchi S, Shirakawa K, Tsubaki T. 1980. Myoclonus epilepsy associated with ragged-red fibres (mitochondrial abnormalities): disease entity or a syndrome? Light and electron microscopic studies of two cases and a review of the literature. J NeurolSci 47:117±133.

Gao J, Chi ZF, Liu XW, et al. Mitochondrial dysfunction and ultrastructural damage in the hippocampus of pilocarpine-induced epileptic rat. Neurosci Lett 2007;411:152- 7.

Gibbs JE, Walker MC, Cock HR. Levetiracetam: antiepileptic properties and protective effects on mitochondrial dysfunction in experimental status epilepticus. Epilepsia 2006;47:469-78

Goto Y, Nonaka I, Horai S (1990) A mutation in the tRNA(Leu)(UUR) gene associated with the MELAS subgroup of mitochondrial encephalomyopathies. Nature 348:651–653

Goto, Y., Nonaka, I., Horai, S., 1991. A new mtDNA mutation associated withmitochondrial myopathy, encephalopathy, lactic acidosis and stroke-like episodes (MELAS).Biochim.Biophys.Acta 1097, 238–240.

Goto, Y., Tsugane, K., Tanabe, Y., Nonaka, I., Horai, S., 1994. A new point mutation atnucleotide pair 3291 of the mitochondrial tRNA(Leu(UUR)) gene in a patient with mitochondrial myopathy, encephalopathy, lactic acidosis, and stroke-like episodes(MELAS). Biochem. Biophys. Res. Commun. 202, 1624–1630.

Gray, M. W., Origin and evolution of mitochondrial DNA. Annu. Rev. Cell Biol. 1989, 5, 25–50.

Gupta S. Molecular steps of death receptor and mitochondrial pathways of apoptosis. Life Sci. 2001 Nov 9;69(25-26):2957-64. Review.

Hammans SR, Sweeney MG, Brockington M, Morgan-Hughes JA, Harding AE. Mitochondrial encephalopathies: molecular genetic diagnosis from blood samples. *Lancet* 1991; 337: 1311–13.

Hanna, M.G., Nelson, I.P., Morgan-Hughes, J.A.,Wood, N.W., 1998. MELAS: a new diseaseassociated mitochondrial DNA mutation and evidence for further genetic heterogeneity.J. Neurol. Neurosurg. Psychiatry 65, 512–517.

Harrison TJ, Boles RG, Johnson DR, LeBlond C, Wong LJ. Macular pattern retinal dystrophy, adult-onset diabetes, and deafness: a family study of A3243G mitochondrial heteroplasmy. Am J Ophthalmol 1997;124:217- 21.

Hirano M, DiMauro S. Clinical features of mitochondrial myopathies and encephalomyopathies. In: Lane RJM, ed. Handbook of muscle disease. New York: Marcel Dekker Inc., 1996:479–504.

Hirano M, Kunz WS, DiMauro S (2008) In epilepsy—a comprehensive textbook: mitochondrial diseases. In: Engel J, Pedley TA (eds) Lippincott Williams & Wilkins, Philadelphia, Vol. III, pp 2621–2630

Houshmand M, Larsson NG, Holme E, Oldfors A, Tulinius MH, Andersen O. Automatic sequencing of mitochondrial tRNA genesin patients with mitochondrial encephalomyopathy. BiochimBiophysActa 1994;1226:49–55.

Howell N, Chinnery PF, Ghosh SS, Fahy E, Turnbull DM. Transmission of the human mitochondrial genome. Hum Reprod 2000;15(Suppl. 2):235- 45.

Jaksch, M., Klopstock, T., Kurlemann, G., Dörner, M., Hofmann, S., Kleinle, S., Hegemann,S., Weissert, M., Müller-Höcker, J., Pongratz, D., Gerbitz, K.D., 1998. Progressivemyoclonus epilepsy and mitochondrial myopathy associated with mutations in thetRNA(Ser(UCN)) gene. Ann. Neurol. 44, 635–640

James AM, Wei YH, Pang CY, Murphy MP (1996) Altered mitochondrial functions in fibroblasts containing MELAS or MERRF mitochondrial DNA mutations. Biochem J 318:401–407

James AM, Sheard PW, Wei YH, Murphy MP (1999) Decreased ATP synthesis is phenotypically expressed during increased energy demand in fibroblasts containing mitochondrial tRNA mutations. Eur J Biochem 259:462–469

Kann O, Kovács R, Njunting M, Behrens CJ, Otahal J, Lehmann TN, Gabriel S, Heinemann U (2005) Brain 128:2396–2407

Kasamatsu H, Vinograd J. Replication of circular DNA in eukaryotic cells. Annu Rev Biochem. 1974;43(0):695-719. Review

Krajewski S, Krajewska M, Ellerby LM, Welsh K, Xie Z, Deveraux QL, Salvesen GS, Bredesen DE, Rosenthal RE, Fiskum G, Reed JC (1999) ProcNatlAcadSci USA 96:5752–5757

Kudin AP, Kudina TA, Seyfried J, et al. Seizure-dependent modulation of mitochondrial oxidative phosphorylation in rat hippocampus. Eur J Neurosci 2002;15:1105-14.

Kunz WS, Goussakov IV, Beck H, et al. Altered mitochondrial oxidative phosphorylation in hippocampal slices of kainate-treated rats. Brain Res 1999;826:236-42.

Kunz WS (2002) The role of mitochondria in epileptogenesis. CurrOpinNeurol 15:179–184

Kunz WS, Kudin AP, Vielhaber S, Blümcke I, Zuschratter W, Schramm J, Beck H, Elger CE (2000) Ann Neurol 48:766–773

Liu CY, Lee CF, Wei YH (2009) Role of reactive oxygen specieselicited apoptosis in the pathophysiology of mitochondrial and neurodegenerative diseases associated with mitochondrial DNA mutations. J Formos Med Assoc 108:599–611

Leonard JV, Schapira AHV. Mitochondrial respiratory chain disorders I: mitochondrial DNA defects. Lancet 2000;355:299–304

Longo N. Mitochondrial encephalopathy.NeurolClin 2003;21:817–31.

Majamaa K, Moilanen JS, Uimonen S, Remes AM, Salmela PI, Karppa M, et al. Epidemiology of A3243G, the mutation for mitochondrial encephalomyopathy, lactic acidosis, and strokelike episodes: prevalence of the mutation in an adult population. Am J Hum Genet 1998;63:447- 54.

Manfredi, G., Schon, E.A., Moraes, C.T., Bonilla, E., Berry, G.T., Sladky, J.T., DiMauro, S.,1995. A new mutation associated with MELAS is located in a mitochondrial DNA polypeptide-coding gene. Neuromuscul.Disord. 5, 391–398.

Manfredi, G., Schon, E.A., Bonilla, E., Moraes, C.T., Shanske, S., DiMauro, S., 1996.Identification of a mutation in the mitochondrial tRNA(Cys) gene associated with mitochondrial encephalopathy. Hum. Mutat. 7, 158–163.

Mancuso, M., Filosto, M., Mootha, V.K., Rocchi, A., Pistolesi, S., Murri, L., DiMauro, S.,Siciliano, G., 2004. A novel mitochondrial tRNAPhe mutation causes MERRFsyndrome. Neurology 62, 2119–2121.

Minassian BA, Sainz J, Delgado-Escueta AV. Genetics of myoclonic and myoclonus epilepsies. ClinNeurosci1995;3:223–35.

Mitani M, Jinnai K, Takahashi K, Koide R, Tsuji S. A case of NARP (neurogenic muscle weakness, ataxia, and retinitispigmentosa) with a T-to-C point mutation at nt 8993 of mitochondrial DNA. ClinNeurol 2000;40:600–4.

Montirosso R, Brambilla D, Felisari G et al. Electrophysiological analysis of cognitive slowing in subjects with mitochondrial encephalomyopathy. J NeurolSci 2002;194:3–9.

Morten, K.J., Cooper, J.M., Brown, G.K., Lake, B.D., Pike, D., Poulton, J., 1993. A new pointmutation associated with mitochondrial encephalomyopathy. Hum. Mol. Genet. 2,2081–2087.

Naini, A.B., Lu, J., Kaufmann, P., Bernstein, R.A., Mancuso, M., Bonilla, E., Hirano, M.,DiMauro, S., 2005.Novel mitochondrial DNA ND5 mutation in a patient withclinical features of MELAS and MERRF. Arch. Neurol. 62, 473–476.

Naviaux RK, Nguyen KV (2004) Ann Neurol 55:706–712

Nishigaki, Y., Tadesse, S., Bonilla, E., Shungu, D., Hersh, S., Keats, B.J., Berlin, C.I.,Goldberg, M.F., Vockley, J., DiMauro, S., Hirano, M., 2003. A novel mitochondrialtRNA(Leu(UUR)) mutation in a patient with features of MERRF and Kearns–Sayresyndrome. Neuromuscul.Disord. 13, 334–340.

Nishimura Y., T. Yoshinari, K. Naruse, T. Yamada, K. Sumi, H. Mitani, T. Higashiyama, T. Kuroiwa, Active digestion of sperm mitochondrial DNA in single living sperm revealed by optical tweezers, Proc. Natl. Acad. Sci. U. S. A.103 (2006) 1382–1387.

Nishino, I., Komatsu, M., Kodama, S., Horai, S., Nonaka, I., Goto, Y.,1996. The 3260mutationin mitochondrial DNA can cause mitochondrial myopathy, encephalopathy, lacticacidosis, and strokelike episodes (MELAS). Muscle Nerve 19, 1603–1604.

Ohinata J, Hasegawa T, Kohyama J. A case of childhood onset myoclonus epilepsy with ragged-red fibers - with special reference to various clinical manifestations. No To Hattatsu 2002;34:427-30.

Ojala D, Montoya J, Attardi G. tRNA punctuation model of RNA processing in human mitochondria. Nature. 1981 Apr 9;290(5806):470-4.

Ozawa M, Goto Y, Sakuta R, Tanno Y, Tsuji S, Nonaka I (1995) The 8,344 mutation in mitochondrial DNA: a comparison between the proportion of mutant DNA and clinico-pathologic findings. NeuromusculDisord 5:483–488

Patel MN. Oxidative stress, mitochondrial dysfunction, and epilepsy. Free Radic Res 2002;36:1139–46.

Pulkes, T., Liolitsa, D., Eunson, L.H., Rose, M., Nelson, I.P., Rahman, S., Poulton, J.,Marchington, D.R., Landon, D.N., Debono, A.G., Morgan-Hughes, J.A., Hanna, M.G., 2005. New phenotypic diversity associated with the mitochondrial tRNA(SerUCN)gene mutation. Neuromuscul.Disord. 15, 364–371.

Ravn, K., Wibrand, F., Hansen, F.J., Horn, N., Rosenberg, T., Schwartz, M., 2001. An mtDNAmutation, 14453G–NA, in the NADH dehydrogenase subunit 6 associated withsevere MELAS syndrome. Eur. J. Hum. Genet. 9, 805–809.

Reddy PH, Beal MF. Are mitochondria critical in the pathogenesis of Alzheimer's disease?Brain Res Brain Res Rev. 2005 Nov;49(3):618-32. Review.

Riggs JE, Schochet SS Jr, Fakadej AV et al. Mitochondrial encephalomyopathy with decreased succinate-cytochromec reductase activity. Neurology 1984;34:48–53.

.Roger AJ, Clark CG, Doolittle WF (1996) A possible mitochondrial gene in the early-branching amitochondriateprotist *Trichomonasvaginalis.* ProcNatlAcadSci USA 93:14618–14622

Ruiz-PesiniE, C. Diez-Sanchez, M.J. Lopez-Perez, J.A. Enriquez, The role of the mitochondrion in sperm function: is there a place for oxidative phosphorylationor is this a purely glycolytic process? Curr.Top. Dev. Biol. 77 (2007) 3–19.

Sakuta, R., Nonaka, I., 1989. Vascular involvement in mitochondrial myopathy. Ann.Neurol. 25, 594–601.

Santorelli FM, Mak SC, El-Schahawi M, et al. Maternally inherited cardiomyopathy and hearing loss associated with a novel mutation in the mitochondrial DNA tRNALys gene (G8363A). *Am J Hum Genet* 1996; 58: 933–39.

Santorelli, F.M., Tanji, K., Kulikova, R., Shanske, S., Vilarinho, L., Hays, A.P., DiMauro, S.,1997. Identification of a novel mutation in the mtDNA ND5 gene associated withMELAS. Biochem.Biophys. Res. Commun. 238, 326–328.

Sato,W., Hayasaka, K., Shoji, Y., Takahashi, T., Takada, G., Saito, M., Fukawa, O.,Wachi, E.,1994. A mitochondrial tRNA(Leu)(UUR) mutation at 3,256 associated withmitochondrial myopathy, encephalopathy, lactic acidosis, and stroke-like episodes(MELAS). Biochem. Mol. Biol. Int. 33, 1055–1061.

Schwartz, M., J. Vissing, Paternal inheritance of mitochondrial DNA, N. Engl. J. Med. 347 (2002) 576–580.

Schon EA, Hirano M, DiMauro S. Molecular genetic basis of the mitochondrial encephalopathies. In: Schapira AHV, DiMauro S,editors. Mitochondrial disorders in neurology 2. Boston: Bufferworth Heinemann; 2002. p. 69–113.

Schuelke, M., Bakker, M., Stoltenburg, G., Sperner, J., von Moers, A., 1998.Epilepsiapartialis continua associated with a homoplasmic mitochondrial tRNA(Ser(UCN))mutation. Ann. Neurol. 44, 700–704.

Servidei S. Mitochondrial encephalomyopathies: gene mutation. NeuromusculDisord 2002;12:524–9.

Shah NS, Mitchell WG, Boles RG. Mitochondrial disorders: a potentially under-recognized etiology of infantilespasms. J Child Neurol 2002;17:369–72.

Shoffner JM, Lott MT, Lezza A, Seibel P, Ballinger SW, Wallace DC. Myoclonic epilepsy and ragged-red fiber disease (MERRF) is associated with a mitochondrial DNA tRNALys mutation. *Cell* 1990; 61: 931–37.

Shoffner JM. Oxidative phosphorylation diseases. In: Scriver CR, Beaudet AL, Sly WS, Valle D, editors. The metabolic and molecular bases of inherited disease, 8th ed. New York7 McGraw-Hill, 2001. p. 2367– 424.

Shtilbans, A., El-Schahawi, M., Malkin, E., Shanske, S., Musumeci, O., DiMauro, S., 1999.Anovel mutation in the mitochondrial DNA transfer ribonucleic acid Asp gene in a childwith myoclonic epilepsy and psychomotor regression. J. Child Neurol. 14, 610–613.

Shtilbans, A., Shanske, S., Goodman, S., Sue, C.M., Bruno, C., Johnson, T.L., Lava, N.S.,Waheed, N., DiMauro, S., 2000. G8363A mutation in the mitochondrial DNA transfer ribonucleicacidLys gene: another cause of Leigh syndrome. J. Child Neurol. 15,759–761.

Silvestri G, Moraes CT, Shanske S, Oh SJ, DiMauro S. A new mtDNA mutation in the tRNALys gene associated with myoclonic epilepsy and ragged-red fibers (MERRF). *Am J Hum Genet* 1992; 51: 1213–17.

Smeitink J, van den Heuvel L, DiMauro S. The genetics and pathology of oxidative phosphorylation. Nat Rev Genet 2001;2:342 - 52.

So N, Berkovic SF, Andermann F, Kuzniecky R, Gendron D, Quesney LF. Myoclonus epilepsy and ragged-red fibers (MERRF). Electrophysiological studies and comparison with the other progressive myoclonus epilepsies. *Brain* 1989; 112: 1261–76.

Spees, J. L., Olson, S. D., Whitney, M. J., Prockop, D. J., Mitochondrial transfer between cells can rescue aerobic respiration. PNAS 2006, 103, 1283 -1288.

Sutovsky, P., R.D. Moreno, G. Schatten, Ubiquitin tag for sperm mitochondria, Nature 402 (1999) 371–372.

Szewczyk, A.,Wojtczak, L., Mitochondria as a pharmacological target. Pharmacol. Rev. 2002, 54, 101–127.

Taniike, M., Fukushima, H., Yanagihara, I., Tsukamoto, H., Tanaka, J., Fujimura, H., Nagai,T., Sano, T., Yamaoka, K., Inui, K., 1992. Mitochondrial tRNA(Ile) mutation in fatalcardiomyopathy. Biochem.Biophys. Res. Commun. 186, 47–53.

Taylor, R.W., Chinnery, P.F., Haldane, F., Morris, A.A., Bindoff, L.A., Wilson, J., Turnbull,D.M., 1996. MELAS associated with a mutation in the valine transfer RNA gene ofmitochondrial DNA. Ann. Neurol. 40, 459–462.

Taylor, R.W., Singh-Kler, R., Hayes, C.M., Smith, P.E., Turnbull, D.M., 2001. Progressivemitochondrial disease resulting from a novel missense mutation in the mitochondrial DNA ND3 gene. Ann. Neurol. 50, 104–107.

Taylor, R.W., Schaefer, A.M., McDonnell, M.T., Petty, R.K., Thomas, A.M., Blakely, E.L.,Hayes, C.M., McFarland, R., Turnbull, D.M., 2004. Catastrophic presentation of mitochondrial disease due to a mutation in the tRNA(His) gene. Neurology 62,1420–1423

Tiranti, V., Carrara, F., Confalonieri, P., Mora, M., Maffei, R.M., Lamantea, E., Zeviani, M.,1999. A novel mutation (8342G–NA) in the mitochondrial tRNA(Lys) geneassociated with progressive external ophthalmoplegia and myoclonus. Neuromuscul.Disord. 9, 66–71.

Toyono M, Nakano K, Kiuchi M et al. A case of MERRF associated with chronic pancreatitis. NeuromusculDisord 2001;11:300–4.

Tsuji M, Kuroki S, Maeda H et al. Leigh syndrome associated with West syndrome. Brain Dev 2003;25:245–50.

Tzen CY, Wu TY, Liu HF. Sequence polymorphism in the coding region of mitochondrial genome encompassing position 8389–8865. Forensic Sci Int 2001;120: 204– 9.

Wallace DC (1999) Mitochondrial diseases in man and mouse. Science 283:1482–1488.

Wallace DC, Lott MT, Brown MD, Kerstann K. Mitochondria and neuro-ophthalmologic diseases. In: Scriver CR, Beaudet AL, Sly WS, Valle D, editors. The metabolic & molecular bases of inherited disease, 8th ed. New York7 McGraw-Hill, 2001. p. 2425–509.

Wallace, D. C., A mitochondrial paradigm of metabolic and degenerative diseases, aging, and cancer: A dawn for evolutionary medicine. Annu. Rev. Genet. 2005, 39, 359 - 407.

Van Goethem G, Mercelis R, Lofgren A et al. Patient homozygous for a recessive POLG mutation presents with features of MERRF. Neurology 2003;61:1811–3.

Varlamov, D.A., Kudin, A.P., Vielhaber, S., Schröder, R., Sassen, R., Becker, A., Kunz, D.,Haug, D., Rebstock, J., Heils, A., Elger, C.E., Kunz,W.S., 2002. Metabolic consequencesof a novel missense mutation of the mtDNA CO I gene. Hum. Mol. Genet. 11,1797–1805.

Vellai T, Takács K, Vida G. A new aspect to the origin and evolution of eukaryotes.J MolEvol. 1998 May;46(5):499-507.

Veltri, K. L., Espiritu, M., Singh, G., Distinct genomic copy number in mitochondria of different mammalian organs. J. Cell. Physiol. 1990, 143, 160–164.

Virgilio R, Ronchi D, Bordoni A, Fassone E, Bonato S, Donadoni C, Torgano G, Moggio M, Corti S, Bresolin N, Comi GP (2009) Mitochondrial DNA G8363A mutation in the tRNALys gene: clinical, biochemical and pathological study. J NeurolSci 281:85–92, Review

Zeviani M, Di Donato S. Mitochondrial disorders. Brain 2004;127:2153–72.

Zeviani, M., Muntoni, F., Savarese, N., Serra, G., Tiranti, V., Carrara, F., Mariotti, C.,DiDonato, S.,1993. A MERRF/MELAS overlap syndrome associated with a new pointmutation in the mitochondrial DNA tRNA(Lys) gene. Eur. J. Hum. Genet. 1, 80–87.

Zsurka G, Baron M, Stewart JD, Kornblum C, Bös M, Sassen R, Taylor RW, Elger CE, Chinnery PF, Kunz WS (2008) J Neuropathol Exp Neurol 67:857–866

Zsurka G, Hampel KG, Nelson I, Jardel C, Mirandola SR, Sassen R, Kornblum C, Marcorelles P, Lavoué S, Lombès A, Kunz WS (2010) Neurology 74:507–512

4

The Role of Cell Therapy in the Treatment of Epilepsy: Lessons from Animal Models and Clinical Trials

Magda Giordano
Instituto de Neurobiología, Universidad Nacional Autónoma de México, Mexico

1. Introduction

The notion of replacing brain cells affected by a particular disease or unable to synthesize a molecule crucial for adequate brain function has been around for many years. The first experiments entailed the transplantation of adult tissue into an adult or young animal; they were met with limited success (Björklund & Stenevi, 1984). Later, scientists started working with fetal tissue, because this tissue fares better when dissected, axons are shorter, cells are still dividing, and growth factors are present in the tissue. These studies were more successful and led to clinical trials using human fetal tissue, and autologous transplants of adrenal chromaffin cells, especially for Parkinson´s disease (Freed, 1991). Transplants were first used in this neurodegenerative disorder because it was assumed that the main problem was the lack of dopamine in the striatum, and this neurotransmitter could be readily provided by chromaffin cells from the adrenal medulla or by mesencephalic dopaminergic cells. Initial preclinical studies had shown, using the 6-OHDA model developed by Ungerstedt (Ungerstedt 1968; Ungerstedt & Arbuthnott, 1970), that intrastriatal grafts of mesencephalic cells could reduce the number of ipsilateral or contralateral rotations induced by apomorphine or amphetamine, suggesting that the dopaminergic tone had been restored in the lesioned striatum. These studies led to others using fimbria fornix lesions (e.g., Dunnett et al., 1982), diabetes insipidus model (e.g., Gash & Sladek, 1980), Huntington´s disease models (e.g., Norman et al., 1989), and epilepsy models (e.g., Castillo et al., 2006). In addition to the experiments showing functional effects of the transplants, there were others looking for the mechanisms underlying the effects of the transplans. A series of studies showed that transplanted cells could establish reciprocal anatomical connections with the host (Wictorin, 1992; Murata et al., 1990). A couple of studies using electrophysiology, and markers or cell activation showed that these connections were functional (Xu et al., 1991; Rutherford et al., 1987; Labandeira-Garcia & Guerra, 1994). Neuroscientists involved in this field concluded that neural transplants could affect the host brain by releasing growth factors, and neurotransmitters, and by establishing functional connections with the host brain, thus reestablishing lost circuits.

However, the source of tissue for transplantation was still an issue to be considered. Fetal tissue was not readily available in all countries, and its use implicated ethical and legal issues not easily resolved. In addition, fetal tissue included all kinds of cells, and in spite of the immuno-privileged status of the brain, it could lead to an inflammatory response in the host. Autologous transplants of chromaffin cells (Freed et al., 1990) and xeno-transplants (Fink et al. 2000) had been used as an alternative source of tissue for transplantation. Then, with the advent of new molecular biology techniques, cell lines with particular properties and characteristics were developed. GABAergic cell lines proved easier to develop than dopaminergic cell lines, and given the fact that epilepsy has been considered as a disorder in which there is an imbalance between excitation and inhibition, these cell lines started to be tested in epilepsy animal models. More recently, once it was demonstrated that Cajal's notion that in the adult nervous system neurons no longer divide was incorrect, and that there are neurogenic pools in the adult brain (Nottebohm, 2002), the potential use of these immature cells for transplantation became a possibility. Furthermore, a myriad of studies started looking for factors to differentiate these immature nerve cells into the desired type of nerve cell, dopaminergic, cholinergic, GABAergic, among others (Vazin & Freed, 2010; Mejía-Toiber et al., in press). Cell lines could be developed from these adult but immature cells, thus solving the problem of having a source of tissue for transplantation. Moreover, now we know that cells, such as fibroblasts can be reprogrammed into neuronal cells (e.g., Takahashi & Yamanaka, 2006), thus, in theory the host could eventually replace its own damaged cells. In this brief overview of the field of neural transplantation, we have seen how the sources of tissue for transplantation have expanded, the techniques have been refined, and new possibilities have emerged to try and restore function in the nervous system. Still, questions remain, how is it that the new cells can modify the function of the host nervous system, is it the transplant that changes the host brain and takes some of its functions, or is it the host brain itself that is modified as a result of the presence of the alien cells in its midst. Is it necessary to transplant new cells into the brain, or do we have to learn how to activate the neurogenesis that is already taking place in the adult brain. How can cells be differentiated without posing a risk for the host, which plasmids are safe to us, and which are not. In the following sections we will focus on the advances of neural transplants in animal models of epilepsy, and in the clinical setting in Parkinson's disease.

2. Preclinical studies using cell transplants of fetal tissue and neural stem cells in animal models of epilepsy

Epilepsy is a neurological disorder with a prevalence of about 1% (Morimoto, Fahnestock et al. 2004) characterized by seizures that occur in a spontaneous and recurrent manner. Seizures are classified as generalized and can manifest themselves as uncontrolled muscular activity or as a sudden interruption of physical and mental activity (absence seizures); or as focal seizures, that are classified according to their manifestation, i.e., if they involve psychic or sensory phenomena, motor or autonomic components, loss of awareness, or evolving to a bilateral, convulsive seizure (Berg et al., 2010). Epileptic seizures are the result of abnormal, excessive and synchronic discharges of groups of neurons that occur as a result of changes in synaptic function and intrinsic properties of neurons that upset the balance between inhibitory and excitatory neurotransmission, favoring the latter (Cossart et al., 2001). In the recent document published by the International League Against Epilepsy (ILAE) Commission on Classification and

Terminology (Berg et al., 2010), the underlying type of causes of epilepsy are considered to be genetic, structural-metabolic or unknown.

Epilepsy is one of the neurological disorders that could benefit from transplantation of cells, since some types of epilepsy are focal, and in the case of generalized seizures they can be suppressed by local injections of GABAergic agents into particular areas of the brain such as the substantia nigra, or piriform cortex (Gale, 1992). Indeed, Kokaia et al. (1994) observed a reduction in generalized seizures in rats previously kindled in the amygdala when GABA-releasing polymer matrices were implanted bilaterally and dorsal to the substantia nigra. The effect lasted until GABA release from the polymer matrices was reduced. Thus, local delivery of an inhibitory neurotransmitter could reduce the neuronal excitability in brain regions from which seizures originate or in brain regions from which they propagate to the rest of the brain.

Initially, studies using transplants in epilepsy models used fetal tissue with some success. Barry et al., (1987) (Table 1), evaluated the effect of fetal noradrenergic transplants in the hippocampus using the kindling model of epilepsy. This model consists in the use of repeated subthreshold electrical stimulations of specific regions of the Central Nervous System (CNS). Afterwards, the animal presents focal epileptiform seizures that then generalize to the rest of the brain. The work of Barry et al. (1989) involved first, the administration of 6-hydroxydopamine (6-OHDA) icv, and then the transplant of fetal noradrenergic cells into the hippocampus. The authors of the study found that animals required a greater number of stimulations to induce the various phases of kindling, in comparison with rats that did not receive the transplants. Also the delay in kindling was related to the density of innervation of the transplant in the host hippocampus. They obtained similar results when transplanting cells of the locus coeruleus into the amygdala and piriform cortex (1989) (see Table 1). A study using noradrenergic cells obtained from locus coeruleus (LC) from E13-E14 rats showed that these cells could reinstate noradrenergic transmission in the noradrenaline-depleted hippocampus (Bengzon et al., 1991). In this particular study, they measured noradrenaline-release using microdialysis after electrical stimulation of the hippocampus, and observed that noradrenaline release from intrinsic and grafted LC neurons occurred concurrently with their seizure suppressing action; thus LC grafts in the hippocampus appeared to be functionally integrated into the host brain, at least during generalized kindled seizures (Bengzon et al., 1991).

Fetal GABAergic cells have also been used with varying degrees of success in other epilepsy models. Fine et al. (1990) used the pilocarpine model in rats with ibotenic acid striatal lesions. Fetal GABAergic cells from the ganglionic eminence (E16) were transplanted into the substantia nigra pars reticulata (SNr), and suppressed the motor seizures; however, similar effects were observed after sciatic nerve transplants, suggesting a non-specific effect. Almost a decade later, Löscher et al., (1998) implanted fetal striatal GABAergic neurons into the substantia nigra in fully kindled animals, and evaluated the threshold for focal discharges (ADT), afterdischarge duration and severity, and duration of seizures during ADT. They found a significant increase in ADT and marked reduction in seizure severity compared with pre-transplantation values; however, the seizure-suppressing effect of GABAergic grafts was not permanent but slowly disappeared over the weeks after transplantation (Löscher et al., 1998).

Another decade later, better results were obtained by Rao et al., (2007) and Hattiangady et al., (2008) when these groups evaluated the effects of transplants of hippocampal cells

(E19), and lateral ganglionic eminence (E15) into the hippocampus in a model of spontaneous recurrent motor seizures (SRMS), respectively. Rao et al., (2007) pretreated the cells with brain derived neurotrophic factor, and neurotrophin-3, plus a caspase inhibitor, or with fibroblast growth factor (FGF-2). They observed that hippocampal cells not treated with trophic factors failed to reduce the SMRS, in contrast to those treated with the trophic factors and the caspase inhibitor; greater survival was observed with FGF-2. Hattiangady et al., (2008) pretreated precursor cells with FGF-2 and a caspase inhibitor, and found an important reduction in SRMS induced by kainic acid. In addition they found that 69% of surviving transplanted neurons differentiated into GABAergic cells suggesting that the reduction in seizures is related with increased inhibitory control in the hippocampus.

Stem cells with their properties of self-renewal and multipotentiality (Wang et al., 2007) represent another source for transplantation into the nervous system. Pluripotent stem cells (PSC) can generate cells from all three embryonic germ layers, mesoderm, endoderm and ectoderm. Two types of mammalian PSC have been identified, the embryonic stem (ES) cells derived from the inner cell mass of the blastocyst, and embryonic germ (EG) cells obtained from post-implantation embryos (Yu & Thomson, 2008). Recent studies have identified different means of obtaining desired lineages from these human ES, for example neural stem cells (NSC) (Carpenter et al., 2001; Reubinoff et al., 2001; Zhang et al., 2001), further differentiated into midbrain dopaminergic neurons (e.g. Perrier et al., 2004), neural crest lineages (Lee et al., 2010), and neural progenitor cells from human EG cells (Pan et al., 2005). Various groups have also described differentiation of mouse stem cells into neural precursors, (e.g. Westmoreland et al., 2001; Kim et al., 2002; Barberi et al., 2003; Lang et al., 2004), and found positive functional effects after transplantation (Rodriguez-Gomez et al., 2007).

In terms of their potential use in epilepsy models, it has been shown that NSC derived from the medial ganglionic eminence and transplanted in the hippocampus of adult rats showing spontaneous recurrent motor seizures, reduced motor seizures, but did not restore cognitive impairments (Waldau et al., 2010). The NSC differentiated mostly into astrocytes, neurons, and oligodendrocyte progenitors. About 50% or the cells expressed GDNF and 10% expressed GABA. NSC grafts restored GDNF expression in hippocampal astrocytes. The authors of the study suggest that the addition of new GABA neurons plus GDNF positive cells may underlie the therapeutic effects they observed.

A different group has developed adenosine-releasing ES cells, by disruption of both alleles of adenosine kinase (Adk) which phosphorylates adenosine in eukaryotes and catalyzes the reaction: Adenosine + ATP= ADP + AMP. The cells were encapsulated in semipermeable polymer membranes and implanted into the lateral ventricles of kindled rats (Güttinger et al., 2005). The authors observed transient protection from convulsive seizures and a profound reduction of afterdischarge activity in EEG recordings. However, they suggest that long-term seizure suppression was precluded by limited viability of the encapsulated cells (Güttinger et al., 2005). In a more recent study with male Sprague-Dawley rats (Li et al, 2007) the same group derived NSC from *Adk-/-* or *Adk+/+* ES cells. They implanted them into the hippocampus before kindling, and compared *Adk-/-* cells to adenosine releasing baby hamster kidney cells *Adk-/-* (BHK-AK2), and to wild type NSC. They observed that wild type NSC delayed the development of seizures; BHK-AK2 exerted a moderate protection, whereas *Adk-/-*NSC retarded epileptogenesis during kindling development and prevented the occurrence of generalized seizures. The effect was sustained for 3 weeks; 26 days after grafting, histological analysis revealed dense cellular transplants in the vicinity of the injection tract, with 56% expressing mature neuronal markers (NeuN).

NSC engineered to express enhanced green fluorescent protein under the control of the tau promoter were transplanted one month after pilocarpine treatment in the hippocampus of Wistar male rats (Rüschenschmidt et al., 2005). Electrophysiological recordings 13-34 days after transplantation showed that the NSC developed characteristic intrinsic and synaptic neuronal properties, and received excitatory and inhibitory synaptic inputs; there was no evidence of tumor formation. Jing et al. (2009) described the transplantation into the hippocampus one-week after kainic acid-induced status epilepticus (SE) of NSC obtained from the subventricular zone of green fluorescent protein-expressing Sprague Dawley rats. In this study an infusion of erythropoietin was delivered by means of an osmotic pump into the right lateral ventricle. Erythropoietin (EPO) is a glycoprotein produced primary in the kidney but also produced locally in neural tissues, according to the authors it has shown neuroprotective effects in nervous system disorders including during the process of SE. The results of this study indicated that NSC transplants were able to prevent the development of SRMS through the suppression of aberrant mossy fiber sprouting and by increasing the number of inhibitory neurons. EPO infusion increased survival but not differentiation or migration of NSC; in terms of effects on EEG, no differences were observed between NSC + EPO, and NSC + vehicle groups.

Human NSC have also been used in models of SE. Chu et al (2004) obtained human NSC from the ventricular zone of embryonic brain (15-weeks gestation); one of the clones obtained was infected with a retroviral vector encoding β-galactosidase (β-gal) and puromycin-resistant genes. These cells were injected intravenously in a tail vein of male Sprague-Dawley rats, 24-h after pilocarpine-induced SE; the control group received only vehicle. Six weeks later histological analysis or electrophysiological recordings of hippocampal slices took place. In the transplanted group the authors observed a reduction of convulsive seizures; β-gal+ cells were found in the hippocampal area (CA1, subiculum, hilus of the dentate gyrus, CA3), amygdala, and piriform cortex; in kidney, lungs, and spleen, without evidence of tumor formation. In rats without SE, no cells were found in the brain. Cells were mostly GABA+ and parvalbumin+; field excitatory postsynaptic potentials in CA1 induced by stimulation of Schaffer collaterals were smaller in transplanted animals. The authors concluded that intravenously transplanted human NSC suppress spontaneous recurrent seizures. Using the same model Costa-Ferro et al. (2010) evaluated the therapeutic potential of bone marrow mononuclear cells (BMC) obtained from transgenic mice. BMC cells have been reported to stimulate endogenous glial or neural stem cells, reduce neuronal apoptosis and neurodegeneration, modulate inflammatory responses, release trophic factors and cytokines involved in tissue repair and regeneration, and promote self-repair mechanisms in the brain (Costa-Ferro et al., 2010). Ninety-min after pilorcarpine-induced SE the animals received BMC or saline only via the tail-vain. By 15 days after transplantation, none of the BMC transplanted animals showed SRMS, while all saline-treated animals did; 120 days later only 25% of transplanted animals showed SRMS with a lower frequency and duration than control animals. Transplants attenuated cell loss in the hippocampus and BMC were found distributed in the brain of pilocarpine-treated recipient animals. In addition, long-term potentiation was preserved in the transplanted animals compared to pilocarpine-treated non-transplanted animals. The authors suggested that BMC could prevent the development of chronic seizures, reduce neuronal loss, and influence the reorganization of the hippocampal network.

Maisano et al., (2009) have also used ES-derived NSC in animal models of epilepsy, and have transplanted the YC5 mouse ES line into the CA3 region of the hippocampus one week after kainic acid or pilocarpine administration. The NSC expressed immature stem cell markers shortly after transplantation; with longer survival time (4-8 weeks) cells in the kainic acid model some cells expressed an early marker of granule neurons (Prox1). Eight weeks after transplantation many grafted neurons received synaptophysin-positive synaptic terminals, suggesting their integration into the host hippocampus. The same group used human NSC and observed similar results after transplantation into the kainate-lesioned brain (In: Maisano, et al., 2009). The cells migrated to the upper blade of the dentate gyrus only in mice that had experienced seizures, and expressed neuroblast markers (doubleclecortin, PSA-NCAM). Mouse but not human NSC formed tetrocarcinomas when transplanted into the mouse hippocampus. More recently, the same group has made electrophysiological recordings one month after transplantation into the dentate gyrus in kainate-treated mice. Their results showed that the cells have normal electrophysiological properties, receive syaptic inputs, and have the ability to fire spontaneous potentials. In their 2009 paper, Maisano et al. suggest the use of protocols to enrich for GABAergic precursors, based on the expression of glutamic-acid decarboxylase-67 (GAD67); they suggest the use of conditioned media, gene transfection of transcriptional factors, or sequential treatment with growth factors and molecules to guide progenitor cells toward GABAergic lineages.

In a recent critical review (Shetty & Hattiangady, 2007) the authors state that there is no evidence in support of using stem cells in the treatment of temporal lobe epilepsy yet, although they acknowledge that the field is still in its initial stage of development. This conclusion is still valid at present. Among the strategies that Shetty and Hattiangady (2007) suggest for further advance in the field, two of them are particularly relevant for theme of the present review. First, is the need for rigorous analyses of the efficacy of grafts of ES cells or NSC placed into the hippocampus after the onset of chronic epilepsy for suppressing seizures as well as learning and memory deficits. In particular, the question of the duration of the suppressive effects is particularly relevant, because as can be gathered from the evidence presented above, the grafts of either fetal tissue or NSC have been evaluated for relatively short periods. These analyses should include evidence for the long-term survival of the grafts, and the differentiation of the cells in these grafts into functional principal hippocampal neurons, or GABA-ergic interneurons. Second, is the need for evaluating combination therapy, i.e., NSC or ES cells transplants and delivery of anticonvulsant compounds into the hippocampus during chronic epilepsy. As these authors suggest, this strategy might result in significant seizure suppressing effects. Finally, it should be emphasized that studies using fetal tissue and NSC transplants must include adequate control groups so that the effects of the grafts can be unequivocally attributed to the particular cell type or compound being tested.

Cell type	Model	Site of transplant	Behavioral effects Histological findings	Reference
Noradrenergic (locus coeruleus, E13-14)	NA-depleted rats; kindling 6-11 months after transplant.	Hippocampus	Delayed onset and retarded progression of kindling; correlated with neuron survival	Barry et al., 1987
Noradrenergic (locus coeruleus, E13-14)	NA-depleted rats; kindling 2-3 months after transplant.	Amygdala-pririform cortex	Delayed onset and retarded progression of kindling.	Barry et al., 1989
Noradrenergic (locus coeruleus, E13-14)	NA-depleted rats; kindling 3 months after transplant, then midrodialysis.	Hippocampus	Retarded progression of kindling; restored basal and seizure-induced extracellular noradrenaline levels in hippocampus, cells immunopositive for tyrosine hydroxylase.	Bengzon et al., 1991
GABAergic (ganglionic eminence, E16)	Ibotenic acid lesioned animals; pilocarpine administration 1 month after transplant.	Substantia nigra reticulata	Reduced occurrence of motor limbic seizures, and intensity score; grafts localized in the substantia nigra.	Fine et al., 1990
GABAergic (ganglionic eminence E14)	Transplanted after fully kindled.	Substantia nigra reticulata	Increased afterdischarge threshold, decreased severity; short-lasting effects.	Löscher et al., 1998
GABAergic (lateral ganglionic eminence, E15)	KA-induced SE; transplanted 4 days after SE ; evaluated 9-12 months after SE.	Hippocampus	Reduced number of SRMS; differentiated into GABAergic cells.	Hattiangady et al., 2008

Table 1. Studies using transplants of fetal tissue and neural stem cells into the brain in animal epilepsy models.

Cell type	Model	Site of transplant	Behavioral effects Histological findings	Reference
Hipocampal cells (E19)	KA-induced SE; transplanted after showing spontaneous motor seizures; evaluated 2 monts after grafting.	Hippocampus	Reduced number of SRMS; greater survival of neurons and GABA interneurons in hippocampi if pretreated with neurotrophic factors and caspase inhibitor.	Rao et al., 2007
Neural stem cells (medial ganglionic eminence, E14)	KA-induced SE; transplanted after showing spontaneous motor seizures; evaluated 3 months after grafting. Evaluation of seizures and learning and memory.	Hippocampus	Reduced frequency and duration of SRMS; no improvement in cognitive function; differentiation into neurons (some GABA+), astrocytes and oligodendrocyte progenitors, restored GDNF in hippocampus.	Waldau et al., 2010
Adenosine-releasing ES cells encapsulated in polymer membranes	Kindling model, evaluated 3 days after grafting until 7 days.	Lateral ventricle	Transient protection from convulsive seizures and reduction of afterdischarge activity in EEG recordings.	Güttinger et al., 2005
NSC from *Adk-/-* or *Adk+/+*	Kindling model, grafted before kindling; evaluated for 3 weeks.	Hippocampus	NSC from *Adk-/-* retarded epileptogenesis, prevented occurrence of generalized seizures. Dense cellular transplants, some cells NeuN+.	Li et al., 2007

Table 1. Studies using transplants of fetal tissue and neural stem cells into the brain in animal epilepsy models. (continuation)

Cell type	Model	Site of transplant	Behavioral effects Histological findings	Reference
NSC	Pilocarpine treatment, transplanted one month later, evaluated 13-34 days after transplantation.	Hippocampus	NSC showed intrinsic and synaptic neuronal properties, receive excitatory and inhibitory inputs.	Rüschenschmidt et al., 2005
NSC	KA-induced SE, transplanted one week later, EEG recorded 3 weeks after transplantation.	Hippocampus, with or without EPO (icv)	Reduced frequency of abnormal spikes; attenuates aberrant mossy fiber sprouting; differentiated into GFAP+ astrocytes; EPO enhanced survival.	Jing et al., 2009
hNSC	Pilocarpine-induced SE, 24h later cells injected; 6 weeks later, histology or electrophysiological recordings of hippocampal slices.	Intravenous administration, tail vein	Reduction in convulsive seizures; smaller fEPSP in CA1; labelled cells found in hippocampus and other brain areas, no tumor formation.	Chu et al., 2004
BMC	Pilocarpine-induced SE, 90 min later cells injected; evaluated 15 and 120 days later.	Intravenous administration, tail vein	Short-term suppressed SRMS; long-term only 25% animals with BMC showed SRMS of lower frequency and duration than controls; attenuated cell loss in the hippocampus; long-term potentiation preserved.	Costa-Ferro et al., 2010

Table 1. Studies using transplants of fetal tissue and neural stem cells into the brain in animal epilepsy models.(continuation)

Cell type	Model	Site of transplant	Behavioral effects Histological findings	Reference
NSC and hNSC	KA or pilocarpine administration, transplanted one week later.	Hippocampus CA3	Expression of immature cell makers, and of granule cells after longer survival times. Inputs of synaptohpysin+ synaptic terminals. Mouse NSC formed teratomas. hNSC migrated to dentate gyrus. Neuronal electrophysiological characteristics.	Maisano et al., 2009

Table 1. Studies using transplants of fetal tissue and neural stem cells into the brain in animal epilepsy models. (continuation)

Adk: adenosine kinase, enzyme that phosphorylates adenosine in eukaryotes; BMC: bone marrow mononuclear cells; CA: *Cornu Ammonis*; EEG: electroencephalogram; EPO: erythropoietin; ES: embryonic stem cells; fEPSP: field excitatory postsynaptic potentials; GABA: gamma-aminobutyric acid; GDNF: glial-derived neurotrophic factor; GFAP: glial fibrillary acidic protein; hNSC: human neural stem cells; icv: intracerebroventricular administration; KA: kainic acid; NA: noradrenaline; NeuN: a mature neuronal marker; NSC: neural stem cells; SE: status epilepticus; SRMS: spontaneous recurrent motor seizures.

3. Preclinical studies using cell transplants of cell lines in animal models of epilepsy

The use of fetal tissue for transplantation involves ethical and technical issues that can be circumvented by using cell lines. The advances in molecular biology techniques provided the means to immortalize and genetically modifiy cells to produce specific growth factors, and enzymes. One example of a cell line with intrinsic GABAergic properties is the clone M213-20, derived from the ganglionic eminence of E14-15 Sprague-Dawley rats. This cell line was obtained by immortalizing neuroblasts using the temperature sensitive allele (A58) of the SV40 large T antigen, and was found to have some GABAergic characteristics (Giordano et al., 1993; 1996). This cell line was further modified by transfection with the $hGAD_{67}$ cDNA by means of a plasmid based on the Epstein-Barr virus. From the clones obtained, one was selected, the M213-2O CL-4 that synthesizes and releases significantly more GABA than the parent cell line (Conejero-Goldberg et al., 2000), reuptakes GABA, responds to glutamate, presents calcium transients, and releases the neurotransmitter in a calcium-dependent manner (Mejia-Toiber et al., 2010). This cell line when transplanted into the inferior colliculus increases the latency for audiogenic seizures (Ross, et al., 2002); it increases the latency for tonic-clonic seizures induced by kainic acid, and decreases their severity when transplanted into the SNr (Castillo et al., 2006) (Table 2). In a more recent

Cell type	Model	Site of transplant	Behavioral effects Histological findings	Reference
M213-2O CL-4	Audiogenic seizures.	Inferior colliculus	Inccreases latency to audiogenic seizures.	Ross et al., 2002
M213-2O CL-4	KA-induced SE; transplanted 8 weeks before.	Substantia nigra reticulata	Increases latency for tonic-clonic seizures, reduces their intensity.	Castillo et al., 2006
M213-2O CL-4	KA-induced SRMS; evaluated at 4 and 12 weeks after transplantation.	Substantia nigra reticulata	Reduces the percentage of animals showing SRMS; longer survival times for transplanted rats, GABA content increased in area of graft.	Castillo et al., 2008
M213-2O CL-4	Kindling model; evaluated for 8 weeks.	Substantia nigra reticulata	No improvement; strong tissue reaction in kindled animals.	Nolte et al., 2008
M213-2O CL-4	Genetic model of absence seizures (GAERS)	Substantia nigra reticulata	No reduction in seizures.	Castillo et al., 2010
Cortical cell line CN1.4 with GAD65cDNA	Transplanted, then kindled in amygdala	Piriform cortex	Increases in pre-kindling partial seizure threshold, and increased latency to the first generalized seizure during kindling. GAD65 long-term expression.	Gernert et al., 2002
Cortical cell line CN1.4 with GAD65cDNA	Pilocarpine-induced SE, then transplanted, evaluated 3 days and 7-8 days after surgery	Substantia nigra reticulata	Fewer SRMS, integration into the host, effect diminished if transgene is suppressed.	Thompson & Suchomelova, 2004
Cortical cell line CN1.4 with GAD65cDNA	Transplanted, then hippocampal stimulation; transplanted, then kindling in entorhinal cortex	Dentate gyrus	Increased after discharge threshold; longer latency to first generalized seizure.	Thompson, 2005
GDNF cells encapsulated in semi-permeable membrane	Kindling, then implanted, then rekindled 4 weeks later.	Ventral hippcampus	Lower levels of GDNF reduced duration of afterdischarges, and seizure severity.	Kanter-Schlifke et al., 2009

GAD: glutamate decarboxylase, the synthetic enzyme for the neurotransmitter GABA; GAERS: Genetic Absence Epilepsy Rat from Strasbourg; GDNF: glial derived neurotrophic factor; KA: kainic acid; SRMS: spontaneous recurrent motor seizures.

Table 2. Studies using cell lines in animal models of epilepsy.

study, it was found that intranigral transplants of this GABAergic cell line decrease the percentage of rats showing spontaneous seizures induced by kainic acid, at 4 and 12 weeks after transplantation into the SNr (Castillo et al., 2008) (Table 2). Beneficial effects are not observed in all animal models using nigral transplants of cell line M213-2O CL-4. In Wistar rats in a model of kindling a strong immune reaction was observed (Nolte et al., 2008). This strong immune reaction was only observed in kindled animals transplanted with cell line M213-CL-4. In another study, transplants of this cell line did not reduce absence seizures in the genetic epilepsy model of the Strasbourg rats (GAERS) (Castillo et al., 2010).

A different cell line, CN 1.4, contains GAD_{65} cDNA the other enzyme involved in the synthesis of GABA. The vector used to generate this cell line, produces two gene products, a tetracycline-responsive transactivator (tTA) and neomycin phosphotransferase (Thompson et al., 2000), thus, when doxycycline is present tTA cannot bind to the promoter, and cannot direct transcription (Thompson 2005). Transplants of this cell line into the SNr reduce susceptibility to crisis in the model of kindling and reduce the number of epileptiform spikes in lithium pilocarpine-induced seizures (Gernert et al., 2002; Thompson & Suchomelova, 2004) (Table 1). In the entorhinal cortex-kindling model Thomspon (2005) observed increased GABA levels in the hippocampus 3 and 10 days after transplantation of this cell line. They found that behavioral seizures and afterdischarges were reduced only in the animals with transplants of the GABA cells. GABA levels *in vivo* and *in vitro* decreased when the cells were treated with doxycycline, and so did the behavioral effects.

In a recent study a genetically modified cell line that synthesizes and releases the glial derived neurotrophic factor (GDNF) was encapsulated in a semipermeable membrane and transplanted into the hippocampus. Those animals transplanted with capsules that released a moderate amount of GDNF showed a decrease in the severity of the seizures and in the duration of the afterdischarge (Kanter-Schlifke, et al., 2009).

At present, there are no other cell lines that have been tested in animal models of epilepsy. These studies taken together, have demonstrated that increasing levels of the inhibitory transmitter GABA into the SNr, hippocampus, amygdala, piriform cortex, or inferior colliculus, does reduce seizures in a variety of animal models. The challenge is to take this knowledge and transform it into a therapeutic strategy that may be successful in the clinical setting.

4. Clinical studies using cell transplants: lessons from Parkinson's disease

Preclinical proof-of-concept studies are necessary to show that transplanted cells can survive, differentiate, integrate, and exert functional effects in the animal model of choice. They are also necessary to find the shortcomings and undesirable side effects of these procedures. However, animal models can only go so far in providing information about the use of neural transplants in the clinical setting. These experimental models have evident shortcomings because they cannot reproduce the particular environment of the diseased brain, the progression of the illness, or the survival time of the host, among others. In this sense, only clinical studies can definitively answer the question of whether or not transplants can reduce the symptoms or slow the progression of the disease, and for how long they may give the patient an overall better quality of life.

The clinical studies using neural and adrenal transplants in Parkinson's disease (PD), can provide with a wealth of information regarding the potential of this procedure, its shortcomings, and the factors that still need to be resolved. PD is a progressive neurological disorder characterized by tremor, rigidity, and slowness of movements, associated with cell loss in the substantia nigra, pars compacta, and other brain structures (Tolosa et al., 2006). Substantia nigra pars compacta cells (SNc) produce and release dopamine (DA) in the caudate nucleus and putamen, a neurotransmitter involved in motor behavior. In addition to loss of DA cells in the nigra, other histopahtological signs include the presence of dystrophic neurites, and Lewy body inclusions in the surviving DA cells. Lewy bodies are α-synuclein and ubiquitin-containing intracytoplasmic inclusions (Kövari et al., 2009). PD was the first neurological disorder in which neural transplants were used. The source of tissue for transplantation initially were adrenal medulla chromaffin cells, since they produce and release substantial quantities of catecholamines (Drucker-Colin & Verdugo-Diaz, 2004). In 1990, Freed et al., wrote a thorough review about the status of intracerebral adrenal medulla grafts, they reviewed the results of about ten of the early studies of adrenal grafts for the treatment of Parkinson's disease. Two primary methods of autotransplantation were used then, the first involved transplantation of adrenal medulla into the striatum by stereotaxic injection; the other involved transplantation of the adrenal tissue to cavities in the wall of the lateral ventricle. The conclusions of this review indicated that intrastriatal adrenal medulla grafts caused only a transient improvement, whereas intraventricular grafts appeared to have a more lasting effect. The degree of improvement, though, differed among studies, and ranged from substantial to modest. The major improvements had to do with increases in duration of "on" times, that is the time when the medication is having an effect, and the patient can move. In Parkinson's disease there are fluctuations in the response to the medication, this periods are known as "on", and "off". Great variability was observed from patient to patient, the majority improved only slightly and a few had greater effects. The evidence also suggested that the creation of a cavity on the wall of the ventricle could enhance the trophic effects of the grafts. In this review, the authors advocated the use of quantitative objective measures of motor function, in addition to rating scales only; the inclusion of control trials involving comparisons between patients receiving grafts and controls, non-treated groups, or groups receiving other treatments. They concluded that when adrenal medulla grafts survive the functional effects could be the result of release of dopamine, and possibly other substances. When they do not survive, the functional effects must be attributed to the host brain reaction to injury or to the release of chemical substances with trophic effects outlasting their production, or the production of substances by surviving non-chromaffin cells. At that time, postmortem studies in human patients showed lack of tyrosine hydroxylase (TH) positive cells (tyrosine hydroxylase is the rate-limiting enzyme in the synthesis of dopamine and norepinephrine) but there was not enough data to correlate the clinical outcome to the presence or absence of TH positive cells. In a later review of the field, Freed (1993) addressed the results of fetal mesencephalic transplants in human patients with Parkinson's disease. These studies reported clinical improvement over the course of several months after transplantation. Early changes were, according to the author, qualitatively similar to those observed after adrenal grafts. Positron emission tomography (PET) studies indicated increased 6-[^{18}F]-fluoro-L-dopa (FD) uptake in the region of the graft. FD is a marker that allows monitoring of the uptake and decarboxylation of FD to fluorodopamine (FDA), and the subsequent storage of FDA in synaptic vesicles, thus giving an indication of pre-synaptic DA function (Au et al., 2005). At that time, no controlled studies on mesencephalic grafts had taken place. A decade later, Roitberg et al. (2000) reviewed the clinical studies using neural grafting for Parkinson's and

Huntington's disease. At that time more than 150 procedures for fetal transplantation in Parkinson's disease had been reported over the world. The range of clinical benefits was variable, some patients showed improvement in terms of reductions in "off" periods, reduction of medication, increase in FD uptake in the grafted areas, improvement in activities of daily living scores, while others showed no improvement, and some patients developed dyskinesia contralateral to the implanted side. Some degree of clinical improvement had been observed even 60 months after transplantation. In terms of anatomical characteristics, the authors indicated that TH positive neurons were identified in the graft of a patient that died 18 months postoperatively from an event unrelated to the surgery. Electron microscopic studies indicated synapses between transplanted TH cells and host cells in the putamen.

Several technical improvements were made in the decade between 1990 and 2000 that could account for better outcome of grafting procedures. Among them were a more favorable donor age, considered to be when dopaminergic cells first appear in the subventricular zone just prior to neuritic process extension. Grafts of fetal tissue older than 9 weeks gestational age did not show significant clinical effects or survival of TH positive cells. Another issue was time between obtaining the tissue and grafting, studies showing clinical benefits used tissue within 24-48 h of tissue acquisition (Roitberg et al., 2000). An advantage of solid versus suspension grafts was suggested, and the number of transplanted cells was also important. Apparently the greater the number of replacement cells, the better the clinical effect. Another factor was the location of the transplant, whether caudate nucleus or putamen, Roitberg et al., (2000) suggested that the putamen was a better site for implantation, and that greater improvement could be achieved by bilateral transplants. Importantly, transplants of TH+ cells had been shown to extend neuritic processes up to 5-7 mm from the grafted site, although complete reversal of symptoms had not been achieved in spite of this innervation pattern. The need for immunosuppression had not been firmly established.

In the first decade of this century, the results of two double-blind controlled trials were published. The first in 2001 by Freed et al., reported on the results of operations on 40 patients that began in 1995 and ended in 1998, and included a sham group, that later had the option of receiving the graft. The results of the study were rather sobering, motor aspects improved 18% in the transplanted group as a whole, and 34%, if only patients 60 years of age or younger were considered. Rigidity and bradykinesia were reduced in the younger groups, but no improvement on tremor was observed. FD indicated an increase in radionuclide uptake in the putamen of the transplanted group, without changes in the sham group. One 66-year-old patient died of causes unrelated to the surgical procedure seven months after transplantation, and the postmortem analysis of the brain indicated the presence of TH+ cells with outgrowth of 2-3 mm, without Lewy bodies. Postmortem analysis of the brain of another patient (a 68-year-old man who died three years after the transplantation procedure, also from causes unrelated to the surgery) showed surviving dopamine cells in the tissue, with outgrowth that extended the full width of the putamen. PET-FD had shown 100% improvement in uptake over baseline measures. On a three-year follow-up, there was a 38% improvement in the younger group of patients and 14% of older patients, five patients developed dystonia and dyskinesia. The authors concluded that their results were similar to those of open studies. In 2003 the results of another double-blind controlled study were reported (Olanow et al., 2003) with similar results. Comparisons between placebo and transplanted groups were not significant even though striatal FD uptake was significantly increased in the transplanted groups, and survival of dopamine neurons was observed at postmortem examination of five patients who died during the study from causes unrelated to the transplant. Number of surviving TH+ cells ranged from 30,000-120,000 per side depending if the patient had received a one-donor or a four-donor graft. Activated microglia and immune reactivity was observed in the transplanted group in and around the region of the graft. In addition 56% of transplanted patients developed dyskinesia. The authors concluded that fetal nigral transplantation was not recommended at that time. Goetz et al. (2005) reached a similar conclusion after an evidence-based medical review update on the various treatments for PD from 2001-2004. On the basis of their analyses, the authors concluded that fetal mesencephalic grafts were non-efficacious meaning that evidence showed that the intervention did not have a positive side effect on studied outcomes.

In 2005 Piccini et al., addressed some of the issues pertaining to the clinical outcome after neural transplantation in PD. On the basis of their results with nine patients from a full series of fourteen grafted PD patients, they suggested that clinical outcome is best when more than 100,000 DA neurons are grafted and at least 1/3 to 1/2 of the putamen is reinnervated. This degree of innervation corresponds to 50% of normal FD uptake, although as indicated in the previous studies it does not always match with the level of clinical improvement. This study contributed importantly to the discussion of the mechanisms that underlie the development of dyskinesia, they found no association between graft-induced dyskinesia and DA release under basal or methamphetamine administration. They also concluded that grafts in the putamen do not protect intrinsic DA neurons in the nigra from degenerating, that a better outcome can be found in patients in whom the degeneration of the intrinsic DA system was confined to areas reached by the graft, and that immunosuppression could be stopped without compromising the survival of the grafts or the clinical improvement. From these studies it became clear that the response to the grafts varies between individuals, that factors such as tissue handling and storage, immunosupressive treatment, and patient selection needs to be improved, thus this type of therapy requires that it be tailored individually to each patient (Winkler et al., 2008).

In a follow-up to the study published by Freed et al. in 2001, Ma et al. (2009) reported the results obtained two and four years after transplantation. Interestingly the motor scores of the transplanted patients improved 25% in the 4-year evaluation in the group as a whole. In addition, differences found previously between younger and older patients, and men and women did not persist over time. Increased FD uptake was found in both hemispheres, and it was correlated to clinical outcome. They also observed that better outcome was associated with the degree of FD uptake present preoperatively in the ventrorostral putamen. In the same region they detected progressive loss over the 4-year period, suggesting ongoing neurodegeneration.

Recently, various studies have addressed the issue of the presence of Lewy bodies, and activated microglia in the grafts of patients that received transplants a decade or more before (Li et al., 2008; Kordower et al., 2008a, 2008b). In these studies it was suggested that the presence of Lewy bodies could indicate that the microenvironment of the host brain may affect DA neurons, or that somehow the pathological process can spread to the grafted cells, although the presence of Lewy bodies may not affect the functional effects of the grafts. Importantly, these studies also found survival of TH+ cells in the transplants.

In contrast, Mendez et al. (2008) after evaluating the histopathological characteristics of 3-4, and 9-14 year-old transplants did not find Lewy bodies in the grafts. In this study, they reported that serotonin cells were present, and they suggested that the presence of this type of cell could be involved in the development of dyskinesia. Cooper et al., (2009) evaluated the histological evidence of the studies dealing with post-mortem cases of patients with neural transplants, and concluded that the presence of Lewy bodies could be related to the type of graft, solid tissue versus cell suspension, the former having resulted in greater microglial activation indicating an increased host inflammatory response that could have contributed to the development of PD-like pathology, and to accelerated aging in some transplants in PD patients. In the view of Cooper et al. (2009) the vast majority of transplanted neurons in the studies reviewed, remained healthy and continued to provide substantial clinical benefits for over a decade. They suggest that future studies should look into the use of pluripotent stem (iPS) cells as a source for donor cells. This technology could improve transplant quality and content, by providing sorted pure DA populations. A similar proposal has been expressed in other reviews on the future of cell and gene therapies for PD (Isacson & Kordower, 2008; Wang et al., 2007; Li et al., 2007; Winkler et al., 2005).

In conclusion, the review of the studies of neural transplants in PD shows that this therapy has to be tailored to each patient, that issues such as the transplantation procedure, i.e., solid tissue grafts versus cell suspension grafts, location of the grafts, tissue handling and storage, age of donor, immunosuppression therapy, and patient selection in terms of age, gender, and degree of degeneration as evaluated by PET-FD uptake have to be taken into consideration. They have also shown that fetal grafts can survive for extended periods, and can improve the clinical status of some of the patients for a considerable length of time. However, it does not appear to be a therapeutic alternative suited for the majority of PD patients. The experience obtained in this regard, needs to be taken into consideration before proceeding to the use of cell transplants in epilepsy. Animal studies using models of epilepsy have provided valuable information about the functional effects of transplants however, a drawback of these studies is the duration of the effects; therefore alternatives such as the use of gene therapy are now being considered (Löscher et al., 2008).

5. Closing remarks

Advances in molecular and cell biology have now made it possible to immortalize neural cells, including stem cells, to replace lost cells or replenish the supply of selected molecules (Mejia-Toiber, in press) and have thus provided a new source for neural transplantation, one that could possibly be tailored to each patient. Although unquestionably promising and exciting, there are still some issues to be solved before these cells can be used routinely in the clinic. Several authors have voiced concerns similar to those expressed for transplants using fetal tissue (e.g., Allan et al., 2010; Kim et al., 2004; Li et al., 2008; Lindvall et al., 2004; Muller et al., 2006; Snyder et al., 2004; Storch et al., 2004). We have classified these concerns in two categories. The first one includes the negative effects of transplantation of stem cells into the brain. These include the immune rejection of the transplant, and the effects of prolonged immunosuppression. Other negative effects are the potential for tumor formation after differentiated ES are transplanted resulting either from residual proliferating ES cells or precursors, or by the epigenetic changes resulting from their manipulation and the presence of retroviral vectors. In the case of cell transplantation in PD there is also the concern for graft-induced dyskinesia (Allan et al., 2010).

The second category of concerns includes the need to tailor cell therapy to the pathology of interest. It must be considered if it would be preferable to transplant a homogeneous population, for example, neural cells, versus transplanting a mixed population including cells of glial lineage in order to favor their integration into the host's nervous system to promote functional recovery. Stem cells can provide the host environment with trophic and neuroprotective support to promote the recovery of endogenous cells, to mobilize host progenitors, and to favor inherent neurogenetic programs within the host, in addition to replacing host cells (Snyder et al., 2004). Furthermore, the reciprocal stem cell-host interaction needs to be taken into consideration, because the host environment may affect stem cell behavior by exposing these cells to factors related to the brain pathology of the host that may confer an invasive phenotype (Muller et al., 2006). Indeed, NSC and BMC have been shown to migrate to localized and also widespread lesions after transplantation (e.g., Costa-Ferro, 2010; Chu et al., 2004); at least three processes seem to influence this migratory behavior: inflammation, reactive astrocytosis, and angiogenesis (Muller et al., 2006).

Undoubtedly, all these developments from adrenal to fetal grafts, to the generation of NSC with specific characteristics have increased our knowledge about the neurologic disorders themselves, about the potential for regeneration and restoration of function that the brain has, about the effects of neurotrophic factors, and about brain development. New technical alternatives have been found, the use of stem cells, the possibility of induced PSC, and gene therapy. One should bear in mind that restoring lost functions by replacing damaged cells is not a trivial process if one considers the intricate relationships that exist among nerve cells, and that complex neural circuits underlie sensory, motor, and cognitive functions. After more than two decades of basic and clinical work in neural transplantation, it has become evident that in order to ensure long-term effects neural transplants need to do more than just supply the molecule of interest. However, the positive results obtained in the past together with the recent technical advances indicate that in the future we can expect that therapeutic alternatives will be available in the clinical setting to improve the quality of life of human patients.

6. Acknowledgments

This work was partially supported by CONACYT Grant No. 103907, and DGAPA-UNAM PAPIIT Grant No. 211709 to M. Giordano. The author thanks S. Mendoza, for assistance in the preparation of this manuscript.

7. References

Allan, L.E., Petit, G.H., & Brundin, P. (2010). Cell transplantation in Parkinson's disease: problems and perspectives. *Current Opinion in Neurology* Vol.23, No.4, (August 2010), pp. 426-432, ISSN 1473-6551.

Au, W.L, Adams, F.R., Roitano, A.R., & Stoessl, A.J. (2005). Parkinson´s disease: in vivo assessment of disease progression using positron emission tomography. *Molecular Brain Research,* Vol.134, (November 2004), pp. 24-33, ISSN 0169-328X.

Barberi, T., Klivenyi, P., Calingasan, N.Y., Lee, H., Kawamata, H., Loonam, K., Perrier, A.L., Bruses, J., Rubio, M.E., Topf, N., Tabar, V., Harrison, N.L., Beal, M.F., Moore, M.A. & Studer, L. (2003). Neural subtype specification of fertilization and nuclear transfer embryonic stem cells and application in parkinsonian mice. *Nature Biotechnology,* Vol 21, No. 10, (Oct, 2003), pp. 1200-1207, ISSN 1087-0156.

Barry, D.I., Kikvadze, I., Brundin, P., Bolwig, T.G., Bjorklund, A. & Lindvall, O. (1987). Grafted noradrenergic neurons suppress seizure development in kindling-induced epilepsy. *Proceedings of the Nationall Academy of Science U S A,* Vol. 84, No. 23, (December 1987), pp. 8712-8715, ISSN 0027-8424.

Barry, D.I., Wanscher, B., Kragh, J., Bolwig, T.G., Kokaia, M., Brundin, P., Bjorklund, A. & Lindvall, O. (1989). Grafts of fetal locus coeruleus neurons in rat amygdala-piriform cortex suppress seizure development in hippocampal kindling. *Experimental Neurology,* Vol.106, No. 2, (November 1989), pp. 125-132, ISSN 0014-4886.

Bengzon, J., Brundin, P., Kalen, P., Kokaia, M. & Lindvall, O. (1991). Host regulation of noradrenaline release from grafts of seizure-suppressant locus coeruleus neurons. *Experimental Neurology,* Vol.111, No. 1, (January 1991), pp. 49-54, ISSN 0014-4886.

Berg, A.T., Berkovic, S.F., Brodie, M.J., Buchhalter, J., Cross, J.H., van Emde Boas, W., Engel, J., French, J., Glauser, T.A., Mathern, G.W., Moshe, S.L., Nordli, D., Plouin, P. & Scheffer, I.E. (2010). Revised terminology and concepts for organization of seizures and epilepsies: report of the ILAE Commission on Classification and Terminology, 2005-2009. *Epilepsia,* Vol.51, No. 4, (April 2010), pp. 676-685, ISSN 1528-1167.

Bjorklund, A. & Stenevi, U. (1984). Intracerebral neural implants: neuronal replacement and reconstruction of damaged circuitries. *Annual Review of Neuroscience,* Vol.7 (March 1984), pp. 279-308, ISSN 0147-006X.

Carpenter, M.K., Inokuma, M.S., Denham, J., Mujtaba, T., Chiu, C.P. & Rao, M.S. (2001). Enrichment of neurons and neural precursors from human embryonic stem cells. *Experimental Neurology,* Vol.172, No. 2, (December 2001), pp. 383-397, ISSN 0014-4886.

Castillo, C.G., Mendoza-Trejo, S., Aguilar, M.B., Freed, W.J. & Giordano, M. (2008). Intranigral transplants of a GABAergic cell line produce long-term alleviation of established motor seizures. *Behavioural Brain Research,* Vol.193, No. 1, (November 2008), pp. 17-27, ISSN 0166-4328.

Castillo, C.G., Mendoza, S., Freed, W.J. & Giordano, M. (2006). Intranigral transplants of immortalized GABAergic cells decrease the expression of kainic acid-induced seizures in the rat. *Behavioural Brain Research,* Vol.171, No. 1, (July 2006), pp. 109-115, ISSN 0166-4328.

Castillo, C.G., Mendoza, S., Saavedra, J. & Giordano, M. (2010) Lack of effect of intranigral transplants of a GABAergic cell line on absence seizures. *Epilepsy and Behavior,* Vol.18, No. 4, (August 2010), pp. 358-365, ISSN 1525-5069.

Chu,K., Kim M., Jung, K.-H., Jeon D., Lee, S.-T., Kim, J., Jeong , S.-W., Kim, S.U., Lee, S.K., Shin, H-.S., & Roh, J.-K. (2004). Human neural stem cell transplantation reduces spontaneous recurrent seizures following pilocarpine-induced status epilepticus in adult rats. Brain research, Vol.1023, No. 2, (September 2004), pp. 213-221, ISSN 0006-8993.

Conejero-Goldberg, C., Tornatore, C., Abi-Saab, W., Monaco, M.C., Dillon-Carter, O., Vawter, M., Elsworth, J. & Freed, W. (2000). Transduction of human GAD67 cDNA into immortalized striatal cell lines using an Epstein-Barr virus-based plasmid vector increases GABA content. *Experimental Neurology,* Vol.161, No. 2, (February 2000), pp. 453-461, ISSN 0014-4886.

Cooper, O., Astradsson, A.,Hallett, P., Robertson, H., Mendez, I.,Isacson, O. (2009). Lack of functional relevance of isolated cell damage in transplants of Parkinson's disease patients, *Journal of Neurology,* Vol.256 Suppl. 3, (September 2009), pp. 310-316, ISSN 1432-1459.

Cossart, R., Dinocourt, C., Hirsch, J.C., Merchan-Perez, A., De Felipe, J., Ben-Ari, Y., Esclapez, M. & Bernard, C. (2001). Dendritic but not somatic GABAergic inhibition is decreased in experimental epilepsy. *Nature Neuroscience,* Vol.4, No. 1, (January 2001), pp. 52 62, ISSN 1097-6256.

Costa-Ferro Z.S.M., Vitola A.S., Pedroso M.F., Cunha F.B., Xavier L.L., Machado D.C., Soares M.B.P., Ribeiro-dos-Santos R., & DaCosta J.C. (2010). Prevention of seizures and reorganization of hippocampal functions by transplantation of bone marrow cells in the acute phase of experimental epilepsy. *Seizure,* Vol.19, No.2, (March 2010), pp. 84-92, ISSN 1532-2688.

Drucker-Colin, R. & Verdugo-Diaz, L. (2004). Cell transplantation for Parkinson's disease: present status. *Cellular and Molecular Neurobiology,* Vol.24, No. 3, (June 2004), pp. 301-316, ISSN 0272-4340.

Dunnett, S.B., Low, W.C., Iversen, S.D., Stenevi, U. & Bjorklund, A. (1982). Septal transplants restore maze learning in rats with fornix-fimbria lesions. *Brain Research,* Vol. 251, No. 2, (November 1982), pp. 335-348, 0006-8993.

Fine, A., Meldrum, B.S. & Patel, S. (1990). Modulation of experimentally induced epilepsy by intracerebral grafts of fetal GABAergic neurons. *Neuropsychologia,* Vol.28, No. 6, (January 1990) pp. 627-634, ISSN 0028-3932.

Fink, J.S., Schumacher, J.M., Ellias, S.L., Palmer, E.P., Saint-Hilaire, M., Shannon, K., Penn, R., Starr, P., VanHorne, C., Kott, H.S., Dempsey, P.K., Fischman, A.J., Raineri, R., Manhart, C., Dinsmore, J. & Isacson, O. (2000). Porcine xenografts in Parkinson's disease and Huntington's disease patients: preliminary results. *Cell Transplantation,* Vol 9, No. 2, (March-April 2000), pp. 273-278, ISSN 0963-6897.

Freed, C.R., Greene, P.E., Breeze, R.E., Tsai, W.Y., DuMouchel, W., Kao, R., Dillon, S., Winfield, H., Culver, S., Trojanowski, J.Q., Eidelberg, D. & Fahn, S. (2001). Transplantation of embryonic dopamine neurons for severe Parkinson's disease. *New England Journal of Medicine,* Vol.344, No. 10, (March 2001), pp. 710-719, ISSN 0028-4793.

Freed, W.J. (1993) Neural transplantation: Prospects for clinical use. *Cell Transplantation,* Vol.2, (January 1993), pp 13-31, ISSN 0963-6897.

Freed, W.J., Poltorak, M. & Becker, J.B. (1990). Intracerebral adrenal medulla grafts: a review. *Experimental Neurology,* Vol.110, No. 2, (November 1990), pp. 139-166, ISSN 0014-4886.

Freed, W.J., Poltorak, M., Takashima, H., LaMarca, M.E. & Ginns, E.I. (1991). Brain grafts and Parkinson's disease. *Journal of* Cellular *Biochemistry,* Vol.45, No. 3, (March 1991), pp. 261-267, ISSN0730-2312.

Gale, K. (1992). GABA and epilepsy: basic concepts from preclinical research. *Epilepsia,* Vol.33 Suppl. 5, (January 1992), pp. S3-S12, ISSN 0013-9580.

Gash, D., Sladek, J.R., Jr. & Sladek, C.D. (1980). Functional development of grafted vasopressin neurons. *Science,* Vol.210, No. 4476, (December 1980), pp. 1367-1369, ISSN 0036-8075.

Gernert, M., Thompson, K.W., Loscher, W. & Tobin, A.J. (2002). Genetically engineered GABA-producing cells demonstrate anticonvulsant effects and long-term transgene expression when transplanted into the central piriform cortex of rats. *Experimental Neurology,* Vol.176, No. 1, (July 2002), pp. 183-92, ISSN 0014-4886.

Giordano, M., Takashima, H., Herranz, A., Poltorak, M., Geller, H.M., Marone, M. & Freed, W.J. (1993). Immortalized GABAergic cell lines derived from rat striatum using a temperature-sensitive allele of the SV40 large T antigen. *Experimental Neurology,* Vol 124, No. 2, (December 1993), pp. 395-400, ISSN 0014-4886.

Giordano, M., Takashima, H., Poltorak, M., Geller, H.M. & Freed, W.J. (1996). Constitutive expression of glutamic acid decarboxylase (GAD) by striatal cell lines immortalized using the tsA58 allele of the SV40 large T antigen. *Cell Transplantation,* Vol.5, No. 5, (September-October 1996), pp. 563-575, ISSN 0963-6897.

Goetz, C.G., Poewe, W., Rascol, O. & Sampaio, C. (2005). Evidence-based medical review update: pharmacological and surgical treatments of Parkinson's disease: 2001 to 2004. *Movement Disorders,* Vol.20, No. 5, (May 2005), pp. 523-539, ISSN 0885-3185.

Guttinger, M., Fedele, D., Koch, P., Padrun, V., Pralong, W.F., Brustle, O. & Boison, D. (2005). Suppression of kindled seizures by paracrine adenosine release from stem cell-derived brain implants. *Epilepsia,* Vol.46, No. 8, (August 2005), pp. 1162-1169, ISSN 0013-9580.

Hattiangady, B., Rao, M.S. & Shetty, A.K. (2008). Grafting of striatal precursor cells into hippocampus shortly after status epilepticus restrains chronic temporal lobe epilepsy. *Experimental Neurology,* Vol.212, No. 2, (August 2008), pp. 468-481, ISSN 1090-2430.

Isacson, O., &. Kordower, J.H. (2008) Future of Cell and Gene Therapies for Parkinson's Disease. *Annals of Neurology,* Vol.64, Suppl. 2, (December 2008), pp. S122–S138, ISSN 1531-8249.

Jing, M., Shingo, T., Yasuhara, T., Kondo, A., Morimoto, T., Wang, F., Baba, T., Yuan W.J., Tajiri,N., Uozumi, T., Murakami, M., Tanabe, M., Miyoshi, Y., Zhao, S., & Date, I. (2009). The combined therapy of intrahippocampal transplantation of adult neural stem cells and intraventricular erythropoietin-infusion ameliorates spontaneous recurrent seizures by suppression of abnormal mossy fiber sprouting. *Brain Research,* Vol.1295, (October 2009), pp. 203-211, ISSN 1872-6240.

Kanter-Schlifke, I., Fjord-Larsen, L., Kusk, P., Angehagen, M., Wahlberg, L. & Kokaia, M. (2009). GDNF released from encapsulated cells suppresses seizure activity in the epileptic hippocampus. *Experimental Neurology,* Vol.216, No. 2, (April 2009), pp. 413-419, ISSN 1090-2430.

Kim, J.H., Auerbach, J.M., Rodriguez-Gomez, J.A., Velasco, I., Gavin, D., Lumelsky, N., Lee, S.H., Nguyen, J., Sanchez-Pernaute, R., Bankiewicz, K. & McKay, R. (2002). Dopamine neurons derived from embryonic stem cells function in an animal model of Parkinson's disease. *Nature,* Vol.418, No. 6893, (July 2002), pp. 50-56, ISSN 0028-0836.

Kim, S.U. (2004). Human neural stem cells genetically modified for brain repair in neurological disorders. *Neuropathology,* Vol.24, No. 2, (September 2004), pp. 159-171, ISSN 0919-6544.

Kokaia, M., Aebischer, P., Elmer, E., Bengzon, J., Kalen, P., Kokaia, Z. & Lindvall, O. (1994). Seizure suppression in kindling epilepsy by intracerebral implants of GABA- but not by noradrenaline-releasing polymer matrices. *Experimental Brain Research,* Vol.100, No. 3, (January 1994), pp. 385-394, ISSN 0014-4819.

Kordower, J.H., Chu, Y., Hauser, R.A., Freeman, T.B. & Olanow, C.W. (2008). Lewy body-like pathology in long-term embryonic nigral transplants in Parkinson's disease. *Nature Medicine,* Vol.14, No. 5, (May 2008), pp. 504-506, ISSN 1546-170X.

Kovari, E., Horvath, J. & Bouras, C. (2009). Neuropathology of Lewy body disorders. *Brain Res Bull,* Vol.80, No. 4-5, (October 2009), pp. 203-210, ISSN 1873-2747.

Labandeira-Garcia, J.L. & Guerra, M.J. (1994). Cortical stimulation induces fos expression in intrastriatal striatal grafts. *Brain Research,* Vol.652, No. 1, (July 1994), pp. 87-97, ISSN 0006-8993.

Lang, K.J., Rathjen, J., Vassilieva, S. & Rathjen, P.D. (2004). Differentiation of embryonic stem cells to a neural fate: a route to re-building the nervous system? *Journal of Neuroscience Research,* Vol.76, No. 2, (April 2004), pp. 184-192, ISSN 0360-4012.

Lee, G., Chambers, S.M., Tomishima, M.J. & Studer, L. Derivation of neural crest cells from human pluripotent stem cells. (2010). *Nature Protocols,* Vol.5, No. 4, (April 2010), pp. 688-701, ISSN 1750-2799.

Li, J. Y., Englund, E., Holton, J. L., Soulet, D., Hagell, P., Lees, A. J., Lashley, T., Quinn, N. P., Rehncrona, S., Bjorklund, A., Widner, H., Revesz, T., Lindvall, O., & Brundin, P. (2008). Lewy bodies in grafted neurons in subjects with Parkinson's disease suggest host-to-graft disease propagation. *Nature Medicine,* Vol.14, No. 5, (May 2008), pp. 501-503, ISSN 1546-170X.

Li, T., Steinbeck, J. A., Lusardi, T., Koch, P., Lan, J. Q., Wilz, A., Segschneider, M., Simon, R. P., Brustle, O., & Boison, D. (2007). Suppression of kindling epileptogenesis by adenosine releasing stem cell-derived brain implants. *Brain,*Vol. 130, Pt.5, (May 2007), pp. 1276-1288, ISSN 1460-2156.

Lindvall, O., & Bjorklund, A. (2004) Cell therapy in Parkinson's disease. *NeuroRx,* Vol.1, No. 4, (October 2004), pp. 382-393, ISSN 1545-5343.

Loscher, W., Ebert, U., Lehmann, H., Rosenthal, C. & Nikkhah, G. (1998). Seizure suppression in kindling epilepsy by grafts of fetal GABAergic neurons in rat substantia nigra. *Journal of Neuroscience Research,* Vol. 51, No. 2, (January 1998), pp. 196-209, ISSN 0360-4012.

Ma, Y., Tang, C., Chaly, T., Greene, P., Breeze, R., Fahn, S., Freed, C., Dhawan, V. & Eidelberg, D. (2010). Dopamine cell implantation in Parkinson's disease: long-term clinical and (18)F-FDOPA PET outcomes. *Journal of Nuclear Medicine,* Vol.51, No. 1, (January 2010), pp. 7-15, ISSN 1535-5667.

Maisano, X., Carpentino, J., Becker, S., Lanza, R., Aaron, G., Grabel, L. & Naegele, J.R. (2009). Embryonic stem cell-derived neural precursor grafts for treatment of temporal lobe epilepsy. *Neurotherapeutics,* Vol 6, No. 2, (April 2009), pp. 263-277, ISSN 1933-7213.

Mejía-Toiber, J., Castillo, C.G., & Giordano, M. (in press). Strategies for the development of cell lines for *ex vivo* gene therapy in the central nervous system. *Cell transplantation.*

Mejia-Toiber, J., Marquez-Ramos, J.A., Diaz-Munoz, M., Pena, F., Aguilar, M.B. & Giordano, M. Glutamatergic excitation and GABA release from a transplantable cell line. *Cell Transplant,* Vol 19, No. 10, (June 2010), pp. 1307-1323, ISSN 1555-3892.

Mendez, I., Vinuela, A., Astradsson, A., Mukhida, K., Hallett, P., Robertson, H., Tierney, T., Holness, R., Dagher, A., Trojanowski, J.Q. & Isacson, O. (2008). Dopamine neurons implanted into people with Parkinson's disease survive without pathology for 14 years. *Nature Medicine,* Vol.14, No. 5, (May 2008), pp. 507-509, ISSN 1546-170X.

Morimoto, K., Fahnestock, M. & Racine, R.J. (2004). Kindling and status epilepticus models of epilepsy: rewiring the brain. *Progress in Neurobiology,* Vol.73, No. 1, (May 2004), pp. 1-60, ISSN 0301-0082.

Muller, F. J., Snyder, E. Y., & Loring, J. F. (2006) Gene therapy: can neural stem cells deliver? *Nature reviews. Neuroscience,* Vol.7, No. 1, (January 2006), pp. 75-84, ISSN 1471-003X.

Murata, Y., Chiba, T., Brundin, P., Bjorklund, A. & Lindvall, O. (1990). Formation of synaptic graft-host connections by noradrenergic locus coeruleus neurons transplanted into the adult rat hippocampus. *Experimental Neurology,* Vol.110, No. 3, (December 1990), pp. 258-267, ISSN 0014-4886.

Nolte, M.W., Löscher, W., Herden, C., Freed, W.J. & Gernert, M. (2008). Benefits and risks of intranigral transplantation of GABA-producing cells subsequent to the establishment of kindling-induced seizures. *Neurobiology of Disease,* Vol .1, No. 3, (September 2008), pp. 342-354, ISSN 1095-953X.

Norman, A.B., Lehman, M.N. & Sanberg, P.R. (1989). Functional effects of fetal striatal transplants. *Brain Research Bulletin,* Vol.22, No. 1, (January 1989), pp. 163-172, ISSN 0361-9230.

Nottebohm, F. (2002). Neuronal replacement in adult brain. *Brain Research Bulletin,* Vol.57, No. 6, (April 2002), pp. 737-749, ISSN 0361-9230.

Olanow, C.W., Goetz, C.G., Kordower, J.H., Stoessl, A.J., Sossi, V., Brin, M.F., Shannon, K.M., Nauert, G.M., Perl, D.P., Godbold, J. & Freeman, T.B. (2003). A double-blind controlled trial of bilateral fetal nigral transplantation in Parkinson's disease. *Annals of Neurology,* Vol.54, No. 3, (September 2003), pp. 403-414, ISSN 0364-5134.

Pan, Y., Chen, X., Wang, S., Yang, S., Bai, X., Chi, X., Li, K., Liu, B. & Li, L. (2005). In vitro neuronal differentiation of cultured human embryonic germ cells. *Biochemical and Biophysical Research Communications,* Vol.327, No. 2, (February 2005), pp. 548-556, ISSN 0006-291X.

Perrier, A.L., Tabar, V., Barberi, T., Rubio, M.E., Bruses, J., Topf, N., Harrison, N.L. & Studer, L. (2004). Derivation of midbrain dopamine neurons from human embryonic stem cells. *Proceedings of the National Academy of Science U S A,* Vol.101, No. 34, (August 2004), pp. 12543-12548, ISSN 0027-8424.

Piccini, P., Pavese, N., Hagell, P., Reimer, J., Bjorklund, A., Oertel, W.H., Quinn, N.P., Brooks, D.J. & Lindvall, O. (2005). Factors affecting the clinical outcome after neural transplantation in Parkinson's disease. *Brain,* Vol.128, Pt 12, (December 2005), pp. 2977-2986, ISSN 1460-2156.

Rao, M. S., Hattiangady, B., Rai, K. S., & Shetty, A. K. (2007). Strategies for promoting anti-seizure effects of hippocampal fetal cells grafted into the hippocampus of rats exhibiting chronic temporal lobe epilepsy. *Neurobiology of disease,* Vol.27, No. 2 (August 2007), pp. 117-132, ISSN 0969-9961.

Reubinoff, B.E., Itsykson, P., Turetsky, T., Pera, M.F., Reinhartz, E., Itzik, A. & Ben-Hur, T. (2001). Neural progenitors from human embryonic stem cells. *Nature Biotechnology,* Vol.19, No. 12, (December 2001), pp. 1134-1140, ISSN 1087-0156.

Rodriguez-Gomez, J.A., Lu, J.Q., Velasco, I., Rivera, S., Zoghbi, S.S., Liow, J.S., Musachio, J.L., Chin, F.T., Toyama, H., Seidel, J., Green, M.V., Thanos, P.K., Ichise, M., Pike, V.W., Innis, R.B. & McKay, R.D. (2007). Persistent dopamine functions of neurons derived from embryonic stem cells in a rodent model of Parkinson disease. *Stem Cells,* Vol.25, No. 4, (April 2007), pp. 918-928, ISSN 1066-5099.

Roitberg, B., Shin, P., Sramek, J., & Kordower, J.H. (2000). Neural grafting for Parkinson's and Huntington's disease, In: *Central nervous system diseases: innovative animal models from lab to clinic,* D.F. Emerich, R.L. Dean III, P.R. Sanberg (Eds.), pp. 441-483, Humana Press Ic, 0-89603-724-X, Totowa, NJ.

Ross, K.C., Waldman, B.C., Conejero-Goldberg, C., Freed, W. & Coleman, J.R. (2002). Transplantation of M213-2O cells with enhanced GAD67 expression into the inferior colliculus alters audiogenic seizures. *Experimental Neurology,* Vol.177, No. 1, (September 2002), pp. 338-340, ISSN 0014-4886.

Ruschenschmidt, C., Koch, P.G., Brustle, O. & Beck, H. (2005). Functional properties of ES cell-derived neurons engrafted into the hippocampus of adult normal and chronically epileptic rats. *Epilepsia,* Vol.46 Suppl. 5, pp. 174-183, ISSN 0013-9580.

Rutherford, A., Garcia-Munoz, M., Dunnett, S.B. & Arbuthnott, G.W. (1987). Electrophysiological demonstration of host cortical inputs to striatal grafts. *Neuroscience Letters,* Vol.83, No. 3, (December 1987), pp. 275-281, ISSN 0304-3940.

Shetty, A.K. & Hattiangady, B. (2007). Concise review: prospects of stem cell therapy for temporal lobe epilepsy. *Stem Cells,* Vol.25, No. 10, (October 2007), pp. 2396-2407, ISSN 1549-4918.

Snyder, E. Y., Daley, G. Q., & Goodell, M. (2004). Taking stock and planning for the next decade: realistic prospects for stem cell therapies for the nervous system Journal of neuroscience research. *Journal of neuroscience research,* Vol.76, No. 2, (April 2004), pp. 157-168, ISSN 0360-4012.

Storch, A., Sabolek, M., Milosevic, J., Schwarz, S. C., & Schwarz, J. (2004). Midbrain-derived neural stem cells: from basic science to therapeutic approaches. *Cell and tissue research,* Vol.318, No. 1 (October 2004), pp. 15-22, ISSN 0302-766X.

Takahashi, K. & Yamanaka, S. (2006). Induction of pluripotent stem cells from mouse embryonic and adult fibroblast cultures by defined factors. *Cell,* Vol.126, No. 4, (August 2006), pp. 663-676, ISSN 0092-8674.

Thompson, K.W. (2005). Genetically engineered cells with regulatable GABA production can affect afterdischarges and behavioral seizures after transplantation into the dentate gyrus. *Neuroscience,* Vol.133, No. 4, (June 2005), pp. 1029-1037, ISSN 0306-4522.

Thompson, K., Anantharam, V., Behrstock, S., Bongarzone, E., Campagnoni, A. & Tobin, A.J. (2000). Conditionally immortalized cell lines, engineered to produce and release GABA, modulate the development of behavioral seizures. *Experimental Neurology,* Vol.161, No. 2, (February 2000), pp. 481-489, ISSN 0014-4886.

Thompson, K.W. & Suchomelova, L.M. (2004). Transplants of cells engineered to produce GABA suppress spontaneous seizures. *Epilepsia,* Vol.45, No. 1, (January 2004), pp. 4-12, ISSN 0013-9580.

Tolosa, E., Wenning, G. & Poewe, W. (2006). The diagnosis of Parkinson's disease. *Lancet Neurology,* Vol.5, No. 1, (January 2006), pp. 75-86, ISSN 1474-4422.

Ungerstedt, U. (1968). 6-Hydroxy-dopamine induced degeneration of central monoamine neurons. *European Journal of Pharmacology,* Vol.5, No. 1, (December 1968), pp. 107-110, ISSN 0014-2999.

Ungerstedt, U. & Arbuthnott, G.W. (1970). Quantitative recording of rotational behavior in rats after 6-hydroxy-dopamine lesions of the nigrostriatal dopamine system. *Brain Research,* Vol.24, No. 3, (December 1970), pp. 485-493, ISSN 0006-8993.

Vazin, T. & Freed, W.J. Human embryonic stem cells: derivation, culture, and differentiation: a review. *Restorative Neurology and Neuroscience,* Vol.28, No. 4, (January 2010), pp. 589-603, ISSN 0922-6028.

Waldau, B., Hattiangady, B., Kuruba, R., & Shetty, A. K. (2010) Medial ganglionic eminence-derived neural stem cell grafts ease spontaneous seizures and restore GDNF expression in a rat model of chronic temporal lobe epilepsy. *Stem cells,* Vol. 28, No. 7, (July 2010), pp. 1153-1164, ISSN 1549-4918.

Wang, Y., Chen, S., Yang, D., & Le, W. D. (2007). Stem cell transplantation: a promising therapy for Parkinson's disease. *Journal of neuroimmune pharmacology,* Vol.2, No. 3, (September 2007), pp. 243-250,ISSN 1557-1904.

Westmoreland, J.J., Hancock, C.R. & Condie, B.G. (2001). Neuronal development of embryonic stem cells: a model of GABAergic neuron differentiation. *Biochemical and Biophysical Research Communications,* Vol.284, No. 3, (June 2001), pp. 674-680, ISSN 0006-291X.

Wictorin, K. (1992). Anatomy and connectivity of intrastriatal striatal transplants. *Progress in Neurobiology,* Vol.38, No. 6, (June 1992), pp. 611-639, ISSN 0301-0082.

Winkler, C., Kirik, D., & Bjorklund, A. (2005). Cell transplantation in Parkinson's disease: how can we make it work? *Trends in neurosciences,* Vol.28, No.2, (February 2005), pp. 86-92, ISSN 0166-2236.

Xu, Z.C., Wilson, C.J. & Emson, P.C. (1991). Synaptic potentials evoked in spiny neurons in rat neostriatal grafts by cortical and thalamic stimulation. *J Neurophysiol,* Vol 65, No. 3, (Mar), pp. 477-493, ISSN 0022-3077.

Yu, J., & Thomson, J. A. (2008). Pluripotent stem cell lines. *Genes & development*, Vol.22, No.15, (August 2008), pp. 1987-1997, ISSN 0890-9369.

Zhang, S.C., Wernig, M., Duncan, I.D., Brustle, O. & Thomson, J.A. (2001). In vitro differentiation of transplantable neural precursors from human embryonic stem cells. *Nature Biotechnoogyl,* Vol.19, No. 12, (December 2001), pp. 1129-1133, ISSN 1087-0156.

5

Adverse Metabolic Effects of Antiepileptic Drug Treatment

Karl O. Nakken
National Centre for Epilepsy, Oslo University Hospital, Norway

1. Introduction

Active epilepsy with recurrent seizures is associated with a range of well-documented unfavourable consequences. Nevertheless, adverse metabolic effects of antiepileptic drug (AED) treatments have only recently received attention. Such effects may be subtle, insidious, take many years to become clinically apparent, and may have a negative impact on general health for many decades. Unfortunately, many neurologists are unaware of such AED-related side-effects.

The relationship between epilepsy and metabolic disorders is multi-factorial. Metabolic encephalopathies, including mitochondrial disorders and some of the progressive myoclonic epilepsies, are important causes of seizures in childhood. Acute metabolic disturbances associated with diseases affecting the kidneys, liver, or pancreas may give rise to seizures. Furthermore, alcohol- or drug-withdrawal may also be associated with seizures. From the other perspective, seizures themselves, in particular prolonged seizures such as in convulsive status epilepticus, may lead to a variety of metabolic abnormalities.

In this chapter I will summarize our current knowledge about the adverse metabolic effects of AED treatment and discuss whether these side-effects are so severe that a reconsideration of our prescribing habits would be beneficial.

2. Effects on bone metabolism

Accumulating evidence indicates an association between long-term use of AEDs and disturbed bone metabolism, resulting in decreased bone mineral density (BMD) and an increased risk of fractures (Lee, 2010). This is particularly problematic for people with epilepsy as their propensity to fractures is already elevated due to other drug side-effects (e.g. dizziness, ataxia), co-existing neurological deficits (e.g. cerebral palsy), and seizure-related falls (Mattson & Gidal, 2004). Furthermore, generalized tonic-clonic seizures are, themselves, associated with an increased risk of fractures, especially vertebral compression fractures (Pedersen et al., 1976).

It is common knowledge that steroids have a negative impact on bone metabolism. However, the bone-depleting effects of AEDs are less well-known. In a survey of 624 neurologists, only 28 % were familiar with AEDs being associated with reduced bone mass, and only 9 % of paediatric neurologists and 7 % of adult neurologists offered their patients prophylactic calcium and vitamin D supplements (Valmadrid et al., 2001). In another survey carried out by Epilepsy Action, a British patient advocacy organization, 75 % of members surveyed reported that they had not been informed that osteoporosis was a possible side-effect of long-term AED use. Of those who had been informed, their epilepsy specialist was the primary source of this information (Epilepsy Action, 2003).

Although the results of studies on the impact of AEDs on BMD are diverse, as much as 75 % of epilepsy patients have been found to be osteopenic and up to 25 % osteoporotic (Coppola et al., 2009).

The drugs most consistently associated with skeletal abnormalities are those that affect the cytochrome P450 (CYP450) system (e. g. phenytoin, phenobarbital, carbamazepine, valproate) (Vestergaard et al., 2004; Pack et al., 2005; Souverein et al., 2006; Tsiropoulos et al., 2008). However, drugs that inhibit carbonic anhydrase (topiramate, zonisamide, acetazolamide) have also been suspected to affect bone health by causing metabolic acidosis. Nevertheless, a double-blind, randomized, preliminary study of topiramate as an anti-obesity drug did not indicate changes in bone turnover markers in comparison with placebo controls (Leung & Ramsay, 2006).

Data on the effects of the new generation AEDs on bone health are sparse. Animal studies have demonstrated that levetiracetam reduces bone strength and bone formation without altering bone mass (Nissen-Meyer et al., 2007), but there are no clinical data that either support or negate this observation. Neither lamotrigine nor oxcarbazepine have been found to interfere with bone mineral metabolism (Sheth & Hermann, 2007; Cetinkaya et al., 2009).

The mechanisms underlying the bone-depleting effects of AEDs are probably complex. For many years the main theory was that enzyme-inducing AEDs (e.g. phenobarbital, phenytoin, carbamazepine) accelerated vitamin D hydroxylation to polar inactive metabolites, thereby resulting in hypocalcaemia, secondary hyperparathyroidism, increased bone turnover, and higher rates of bone loss. Although this is still considered an important mechanism, later studies have shown that AEDs may cause bone loss even in the absence of vitamin D deficiency (Farhat et al., 2002; Andress et al., 2002). Furthermore, valproate, a CYP450 inhibitor, has also been shown to have an adverse effect on bone health, probably via completely different mechanisms (Sheth et al., 1995; Sato et al., 2001; Guo et al., 2001; Sheth, 2004). Decreased intestinal absorption of calcium, resistance to parathyroid hormone, calcitonin deficiency, interference with vitamin K metabolism, and a direct drug-effect on bone cell functions have also been suggested as possible mechanisms (Feldkamp et al., 2000; Petty et al., 2007). Other indirect effects of the drugs, such as hormonal changes, increases in homocysteine, reduction in insulin growth factor 1, and the effect of valproate as a histone deacetylase inhibitor, thereby reducing collagen I and osteonectin, may also contribute (Fuller et al., 2010).

3. Effects on lipid metabolism

The CYP450 enzyme system is involved in the synthesis and metabolism of cholesterol (Nebert & Russel, 2002). In particular, CYP51A1 plays a key role in cholesterol synthesis (Gibbons, 2002). Enzyme-inducing AEDs would therefore be expected to increase cholesterol production, and, in keeping with this hypothesis, several cross-sectional studies have demonstrated that patients treated with phenobarbital, phenytoin, or carbamazepine have elevated total cholesterol levels compared with normal controls (Isojärvi et al., 1993; Verotti et al., 1998; Eiris et al., 2000; Nikolaos et al., 2004). Specific studies have shown increases in most of the various lipid fractions, including low-density and high-density lipoproteins and triglycerides. However, the increase in high-density lipoproteins tends to be modest relative to the other lipid fractions (Isojärvi et al., 1993; Nikolaos et al., 2004). A recent study of patients whose AED treatments were switched from the inducing agents, carbamazepine and phenytoin, to the non-inducing lamotrigine and levetiracetam, demonstrated a decline in total cholesterol, averaging 26 mg/dl after 6 weeks (Mintzer et al., 2009). The greatest change was in the atherogenic low-density lipoproteins.

Thus, most studies indicate that the effects of enzyme-inducing AEDs on specific lipid fractions favour an atherogenic profile, while the enzyme-inhibiting agent, valproate, exerts the opposite effect (Verotti et al., 1997; Verotti et al., 1998; Nikolaos et al., 2004).

4. Effects on homocysteine, lipoprotein A, and C-reactive protein levels

The amino acid homocysteine is prothrombotic, and is therefore considered a significant risk factor for cardiovascular mortality (Selhub, 2008), stroke (Spence, 2007), dementia (Ravaglia, 2005), and possibly also pharmacoresistant seizures (Sener, 2006). Whether the increased risk is associated with homocysteine itself, or whether homocysteine is merely a marker, is currently not determined. Homocysteine concentration is inversely related to plasma levels of folate, vitamin B6, and vitamin B12. Almost two-thirds of high homocysteine cases can be attributed to low vitamin status (Selhub, 2008).

Lipoprotein A has also been found to be an independent risk factor for cardiovascular disease (Danesh et al., 2000).

Some studies indicate that enzyme-inducing AEDs may increase the levels of both lipoprotein A and homocysteine (Schwaninger et al., 1999; Schwaninger et al., 2000; Apeland et al., 2001; Bramswig et al., 2003). Moreover, a recent study showed that homocysteine levels were significantly reduced when patients were tapered off phenytoin, but not carbamazepine (Minzer et al, 2009). Thus, it appears that the effects of inducing AEDs may not be entirely uniform.

C-reactive protein (CRP) concentration has been found to be correlated with risk of vascular disease, independent of serum lipids (Ridker et al., 1997). In the aforementioned study, in which patients were switched from the inducing drugs, carbamazepine or phenytoin, to the non-inducing agents, levetiracetam or lamotrigine, a reduction in CRP of almost one third was recorded after 6 weeks (Mintzer et al., 2009).

5. Valproate may cause metabolic syndrome and hyperammonaemia

Metabolic syndrome, as indicated by centripetal obesity, glucose intolerance, hypertension, elevated triglycerides, low high-density lipoprotein cholesterol, and hyperandrogenism/polycystic ovaries, occurs in 41 % of women treated with valproate, compared with 5.3 % of those treated with carbamazepine, and apparently none of those being treated with lamotrigine and topiramate (Kim & Lee, 2007). This syndrome appears to occur exclusively in those who develop obesity during valproate use (Verotti et al., 2010).

However, worth noticing is that it has been estimated that appproximately 25 % of the general population of adults in USA has metabolic syndrome.

Further, valproate and its metabolites interfere with several biochemical pathways in the mitochondria, leading to disruption of the urea cycle and thereby causing hyperammonaemia (Garcia 2009), and this may occur in 20-50 % of patients being treated with valproate. In some patients this is well-tolerated, but in others elevated ammonia can be associated with encephalopathy with confusion, ataxia, reduced cognitive abilities, decline in conscious level, triphasic waves in EEG, and increased seizure frequency (Perucca, 2002).

6. Effects on body weight

Obesity has become epidemic in the western world (Aronne, 2002). People with epilepsy also have an increased rate of obesity, and this may be related to a high prevalence of depression (Gilliam et al., 2003), physical inactivity (Bjørholt et al., 1990), unhealthy diet, and AED treatment. Obesity may have many negative consequences, including insulin resistance, reproductive dysfunction, cardiovascular disorders, gall bladder disease, bone and joint disease, and cancer (Aronne, 2002).

AEDs may be associated with either increases or reductions in body weight (Biton, 2003).

Those AEDs that have most consistently been reported to increase body weight include valproate, carbamazepine, gabapentin, pregabalin, and vigabatrin (Sheth, 2008). Of these, the clinically most important is the valproate-associated increase in body weight. This appears to be cumulative over the course of many years of treatment (Biton et al., 2001), and seems to be an important risk factor for the development of non-alcoholic fatty liver disease, which occurs in 61 % of patients (Luef et al., 2004). Valproate is a fatty acid derivative and competes with free fatty acids for albumin binding, and, as a GABAergic agonist, is known to be involved in insulin secretion from pancreatic beta-cells. Thus, valproate-associated weight gain is probably due to hyperinsulinaemia with relative insulin resistance (Luef et al., 2004). Elevated levels of cortisol, leptin, and neuropeptide Y may also be contributory (Aydin et al., 2005).

Those AEDs most often associated with weight loss include felbamate, topiramate, and zonizamide. A prospective uncontrolled topiramate trial demonstrated that 86 % of patients had lost weight after 12 months of treatment (Ben-Menachem et al., 2003). Those with a body mass index (BMI) > 30 lost 12 % of their body weight, whereas those with BMI < 30 lost 5 %. Body fat loss represented 60-70 % of the weight loss. Serum glucose levels, glucose tolerance test, and blood lipid profiles improved, and serum leptin levels were reduced (Ben-Menachem et al., 2003).

Felbamate is associated with anorexia and loss of between 3 and 5 % of body weight in children, and mostly occurs during the first 3 months of therapy (Bourgeois, 1997).

A recent study on the effect of zonisamide on body weight revealed a mean decrease in body weight by 3.7 %. A weight loss > 5 % was documented in 35 % of patients in the study, and a weight gain > 5 % in 14 %. The weight loss was most prominent in those that were overweight prior to treatment. The weight changes did not appear to be dose-related, and were reversible after discontinuation of therapy (Wellmer et al., 2009).

Phenytoin, lamotrigine, and levetiracetam are assumed to be weight-neutral agents.

7. Some AEDs may induce metabolic acidosis

Metabolic acidosis results either when the kidney is unable to excrete dietary H^+ load or when there is an excessive loss of HCO_3^- secondary to reduced renal tubular reabsorption. The three AEDs that inhibit carbonic anhydrase, acetazolamide, topiramate, and zonisamide, are all associated with varying degrees of renal tubular acidosis. Topiramate causes a mild hyperchloraemic, non-anion gap metabolic acidosis with low levels of bicarbonate (Mirza et al., 2009), typically appearing soon after initiation of therapy. However, a marked reduction in bicarbonate occurs in less than 10 % of patients, and the reduction seems to be dose-related (Mirza et al., 2009).

8. Effects on gonadal steroids

The CYP450 enzymes are involved in both steroidogenesis and the metabolism of endogenous steroids (Nebert & Russel, 2002). As would be expected, studies of both men and women treated with enzyme-inducing AEDs have shown reduced testosterone levels compared with those taking non-inducing AEDs (Herzog et al., 2005; Løfgren et al., 2006; Talbot et al., 2008). However, whether the extent of reduction in testosterone levels is sufficient to compromise sexual functions has not yet been ascertained (Talbot et al., 2008). Nevertheless, decreased sexual function, with reduced sexual desire, orgasmic dysfunction, and low levels of oestradiol has been found in women with epilepsy (Bergen et al., 1992; Morrell et al., 2005).

9. Effects on serum concentrations of sodium

Asymptomatic hyponatraemia (serum sodium < 135 mmol/l) occurs in up to 50 % of patients using oxcarbazepine, and develops gradually during the first months of therapy. Severe hyponatraemia (serum sodium < 125 mmol/l) is found in approximately 3 % of patients with previously normal serum sodium (Schmidt et al., 2001; Holtmann et al., 2002) and may be associated with various symptoms, such as nausea, fatigue, or seizure worsening. Those most at risk of developing oxcarbazepine-associated hyponatraemia are the elderly and those using other sodium-depleting agents, including diuretics, oral contraceptives, or nonsteroidal anti-inflammatory drugs (Schmidt et al., 2001).

Valproate has also been reported to cause a syndrome of inappropriate antidiuretic hormone secretion (SIADH) or hyponatraemia (Beers et al., 2010).

The mechanism by which oxcarbazepine, and to lesser degree carbamazepine, lowers the sodium levels has not yet been fully elucidated.

10. Potential consequences of the metabolically adverse effects of AEDs

As the occurrence of osteoporosis rises with age, and life expectancy has increased, osteoporosis is a considerable health problem in the general population. Currently 50 million people worldwide are estimated to suffer from epilepsy, and this number, along with the rapid increase in use of AEDs for other indications (Landmark, 2008), suggests that millions of people will soon be adversely affected by the osteopenic effects of some AEDs.

The risk of fractures in patients with epilepsy has not been precisely defined, but is undoubtedly greater than in the general population. Both the epilepsy itself and the bone-depleting effects of AEDs are probably contributory factors to the increased risk (Mattson & Gidal, 2004). However, it should be acknowledged that most studies on AED-associated bone disorders have methodological limitations, and thus, their results should be interpreted with caution.

In comparison with the general population, people with epilepsy appear to have a 2-6 times greater risk of fractures (Andress et al., 2002; Mattson & Gidal, 2004; Sheth et al., 2006), and the fracture risk seems to increase with the cumulative duration of AED exposure, with the strongest association occurring in those with more than 12 years of use (Souverein et al., 2006). A meta-analysis of clinical studies investigating the effects of epilepsy and epilepsy treatment on fracture risk and BMD, found the relative risk to be increased by 2.2 for any fracture, by 5.3 for hip fracture, by 1.7 for forearm fracture, and by 6.2 for spinal fracture. The estimated risks of fractures were higher than would be expected from BMD TZ-scores (Vestergaard, 2005).

As enzyme-inducing AEDs change the lipid profile in an atherogenic direction and also elevate other surrogate vascular risk markers, it could be expected that those using such drugs are at increased risk of developing vascular disease. However, studies on epilepsy and comorbid vascular disease are conflicting. One Finnish study revealed a *lower* prevalence of ischemic heart disease in epilepsy patients than in a control group (Muuronen et al., 1985), while a Norwegian study showed no significant difference in coronary risk profile between epilepsy patients and controls (Nakken & Kornstad, 1998). Other studies have shown a mildly increased mortality from ischemic heart disease among epilepsy patients, with standardized mortality ratios between 1.2 and 2.5 (Annegers et al., 1984; Nilsson et al., 1997).

Those AEDs causing metabolic acidosis (acetazolamide, topiramate, zonisamide) may give rise to hyperventilation, acroparestesias, fatigue, anorexia, kidney stones, osteoporosis, and cardiac arrhythmias. In children, chronic metabolic acidosis may reduce growth rates. While the rate of kidney stones is estimated to be approximately 0.5 % in the general population, with some geographical variations, users of zonisamide and topiramate are found to have 1-4 % risk of developing nephrolithiasis, with men at greater risk than women (Vega et al., 2007).

As with the effects of enzyme-inducing AEDs on the lipid profile, more studies are needed to elucidate more fully the clinical consequences of the drugs' effects on gonadal steroids.

11. How to manage adverse metabolic effects associated with AED use

Low bone mass associated with AED use is largely unrecognized, undetected, and untreated (Sheth, 2004). Further, there are no formal guidelines for monitoring, prevention, and management of bone disease among those patients using AEDs (Lee, 2010).

However, those AEDs that involve the CYP450 enzyme system should be avoided, if possible, in high risk patients (Table 1). Osteoprotective behaviour should be promoted; sunlight exposure and weight-bearing exercise should be encouraged, and known risk factors, like smoking and alcohol consumption, should be avoided.

Table 1. Patients with an increased risk of fractures

- Old age (> 70 years)
- Postmenopausal women
- Using enzyme-inducing AED(s)
- Previously experienced low-energy fractures
- DEXA-values below 2.5 SD of normal
- A combination of risk factors, such as low BMI, smoking, sedentary lifestyle, poor diet, and modest sun exposure
- More than 3 cm reduction of body height in persons < 70 years, more than 5 cm in persons > 70 years

I recommend that patients with epilepsy that are taking AEDs on long-term basis should ensure that their dietary intake of calcium and vitamin D is adequate; vitamin D 800 IU/day and calcium 1000 mg/day. High risk patients should take higher doses; vitamin D 1000-4000 IU/day and calcium 1500 mg/day (Nakken & Taubøll, 2010).

BMD screening is warranted for persons with long-term AED exposure, particularly for those using enzyme-inducing AEDs or valproate, or patients with other risk factors for bone loss. A Dual-Energy X-ray Absorptiometry (DEXA) measurement should be conducted five years after the initiation of AED treatment in all patients, and should be conducted every 2-3 years in high risk patients.

Hormonal replacement therapy may be useful in menopausal women with other significant climacteric symptoms, including hot flashes. However, oestrogen may in some women reduce the seizure threshold.

The role of antiresorptive agents, like bisphosphonates, in the treatment of AED-associated bone loss is currently unresolved. However, based on general treatment principles for osteoporosis, I suggest that the use of bisphosphonates should be discussed for patients with DEXA T-scores that are below –2.5, and for those with T-scores between –1 and –2.5 who have experienced low energy fractures.

Serum sodium should be measured regularly in patients treated with oxcarbazepine, and combination with other sodium-depleting drugs should be avoided. If severe hyponatraemia (serum sodium < 125 mmol/l) should occur, then dose reduction or switching to another AED is recommended.

Patients being treated with valproate should be followed up closely with respect to weight changes, and valproate should be avoided, if possible, in patients with an obesity problem. If valproate-associated metabolic syndrome occurs, another AED should be used. If patients treated with valproate develop signs that are consistent with encephalopathy, particularly in the presence of asterixis and/or delta slowing on EEG, checking for hyperammonaemia is a reasonable precaution (Perucca, 2002). Hyperammonaemia develops in the context of normal liver functions and is associated with carnitine deficiency. Thus, carnitine supplementation has been recommended (Hamed & Abdella, 2009).

Topiramate or zonizamide should not be offered to patients with a previous history of anorexia or kidney stones, or those on a ketogen diet (Paul et al., 2010). Increasing fluid intake and urine output can help in reducing the risk of kidney stone formation.

12. Conclusion

The adverse metabolic effects of AEDs are probably currently underestimated, and thus represent an area of legitimate concern. As most of these effects develop insidiously over many years, they might either be overlooked or not associated with the drug therapy. Most adverse metabolic effects are associated with the older generation of AEDs, especially those with enzyme-inducing or enzyme-inhibiting properties. Although the side-effect profiles of the new generation of AEDs are not completely elucidated, many of these drugs do not affect liver enzymes. Assuming that the seizure reducing effects of the new AEDs are comparable to those of the old ones, as indeed has been indicated in some studies (Brodie et al., 1999; Brodie et al., 2007; Marson et al., 2007), and have a preferable adverse effect profile, the new drugs should be selected as first-line treatment in patients with newly diagnosed epilepsy.

13. References

Andress, D.L.; Ozuna, J.; Tirschwell, D. et al. (2002). Antiepileptic drug-induced bone loss in young male patients who have seizures. *Archives of Neurology* Vol.59, pp. 781-786

Annegers, J.F.; Hauser, W.A. & Shirts, S.B. (1984). Heart disease mortality and morbidity in patients with epilepsy. *Epilepsia* Vol.25, pp. 699-704

Apeland, T.; Mansoor, M.A. & Strandjord, R.E. (2001). Antiepileptic drugs as independent predictors of plasma total homocysteine levels. Epilepsy Research Vol.47, pp. 27-35

Aronne, L.J. (2002). Obesity as a disease: etiology, treatment, and management considerationss for the obese patient. *Obesity Research* Vol.10 (suppl 2), pp. S95-S96

Aydin, K.; Serdaroglu, A.; Okuyaz, C. et al. (2005). Serum insulin, leptin, and neuropeptide y levels in epileptic children treated with valproate. *Journal of Child Neurology* Vol.20, pp. 848-851

Beers, E.; van Puienbrock, E.P.; Bartelink, I.H. et al. (2010). Syndrome of inappropriate antidiuretic hormone secretion (SIADH) or hyponatremia associated with valproic acid: four case reports from the Netherlands and a case/non-case analysis of vigibase. *Drug Safety* Vol.33, No.1, pp. 47-55

Ben-Menachem, E.; Axelsen, M.; Johanson, E.H. et al. (2003). Predictors of weight loss in adults with topiramate-treated epilepsy. *Obesity Research* Vol.11, No.4, pp. 556-562

Bergen, D.; Daugherty, S. & Eckenfels, E. (1992). Reduction of sexual activities in females taking antiepileptic drugs. *Psychopathology* Vol.25, pp. 1-4

Biton, V.; Mirza, W.; Montouris, G. et al. (2001). Weight change associated with valproate and lamotrigine monotherapy in patients with epilepsy. *Neurology* Vol.56, pp. 172-177

Biton, V. (2003). Effect of antiepileptic drugs on bodyweight: overview and clinical implications for the treatment of epilepsy. *CNS Drugs* Vol.17, No.11, pp. 781-791

Bjørholt, P.G.; Nakken, K.O.; Røhme, K. et al. (1990). Leisure time habits and physical fitness in adults with epilepsy. *Epilepsia* Vol.31, No.1, pp. 83-87

Bourgeois, B.F. (1997). Felbamate. *Seminars in Pediatric Neurology* Vol.4, pp. 3-8

Bramswig, S.; Sudhop, T.; Luers, C. et al. (2003). Lipoprotein(a) concentrations increases during treatment with carbamazepine. *Epilepsia* Vol.44, pp. 457-460

Brodie, M.J.; Overstall, P.W. & Giorgi, L. (1999). Multicentre, double-blind, randomised comparison between lamotrigine and carbamazepine in elderly patients with newly diagnosed epilepsy. The UK lamotrigine elderly study group. *Epilepsy Research* Vol.37, pp. 81-87

Brodie, M.J.; Perucca, E.; Ryvlin, P. et al. (2007). Comparison of levetiracetam and controlled-release carbamazepine in newly diagnosed epilepsy. *Neurology* Vol.68, pp. 402-408

Cetinkaya, Y.; Kurtulmus, Y.S.; Tutkavul, K. et al. (2009). The effect of oxcarbazepine on bone metabolism. *Acta Neurologica Scandinavica* Vol.120, No.3, pp. 170-175

Coppola, G.; Fortunato, D.; Auricchio, G. et al. (2009). Bone mineral density in children, adolescents, and young adults with epilepsy. *Epilepsia* Vol.50, No.9, pp. 2140-2146

Danesh, J.; Collins, R. & Peto, R. (2000). Lipoprotein(a) and coronary heart disease. Meta-analysis of prospective studies. *Circulation* Vol.102, pp. 1082-1085

Eiris, J.; Novo-Rodrígez, M.I.; Del Río, M. et al. (2000). The effect on lipid and apolipoprotein serum levels of long-term carbamazepine, valproic acid and Phenobarbital therapy in children with epilepsy. *Epilepsy Research* Vol.41, pp. 1-7

Epilepsy Action (UK) (2003). Anti-epileptic drugs and the risk of osteoporosis and osteomalacia: How much information do patients taking anti-epileptic drugs feel they receive about side effects of this medication? *British Epilepsy Association, Leeds, UK.* Available from: http://www.epilepsy.org.uk/campaigns/surveys/osteoporosis

Farhat, G.; Yamout, B.; Mihati, M.A. et al. (2002). Effect of antiepileptic drugs on bone density in ambulatory patients. *Neurology* Vol.58, pp. 1348-1353

Feldkamp, J.; Becker, A.; Witte, O.W. et al. (2000). Long-term anticonvulsant therapy leads to low bone mineral density - evidence for direct drug effects of phenytoin and carbamazepine on human osteoblast-like cells. *Experimental and Clinical Endocrinology & Diabetes* Vol.108, pp. 37-43

Fuller, H.R.; Man, N.T.; Lam le, T. et al. (2010). Valproate and bone loss: iTRAQ proteomics show that valproate reduces collagens and ostenectin in SMA cells. *Journal of Proteome Research* Vol.9, No.8, pp. 4228-4233

Garcia, M.; Huppertz, H.J.; Ziyeh, S. et al. (2009). Valproate-induced metabolic changes in patients with epilepsy: assessment with H-MRS. *Epilepsia* Vol.50, No.3, pp. 486-492

Gibbons, G.F. (2002). The role of cytochrome P450 in the regulation of cholesterol biosynthesis. *Lipids* Vol.37, pp. 1163-1170

Gilliam, F.; Hecimovic, H. & Sheline, Y. (2003). Psychiatric comorbidity, health, and function in epilepsy. *Epilepsy & Behavior* Vol.4, suppl 4, S26-S30

Guo, C-Y.; Ronen, G.M. & Atkinson, S.A. (2001). Long-term valproate and lamotrigine treatment may be a marker for reduced growth and bone mass in children with epilepsy. *Epilepsia* Vol.42, pp. 1141-1147

Hamed, S.A. & Abdella, M.M. (2009). The risk of asymptomatic hyperammonemia in children with idiopathic epilepsy treated with valproate: relationship to carnitine status. *Epilepsy Research* Vol.86, No.1, pp. 32-41

Herzog, A.G.; Drislane, F.W.; Schomer, D.L. et al. (2005). Differential effects of antiepileptic drugs on sexual function and hormones in men with epilepsy. *Neurology* Vol.65, pp. 1016-1020

Holtmann, M.; Krause, M.; Opp, J. et al. (2002). Oxcarbazepine-induced hyponatremia and the regulation of serum sodium after replacing carbamazepine with oxcarbazepine in children. *Neuropediatrics* Vol.33, No.6, pp. 298-300

Isojarvi, J.I.; Pakarinen, A.J. & Myllyla, V.V. (1993). Serum lipid levels during carbamazepine medication. A prospective study. *Archives of Neurology* Vol.50, pp. 590-593

Kim, J.Y. & Lee, H.W. (2007). Metabolic and hormonal disturbances in women with epilepsy on antiepileptic drug monotherapy. *Epilepsia* Vol.48, pp. 1366-1370

Landmark, C.J. (2008). Antiepileptic drugs in non-epilepsy disorders: relations between mechanisms of action and clinical efficacy. *CNS Drugs* Vol.22, No.1, pp. 27-47

Lee, R.H.; Lyles, K.W. & Colón-Emeric, C. (2010). A review of the effect of anticonvulsant medications on bone mineral density and fracture risk. *The American Journal of Geriatric Pharmacotherapy* Vol.8, No.1, pp. 34-46

Leung, A. & Ramsay, E. (2006). Effect of topiramate on bone resorption in adults. *American Epilepsy Society* (Abstract) Vol.2, p. 150

Löfgren, E.; Tapanainen, J.S.; Koivunen, R. et al. (2006). Effects of carbamazepine and oxcarbazepine on the reproductive endocrine function in women with epilepsy. *Epilepsia* Vol. 47, pp. 1441-1446

Luef, G.J.; Waldmann, M.; Sturm, W. et al. (2004). Valproate therapy and nonalcoholic fatty liver disease. *Annals of Neurology* Vol.55, pp. 729-732

Marson, A.G.; Al-Kharusi, A.M.; Alwaidh, M. et al. (2007). The SANAD study of effectiveness of carbamazepine, gabapentin, lamotrigine, oxcarbazepine, or topiramate for treatment of partial epilepsy: an unblinded randomised controlled trial. *Lancet* Vol.369, pp. 1000-1015

Mattson, R.H. & Gidal, B.E. (2004). Fractures, epilepsy, and antiepileptic drugs. *Epilepsy & Behavior* Vol.5, pp. S36-S40

Mintzer, S.; Boppana, P.; Toguri, J. et al. (2006). Vitamin D levels and bone turnover in epilepsy patients taking carbamazepine or oxcarbazepine. *Epilepsia* Vol.47, pp. 510-515

Mintzer, S.; Skidmore, C.T.; Abidin, C.J. et al. (2009). Effects of antiepileptic drugs on lipids, homocystein, and C-reactive protein. *Annals of Neurology* Vol.65, No.4, pp. 448-456

Mirza, N.; Marson, A.G. & Pirmohamed, M. (2009). Effect of topiramate on acid-base balance: extent, mechanism and effects. *British Journal of Clinical Pharmacology* Vol.68. No.5, pp. 655-661

Morrell, M.J.; Flynn, K.L.; Done, S. et al. (2005). Sexual dysfunction, sex steroid hormone abnormalities, and depression in women with epilepsy treated with antiepileptic drugs. *Epilepsy & Behavior* Vol.6, pp. 360-365

Muuronen, A.; Kaste, M.; Nikkila, E.A. et al. (1985). Mortality from ischaemic heart disease among patients using anticonvulsive drugs: a case control study. *British Medical Journal* (Clinical Research Edition) Vol.291, pp. 1481-1483

Nakken, K.O. & Kornstad, S. (1998). Do males 30-50 years of age with chronic epilepsy and on long-term anticonvulsant medication have lower-than-expected risk of developing coronary heart disease? *Epilepsia* Vol.39, pp. 326-330

Nakken, K.O. & Taubøll, E. (2010). Bone loss associated with use of antiepileptic drugs. *Expert Opinion on Drug Safety* Vol.9, No.4, pp. 561-571

Nebert, D.W. & Russel, D.W. (2002). Clinical importance of the cytochromes P450. *Lancet* Vol.360, pp. 1155-1162

Nikolaos, T.; Stylianos, G.; Chryssoula, N. et al. (2004). The effect of long-term antiepileptic treatment on serum cholesterol (TC, HDL, LDL) and triglyceride levels in adult epileptic patients on monotherapy. *Medical Science Monitor* Vol.10, pp. MT50-MT52

Nilsson, L.; Tomson, T.; Farahmand, B.Y. et al. (1997). Cause-specific mortality in epilepsy: a cohort study of more than 9,000 patients once hospitalized for epilepsy. *Epilepsia* Vol.38, pp. 1062-1068

Nissen-Meyer, L.S.H.; Svalheim, S.; Taubøll, E. et al. (2007). Levetiracetam, phenytoin and valproate act differently on rat bone mass, structure and metabolism. *Epilepsia* Vol.48, No.10, pp. 1850-1860

Pack, A.L.; Morrell, M.J.; Marcus, R. et al. (2005). Bone mass and turnover in women with epilepsy on antiepileptic drug monotherapy. *Annals of Neurology* Vol.57, pp. 252-257

Paul, E.; Conant, K.D.; Dunne, I.E. et al. (2010). Urolithiasis on the ketogenic diet with concurrent topiramate or zonisamide therapy. *Epilepsy Research* Vol.90, No.1-2, pp. 151-156

Pedersen, K.K.; Christiansen, C.; Ahlgren, P. et al. (1976). Incidence of fractures of the vertebral spine in epileptic patients. *Acta Neurologica Scandinavica* Vol.54, pp. 200-203

Perucca, E. (2002). Pharmacological and therapeutic properties of valproate: a summary after 35 years of clinical experience. *CNS Drugs* Vol.16, pp. 695-714

Petty, S.J.; O'Brien, T.J.; Wark, J.D. (2007). Anti-epileptic medication and bone health. *Osteoporosis International* Vol.18, pp. 129-142

Ravaglia, G.; Forti, P.; Maioli, F.; et al. (2005). Homocysteine and folate as risk factors for dementia and Alzheimer disease. *The American Journal of Clinical Nutrition* Vol.82, pp. 636-643

Ridker, P.M.; Cushman, M.; Stampfer, M.J. et al. (1997). Inflammation, aspirin, and risk of cardiovascular disease in apparently healthy men. *The New England Journal of Medicine* Vol.336, pp. 973-979

Sato, Y.; Kondo, I.; Ishida, S. et al. (2001). Decreased bone mass and increased bone turnover with valproate therapy in adults with epilepsy. *Neurology* Vol.57, pp. 445-449

Schmidt, D.; Arroyo, S. & Baulac, M. (2001). Recommendation on the clinical use of oxcarbazepine in the treatment of epilepsy: a consensus view. *Acta Neurologica Scandinavica* Vol.104, No.3, pp. 167-170

Schwaninger, M.; Ringleb, P.; Winter, R. et al. (1999). Elevated plasma concentrations of homocysteine in antiepileptic drug treatment. *Epilepsia* Vol.40, pp. 345-350

Schwaninger, M.; Ringleb, P.; Annecke, A. et al. (2000). Elevated plasma concentrations of lipoprotein (a) in medicated epileptic patients. *Journal of Neurology* Vol.247, pp. 687-690

Selhub, J. (2008). Public health significance of elevated homocysteine. *Food and Nutrition Bulletin* Vol.29, (2 Suppl), pp. S116-125

Sener, U.; Zorlu, Y.; Karaguzel, O. et al. (2006). Effect of common anti-epileptic drug monotherapy on serum levels of homocysteine, vitamin B12, folic acid and vitamin B6. *Seizure* Vol.15, No.2, pp. 79-85

Sheth, R.D.; Wesolowski, C.A.; Jacob, J.C. et al. (1995). Effect of carbamazepine and valproate on bone mineral density. *The Journal of Pediatrics* Vol.127, pp. 256-262

Sheth, R.D. (2004). Metabolic concerns associated with antiepileptic medications. *Neurology* Vol. 63, pp. S24-S29

Sheth, R.D. (2004). Bone health in pediatric epilepsy. Epilepsy & Behavior Vol.5, pp. S30-S35

Sheth, R.D.; Gidal, B.E. & Hermann, B.P. (2006). Pathological fractures in epilepsy. *Epilepsy & Behavior* Vol.9, No.4, pp. 601-605

Sheth, R.D. & Hermann, B.P. (2007). Bone mineral density with lamotrigine monotherapy for epilepsy. *Pediatric Neurology* Vol.37, pp. 250-254

Sheth, R.D. & Montouris, G. (2008). Metabolic effects of AEDs: impact on body weight, lipids and glucose metabolism. *International Review of Neurobiology* Vol.83, pp. 329-346

Souverein, P.C.; Webb, D.J,.; Weil, J.G. et al. (2006). Use of antiepileptic drugs and risk of fractures: case-control study among patients with epilepsy. *Neurology* Vol.66, No.9, pp. 1318-1324

Spence, J.D. (2007). Homocysteine-lowering therapy: a role in stroke prevention? *Lancet Neurology* Vol.6, pp. 830-838

Talbot, J.A.; Sheldrick, R.; Caswell, H. et al. (2008). Sexual function in men with epilepsy: how important is testosterone? *Neurology* Vol.70, pp. 1346-1352

Tsiropoulos, I.; Andersen, M.; Nymark, T. et al. (2008). Exposure to antiepileptic drugs and the risk of hip fracture: a case-control study. *Epilepsia* Vol.49, No.12, pp. 2092-2099

Valmadrid, C.; Voorhees, C.; Litt, B. et al. (2001). Practice patterns of neurologists regarding bone and mineral effects of antiepileptic drug therapy. *Archives of Neurology* Vol.58, pp. 1369-1374

Vega, D.; Maalouf, N.M. & Sakhaee, K. (2007). Increased propensity for calcium phosphate kidney stones with topiramate use. *Expert Opinion on Drug Safety* Vol.6, No.5, pp. 547-557

Verotti, A.; Domizio, S.; Angelozzi, B. et al. (1997). Changes in serum lipids and lipoproteins in epileptic children treated with anticonvulsants. *Journal of Paediatrics & Child Health* Vol.33, 242-245

Verotti, A.; Basciani, F.; Domizio, S. et al. (1998). Serum lipids and lipoproteins in patients treated with antiepileptic drugs. *Pediatric Neurology* Vol.19, pp. 364-367

Verotti, A.; Manco, R.; Agostinelli, S. et al. (2010). The metabolic syndrome in overweight epileptic patients treated with valproic acid. *Epilepsia* Vol.51, No.2, pp. 268-273

Verotti, A.; D'Egidio, C.; Mohn, A. et al. (2010). Weight gain following treatment with valproic acid: pathogenetic mechanisms and clinical implications. *Obesity Reviews* (Epub ahead of print: doi: 10.1111/j.1467-789X.2010.00800.x)

Vestergaard, P.; Rejnmark, L. & Mosekilde L. (2004). Fracture risk associated with use of antiepileptic drugs. *Epilepsia* Vol.45, No.11, pp. 1330-1337

Vestergaard P. (2005). Epilepsy, osteoporosis and fracture risk – meta-analysis. *Acta Neurologica Scandinavica* Vol.112, No.5, pp. 277-286

Wellmer, J.; Wellmer, S. & Bauer, J. (2009). The impact of zonisamide on weight. A clinical study in 103 patients with epilepsy. *Acta Neurologica Scandinavica* Vol.119, No.4, pp. 233-238

6

Population Pharmacokinetic Analysis of Therapeutic Drug Monitoring Data in Optimizing Pharmacotherapy of Antiepileptic Drugs

Katarina Vučićević[1], Branislava Miljković[1], Sandra Vezmar Kovačević[1], Zoran Todorović[2], Milica Prostran[2] and Iztok Grabnar[3]

[1]*Department of Pharmacokinetics and Clinical Pharmacy, Faculty of Pharmacy, University of Belgrade,*
[2]*Department of Pharmacology, Clinical Pharmacology and Toxicology, School of Medicine, University of Belgrade,*
[3]*Chair of Biopharmaceutics and Pharmacokinetics, Faculty of Pharmacy, University of Ljubljana,*
[1,2]*Serbia*
[3]*Slovenia*

1. Introduction

Epilepsy is an episodic disease; hence the aim of the therapy is to minimize frequency of epileptic seizures and to improve the quality of patients' life with minimal adverse effects of antiepileptic drugs (AEDs) (Gidal & Garnett, 2005). Therapeutic Drug Monitoring (TDM) is a concept of individualisation of therapy based on drug concentration data, and application of pharmacokinetic (PK) and pharmacodynamic (PD) principles. It is not only a process of measuring drug concentration levels in biological fluids, but putting them into service of an optimized individual pharmacotherapy. The aim of TDM is to accomplish the optimal therapeutic drug response with minimal adverse drug effects e.g. better pharmaceutical care of patients (Bauer, 2008; Pokrajac, 2008).

Due to marked inter- and intraindividual PK characteristics of AEDs, TDM is indicated since the beginning of 1960s during the therapy of phenitoin (Buchthal et al., 1960). Shortly afterwards, it was recommended to monitor other AEDs, and correlate their concentrations with therapeutic effects (Kutt & Penry, 1974; Patsalos et al., 2008). Since PK and PD of AEDs demonstrate large interindividual variability, which is sometimes hard to identify, TDM of AEDs is incorporated into the therapy of epilepsy (Bauer, 2008; Commission on Antiepileptic Drugs, 1993; Dhillon & Kostrzewski, 2006). AEDs are being monitored also nowadays, but much of the available TDM data is insufficient due to inappropriate indication for performing the test, timing of samples collection, length of unchanged dosing regimen before measuring drug concentration, and unreliable documentation. Hence, TDM should be performed only if there is a clear indication: after initiation of treatment or after dose adjustment when the clinician decides to aim at preselected target concentration for that patient, to establish individual therapeutic range after achievement of desired clinical response, when there is suspicion of signs or symptoms of concentration-related toxicity, when seizures persist despite apparently adequate dosage, if there is an alteration of PK (e.g. combination therapy, impairment of liver and/or renal function, paediatric population of patients, pregnancy), if there is change in drug formulation/switching to generic formulations, if there is unexpected change in clinical response, and if *non-compliance* is suspected (Patsalos et al., 2008). Throughout TDM, it is crucial to be aware of the dosing regimen, the duration of therapy, sample timing, as well as to keep high-quality recordings in patients' charts. In routine TDM of AEDs, it is recommended to obtain samples in steady-state corresponding to expected peak (maximum) and trough (minimum) concentration. Information from TDM must be interpreted in an adequate way since they could be used in rational pharmacotherapy of epilepsy (Bauer, 2008; Patsalos et al., 2008).

Owing to the fact that different factors affect individual PK parameters of AEDs, and consequently also the dosing regimen and clinical effects of a drug, identification of sources of intra- and interindividual variability among patients is essential for optimal drug therapy. Population modelling is a powerful tool to study whether demographic parameters (e.g. age, weight), pathophysiological conditions (e.g. other health problems, impairment of liver or/and renal function, concomitant therapy), and other sources of variability influence the dose-concentration relationship, and if so, to what extent. It is usually emphasized that population analysis is the analysis of variability, and it is more precise in determination of variability of PK parameters in the specific population over traditional PK analysis (Food and Drug Administration [FDA], 1999; Sheiner et al., 1977). Since many factors contribute to PK variability of AEDs, due to features of TDM data (1-2 plasma samples per patient), and characteristics of population analysis, population approach has irreplaceable role in PK analysis of TDM data. In this chapter, it the importance and advantages of population PK analysis in routine TDM of AEDs will be emphasized, the protocol of population studies explained, as well as the process of collecting and manipulating data, and finally the importance and application of the final population model in the clinical practice will be thoroughly discussed.

2. Traditional versus population pharmacokinetic approach

Traditional (classical) PK analysis refers to two-stage analysis using compartmental or noncompartmental PK approach. An accurate estimation of PK parameters requires frequent data sampling and concentration measurement in individual patients. In contrast, the population approach is based on one or more samples from an individual patient which are evaluated using model-dependent (compartmental) data analysis which, additionally, takes into account drug variability using specific statistical analysis. Hence, there are marked differences between these two approaches (Table 1). The subjects of traditional PK analysis are usually healthy volunteers or highly selected patients, whom drugs are being given by relatively simple dosing regimens (e.g. single bolus dose or single infusion). Protocol of the study with restrictive inclusion/exclusion criteria requires many samples per patient (sometimes as much as 10) – rich/dense data, which allows obtaining the individual PK profile of the drug. Sampling schedule is usually designed to obtain samples in short intervals and is the same for each individual in the study. Interindividual variability in PK is minimized in this way, and traditional controlled PK study focuses on the effect of a single factor on PK of a drug (FDA, 1999). In the first step of a two-stage approach, individual PK parameters are estimated through non-linear regression (e.g. one-compartment model) using individual dense concentration-time data. The individual values of PK parameters are used for the second stage, by calculating descriptive statistics typically average parameters values, standard deviation, coefficient of variation, or variance (Ette & Williams, 2004b).

Moreover, the dependencies between PK parameters and factor(s) that are not controlled by study design are calculated using classical statistic approaches such as linear stepwise regression, covariance analysis (Sun et al., 1999).

CHARACTERISTICS	TRADITIONAL (TWO-STAGE) ANALYSIS	POPULATION (NONLINEAR MIXED EFFECTS) ANALYSIS
Nature of the analysis	Pharmacokinetic model is fit to the data to each individual, whereas parameters are summarized	Pharmacokinetic model is fit to the data from all individuals, whereas based on empirical Bayes approach individual parameters are calculated
Experimental design	Stringent/controlled design is necessary	Stringent or non-stringent study design
Study population	Healthy volunteers or highly selected patients	Target patient population
Study size	Small	Large
Sampling data	Frequent sampling (usually 1-6 per patient - rich data)	Rich or sparse (1-2 samples) data within individuals with possibility of uneven number of data from different individuals
Interindividual variability	Minimized due to restrictive inclusion/exclusion criteria	Possible to identify sources of interindividual variability

Table 1. Characteristics of traditional and population pharmacokinetic analysis of data

On the other hand, in the population PK analysis individual patient is not the centre of the study; hence the aim is to develop population profile of a drug, whereas based on empirical Bayes approach individual parameters values are calculated. Study design allows large heterogeneous (e.g. by age, body weight, etc.) study population of patients from whom small number of samples - sparse/poor data are available. Sparse sampling in population PK analysis enables obtaining data from patient populations who are difficult to study due to ethical barriers, such as neonates, severely ill patients (Sheiner et al., 1977).
The protocol of the study is unbalanced, and it gives the opportunity to analyze data from individuals which differ in the number of samples per patient (FDA, 1999). Great advantage of population studies is that patients with insufficient data can be included in the study, whereas these subjects are usually excluded in traditional PK studies. Usual solutions to this problem include case imputation sample mean, median or estimation via linear regression values (e.g. total body weight can be predicted based on patients' age and gender) (Bonate, 2005). Concentrations bellow the limit of quantification (LOQ) of the assay are handled similarly. The usual strategy is not to exclude these data but to give them the value of LOQ/2. In order not to have doubts if the low concentrations is indication of noncompliance, the recommendation is to record the concentration even if it is below LOQ. This matter is a subject of much discussion, and there is no consensus on handling below LOQ data (Barrett, 2002; European Medicines Agency [EMEA], 2007). These alternative ways of treating problematic data give the possibility to maximally exploit the data, which is not possible in the traditional analysis. The milestone of population approach is the possibility to determine sources of variability with are usually consequence of a complex interaction of more factors (Vučićević et al., 2005; Sheiner et al., 1977). It is usually regarded as an analysis which is a study of drug variability, not only from a qualitative but also from quantitative aspect.

The population approach to PK analysis of data was originally proposed for application to routinely collected clinical - TDM data (Sheiner et al., 1977), i.e. sparse and unbalanced observations from a large group of heterogeneous individuals. TDM data are heterogeneous (according to patients' characteristics, therapy, dosing regimens), but they are representative of the actual population of patients taking the drug of interest since they are gathered directly from such patients, and from the ethical perspective there is a justifiable purpose of patients' care. At the same time, heterogeneous data are the source of the information of drug behaviour (Barrett, 2002; Sheiner et al., 1977), and discovery of unexpected but important influences of various factors on PK is possible. However, in order to evaluate the effect of one factor on PK parameter, number of covariates in the studied group must be sufficient, so the results of the study would lead us to significant conclusions about the effect of the specific covariate on the PK parameter. In other words, if we want to estimate the effect of valproic acid (VPA) co-therapy on carbamazepine (CBZ) PK, the results of our study suggest that at least 10-20% of patients co-treated with VPA are needed (Vučićević et al., 2007, 2009). This is necessary in order to obtain a sufficient level of certainty in the results of the analysis. Thus, an analysis of routine TDM data possesses several advantages in terms of data availability, representativeness of patients, and richness of the data set. Therefore, it is not overestimated to claim that routine TDM data on AED is a very attractive and often unused source of drug information with a strong potential. The advantage is mainly in the quantity of samples, and the fact that they represent the population of all patients who are treated with that drug in a certain setting. Moreover, the study protocol is not as strict as in traditional PK studies and therefore much more viable in the daily routine, from the perspective of ethics (blood sampling is an invasive procedure which is not justified only for research purposes) and time management. Owing to the characteristics of population approach, and characteristics of routine data, population modelling serves as a logical extension of TDM of AEDs with possibility of identification and quantification of factors that contribute to PK variability (Sheiner et al., 1977).

3. Methodological aspects of population pharmacokinetic analysis

Term population analysis is used as a synonym for nonlinear mixed effects modelling. The same phrase, abbreviated, is used for the name of the widely used population pharmacokinetic analysis software - NONMEM® (ICON Developments, USA). In this section main methodological aspects will be addressed.

3.1 Nonlinear mixed effects models

The basis of nonlinear mixed effects modelling is one stage approach, which means that all parameters are being estimated simultaneously. The purpose of this analysis is to estimate: population and individual PK parameters, interindividual and residual variability, and to identify and investigate sources of variability that influence PK of a drug. All aspects are of great interests since they are required for the optimal dosage regimen design for individual patients, and they provide quantitative PK characteristics of a drug. Potential factors affecting PK behaviour of a drug (covariates) are:

- Demographic such as age, gender, body weight, race.
- Genetic due to polymorphism of cytochrome P (CYP) 450 isoenzymes (CYP2D6, CYP2C9, CYP2C19, etc.) involved in the metabolism of AEDs.
- Physiological and pathophysiological including pregnancy, gastrointestinal diseases, decreased function of elimination organs (liver, kidneys), acute and chronic diseases.

- Concomitant therapy as a result of drug-drug interactions, since two or more AEDs can be included in the therapy of epilepsy.
- Enviromental factors like smoking, alcohol intake or diets.
- Other factors such as drug formulation, biological rhythms, compliance (Ette & Williams, 2004a; Sun et al., 1999).

The main components of population PK model are given on Fig.1.

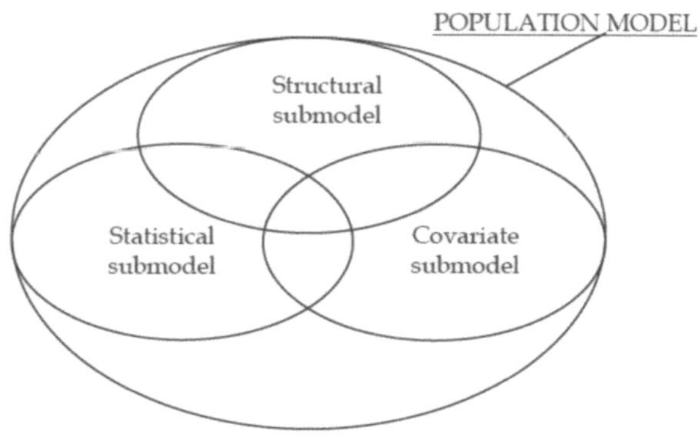

Fig. 1. Components of a nonlinear mixed effect (population) model

Term "mixed" stands for combination of fixed and random effects. Parameters of fixed effects represent population PK parameter values which are actually values of central tendency or typical values of parameters. These parameters are components of a structural PK model which refers to compartmental PK model. For example, intravenously given drug on a Fig. 1 follows one-compartment model with first-order elimination, and structural model is:

$$C_p = \frac{D}{V_d} \cdot e^{-\frac{CL}{Vd} \cdot t} \quad (1)$$

Dependent variable is observed drug concentration (Cp), whereas clearance (CL) and volume of distribution (Vd) are fixed parameters since they quantitatively describe the effect of a given dose (D) in specific time (t) on a drug level. Fixed effects parameters have symbols *theta* (θ). Population (typical) values of PK parameters (TV) can be explained in terms of covariates. As presented on Fig.2, patients' CL is defined in terms of a linear function of body weight (WT), given by:

$$TVCL = \theta_1 + \theta_2 \cdot WT \quad (2)$$

Parameters of random effects include: interindividual (between subject) variability which is partially but not completely possible to describe using available covariates and residual variability consisting of intraindividual (within subject) variability, measurement error, model misspecification, etc.

Since each individual in the population has specific value of a PK parameter which differs to some extent from the population typical value, it is described in terms of interindividual unexplained variability. This variability is described using parameter *eta* (η), and a variety of error models can be used. As given in Fig. 2, all *eta*s in the studied population for a specific PK parameter (e.g. η_{CL}) are assumed to be normally distributed with a mean value of zero, and variance of ω^2_{CL}.

Residual error refers to the deviation of measured (observed) drug concentration from the predicted level in a specific time using structural PK model. This parameter uses the symbol *epsilon* (ε). All parameter values for residual variability are assumed to be normally distributed with a variance of σ^2 (Fig. 2).

Covariates, as previously mentioned, represent any variable/factor specific for a patient which can influence PK of a drug. Covariate submodels are integrated part of a structural part of a population model (Fig.1). A relationship between PK parameters and covariates depends on its nature, and range values (Jonsson & Karlsson, 1998; Mentre & Mallet, 1994). Therefore, there are:

- Categorical covariates that are qualitative, and they can be dichotomous with two values (e.g. gender: male or female; mono- or combination therapy) or polychotomous with more than two values (e.g. patients' race: white, black or yellow).
- Continuous covariates which have defined scale of its values and they are quantitative, such as body weight, age, creatinine clearance etc. Relationship between this covariate and PK parameter can be linear or nonlinear.

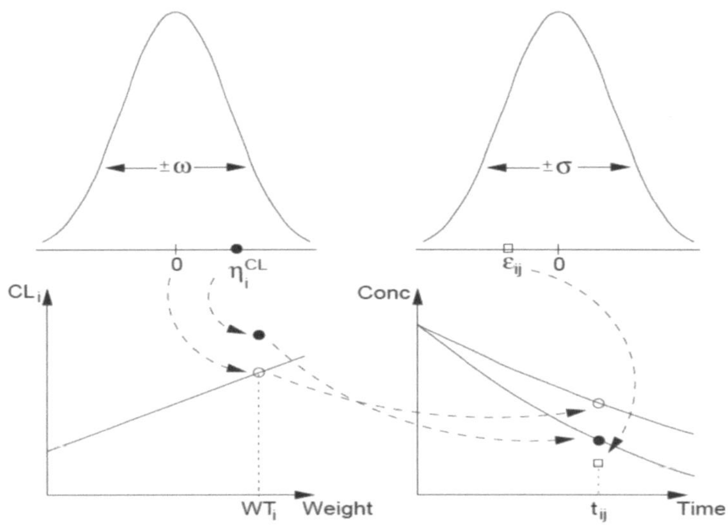

Fig. 2. Schema of nonlinear mixed effect model. Interindividual variability (left) and residual variability (right). Population (○) and individual (●) pharmacokinetic parameter/predicted and observed concentration (□) (Beal & Sheiner, 1989-2006)

Selection of an adequate model describing effect of a factor on PK parameter depends on preliminary modelling results. These results include individual values of PK parameters based on a distribution of base model parameters (empirical Bayes estimates), and its graphical dependences of covariates. Details of a modelling process will be explained in the following section.

3.2 Population model building and validation techniques

Since the aim of the population analysis is to describe interindividual variability in PK parameters, it can be done through the most commonly used stepwise covariates model building method, also known as forward inclusion-backward exclusion method. After defining the structural and statistical models (which form base model), influence of each covariate on PK parameter is examined (Bonate, 2005; Jonsson & Karlsson, 1998).

Software NONMEM® fits data to defined structural and error models according to principles based on maximum likelihood which is expressed via objective function value (OFV). Software performs iterative search of a parameters values that maximizes the probability of input data leading to minimization of OFV. OFV is proportional to double negative logarithm of data probability. Logarithm of data probability follows chi-squared (χ^2) distribution (Beal & Sheiner, 1989-2006).

Apart from finding important covariates, the functional relationship also has to be specified. There are several suggestions on covariate model building (Bonate, 2005; Jonsson & Karlsson, 1998; EMEA, 2007), but no consensus has been reached. Mainly graphics which demonstrate correlation of individual empirical Bayes parameter estimates of the base model versus selected covariates are used for identification of candidate covariates.

Each covariate was added in the base model, and examined for its effect on PK parameter by evaluating the drop in OFV. Each covariate was ranked against the base model by minimum decrease in OFV of 3.84 (χ^2 distribution, $p<0.05$ for 1 degree of freedom), and only significant covariates were introduced into the full model. The final model was determined by removing the covariates one by one from the full model, and a difference in the OFV more than 6.63 (χ^2 distribution, $p<0.01$ for 1 degree of freedom) was required to maintain covariate in the model (Beal, 2002; Beal & Sheiner, 1989-2006). Maintaining/excluding one covariate in/from the model in based on the combination of several considerations: statistical, graphical, and clinical relevance of the obtained relationship (Wählby et al., 2001). Additional indicators for the retention of a covariate in the model are decrease in interindividual and residual variability, minimal correlation between parameters, improvement in the precision of the parameter estimates, small standard errors of parameter estimates, gradients for each estimated parameter in final iteration step should be between 10^{-3} and 10^{2}. In each model-building step improvement of the model is assessed by the goodness-of-fit plots, including the agreement between the observed and predicted drug concentrations, reduction in the range of weighted residuals, and uniformity of the distribution of weighted residuals when plotted against predicted concentrations (Barrett, 2002; Beal & Sheiner, 1989-2006).

One of the most demanding tasks is the demonstration whether the final population PK model accurately represent the studied population. Depending on the objective of the analysis, the need for model validation may vary. There are generally two types of validation:

- Internal which is performed in the group of patients used for model development. Methods commonly used are data splitting, bootstrap, cross-validation.
- External which includes a separate, independent group of patients not included in model development (Bonate, 2006).

However, if developed population PK model is going to be used for dosage recommendations the predictive performance needs to be tested (Sun et al., 1999). To evaluate the performance of the final model in predicting drug concentrations, a second, validation group of patients is studied. Hence, external validation is performed. The measured drug concentrations in this group must be compared with the corresponding predicted values obtained using the final population PK model, patients' covariates and dosing information. Predictive performance of the model is assessed by calculating the mean error and its 95% confidence interval (CI) as an estimate of bias, and the root mean squared prediction error and 95% CI as an estimate of precision. CIs including the value of zero were considered unbiased (Sheiner & Beal, 1981; Wu, 1995).

3.3 Population pharmacokinetic modelling of routine therapeutic drug monitoring data

As previously stated, routine TDM data are particularly attractive and available source of information since they represent PK behaviour of a drug in the group of patients receiving the drug for the therapeutic purposes. From economical perspective, an analysis of routine data is reasonable, since it reduces experimental costs (Sheiner et al., 1977). Nevertheless, the drug dosing history is often poorly recorded and the level of noncompliance is underestimated, which leads to biased estimation of population model parameters.

During TDM of AEDs, sampling enables mainly the collection of trough and to less extent peak drug concentrations. Commonly, from each patient a single blood sample is obtained at or close to trough concentration, shortly before the next dose. The relationship of patients' characteristics and minimum drug level can be explored by simple statistical analysis, but calculation of PK parameters seems almost impossible using traditional PK approach. Whereas, with population PK analysis it is possible to estimate PK parameters and two levels of variability (Sheiner et al., 1977).

However, the nature of the data influences the parameters that can be estimated in the analysis (Sun et al., 1999). In other words, a certain PK parameter cannot be calculated with any degree of a precision unless data used for analysis reflect the parameter. As reported by Sheiner & Beal, 1983, the use of mostly trough samples in the sampling design results in a good precision of the CL and its variability, and poorer precision of Vd and its variability. For that reason Vd is usually not estimated in population analysis of TDM data. Moreover, insufficient sampling during the absorption phase of *per os* given drugs, does not allow estimation of the parameters of the absorption process (rate constant of absorption); hence its values should be fixed to the literature value (Booth & Gobburu, 2003; Jiao et al., 2004; Wade et al., 1993). It has been shown (Wade et al., 1993) when no data were available from the absorption phase, misspecification of rate constant of absorption had no effect on other estimated parameters of the model. When doing this, a sensitivity analysis can be performed in order to confirm the effect of fixed parameter value on the final model parameter estimates. These methodological issues have been extensively applied during population PK analysis during the modelling of routine sparse TDM data of AEDs (Yukawa, 1999).

If an absolute bioavailability of a drug is either unknown or very variable, it is possible to refer to apparent PK parameter values. Therefore, in the population PK studies of AEDs data, the only PK parameter which can be estimated with good precision from routine TDM data (mainly trough concentrations) is the apparent clearance (CL/F). Clearance is a vital PK parameter in dosage adjustment regimen, since the most widely used method of AEDs dosage adjustment is based upon the fact that in steady-state the rate of drug administration equals the rate of drug elimination (determined by a product of CL/F and the average steady-state drug concentration), given by equation (3).

$$R = \frac{D}{\tau} = CL / F \cdot C^{ss} \tag{3}$$

As reported (Sheiner & Beal, 1983) there is no significant loss in estimating CL/F and its variability by population modelling from routine type of data compared to better designed studies where more samples per patient are available.

4. Importance and application of population pharmacokinetic models from therapeutic drug monitoring of antiepileptic drugs

When a drug is marked and used for the treatment of a disease or condition, the main goal of therapy is to optimize dosage regimen in the individual patient. Degree of PK and/or PD variability of a drug influences the applicability of average dosing regimen for an individual patient. Since AEDs show marked PK variability, poor correlation between plasma levels and dose was observed (Bauer, 2008; Miljković et al., 1991). Therefore, interindividual variability in drug disposition as well as in drug's response is often the reason for adverse drug reactions, as well as lack of therapeutic efficacy. Various factors contribute to large differences in plasma drug concentrations at steady-state among patients receiving the same dose, and consequently affect individual PK parameters of AEDs. For instance, patients' age or body weight are the commonly identified factors that affect AEDs' elimination since they show functional and physiological status of organs (e.g. liver, kidneys) involved in metabolism and/or excretion of a drug. Among other factors patients' race, gender, smoking status, drug formulation were found to affect PK parameters of some AEDs.

Consequently, evaluation and management of the variability is the aim of rational drug therapy with its individual approach to each patient. Understanding the factors which can influence AEDs PK characteristics throughout population modelling technique in combination with TDM is a valuable tool in designing a safe and effective dosing regimen for epileptic patients.

Therapy of epilepsy usually begins with one AED depending on the type of the seizure. When increasing the dose or substituting a drug with another AED does not give a desired therapeutic effect, a combination of AEDs might be considered. When another drug is added on, PK and/or PD drug-drug interactions may occur, leading to greater variability. However, the extent to which corresponding parameters are changed, indicate the need for the change of dosage regimen. It is a well known that some AEDs such as CBZ and PB are inducers of CYP450 isoenzymes, thus consequently affect PK parameters of elimination of AEDs that show CYP450 dependent elimination. In addition, VPA inhibits the metabolism of lamotrigine and PB, and a reduction in the dosage of the latter drugs is usually indicated when VPA is added on (Patsalos & Perucca, 2003a, 2003b; Perucca, 2006). To conclude, many drug-drug interactions between AEDs and AEDs with non-AEDs are proven by controlled PK studies; however population PK studies allow quantification of such interactions using sparse data. Drug interactions represent constant concern in the clinical practice owing to the fact that the treatment of epilepsy usually requires polytherapy, and that interindividual variability in PK can be caused by drug interactions (Patsalos & Perucca, 2003a, 2003b; Perucca, 2006). Therefore, it is logical the importance of population approach to identify and quantitatively describe drug-drug interactions in the clinical practice (Vučićević et al., 2007a, 2008, 2009a). It has been found that population PK analysis was powerful tool in detecting interaction, but also showed its' superiority over traditional PK approach (Grasela et al., 1987; Zhou, 2006). In the traditional PK studies it is possible to observe, under controlled conditions of the study, if one drug statistically significant changes the average PK parameter of another. Consequently, population-based analysis is particularly important to quantify known or suspected drug-drug interactions, as well as to detect any unexpected interactions. Several examples of developed population PK models for AEDs from routine TDM data in adult population are given in Table 2. Traditionally, TDM has mainly focused on the older antiepileptic drugs, such as CBZ, phenobarbital, phenytoin, primidone, and VPA, which all have been in clinical use for several decades. For that reason, population PK models are numerous, and some of them are presented in Table 2. Based on these population PK models, it is possible to observe quantitative effect of concomitant drugs in therapy with CBZ, or VPA.

DRUG	POPULATION PHARMACOKINETIC MODEL	REFERENCE
Carbamazepine		
$CL/F[l/h]=5.35\cdot\left(\frac{DCBZ}{15}\right)^{0.591}\cdot\left(1+0.414\cdot\frac{DPB}{2}\right)\cdot\left(\frac{WT}{70}\right)^{0.564}\cdot1.18^{VPA}$, where *DCBZ* and *DPB* are daily doses of carbamazepine and phenobarbitone in mg/kg; *VPA*=1 if valproic acid dose is greater 750 mg/day, or 0 if else		Vučićević et al., 2007b
$CL/F[l/h]=0.141\cdot DCBZ^{0.406}\cdot WT^{0.117}\cdot1.23^{VPA}\cdot1.44^{PHT}\cdot1.26^{PB}$, where *DCBZ* is daily dose of carbamazepine in mg; *VPA*=1, *PHT*=1, *PB*=1 if valproic acid dose greater than 18 mg/kg, phenytoin, phenobarbitone are present in therapy, or 0 if else		Jiao et al., 2004
$CL/F[ml/h\cdot kg]=64.9\cdot DCBZ^{0.465}\cdot WT^{-0.336}\cdot1.03^{VPA}\cdot1.44^{POLY}\cdot1.16^{PB}$, where *DCBZ* is daily dose of carbamazepine in mg/kg; *VPA*=1, *PB*=1, *POLY*=1 if valproic acid, phenobarbitone or more than two AEDs are present in therapy, or 0 if else		Yukawa & Aoyama, 1996
$CL/F[l/day\cdot kg]=40.7\cdot AGE^{0.494}\cdot WT^{-1.17}\cdot1.44^{PB}$, where AGE is in years, *PB*=1 if phenobarbitone is present in therapy, or 0 if else		Chan et al., 2000
$CL/F[l/h]=(0.0134\cdot WT+3.58)\cdot1.42^{PHT}\cdot1.17^{PB/FEL}\cdot1.62^{PHT+PB/FEL}\cdot0.749^{AGE}$, where *PHT*=1, *PB/FEL*=1, *PHT+PB/FEL*=1, *AGE*=1 if patient is treated with phenytoin, phenobarbitone or felbamate, phenytoin and phenobarbitone/felbamate, or is older than 70 years, or 0 if else		Graves et al., 1998
Valproic acid		
$CL/F[l/h]=0.517\cdot\left(\frac{WT}{70}\right)^{0.556}\cdot1.43^{VPA}\cdot0.765^{TPR}$, where *VPA*=1 if *VPA* dose is greater 1000 mg/day, and *TPR*=1 in co-therapy with topiramate, or 0 if else.		Vučićević et al., 2009b
$CL/F[l/h]=0.105+0.151\cdot CBZ+0.000248\cdot DVPA+0.0968\cdot\frac{AGE}{20}+0.0803\cdot INDI$, where *DVPA* is valproic acid dose in mg/day; *CBZ*=1 in co-therapy with carbamazepine, or 0 if else; *INDI* is uncontrolled epilepsy		El Desoky et al., 2004
$CL/F[ml/h\cdot kg]=17.2\cdot DVPA^{0.159}\cdot WT^{-0.264}\cdot0.821^{CZP}\cdot0.896^{GEN}$, where *DVPA* is daily valproic acid dose in mg/kg; *CZP*=1 for concomitant therapy with clonazepam, *GEN*=1 for female, or 0 if else		Yukawa et al., 2003
$CL/F[l/h]=0.004\cdot WT\cdot DVPA^{0.304}\cdot1.363^{CBZ}\cdot1.541^{PHT}\cdot1.397^{PB}$, where *DVPA* is daily dose of valproic acid in mg/kg; *CBZ*=1, *PHT*=1, *PB*=1 if carbamazepine, phenytoin, phenobarbitone are present in therapy, or 0 if else		Blanco-Serrano et al., 1999.

Table 2. Population pharmacokinetic models of carbamazepine and valproic acid derived from routine therapeutic drug monitoring data in adult population of epileptic patients

The importance of a population PK models is best shown in an example. It is a well known fact that PB acts as an inductor of CYP450 isoenzymes, thus consequently it effects CBZ elimination (Patsalos & Perucca, 2003a). Since induction process requires synthesis of new enzymes, time course of an induction is a function of enzyme synthesis rate. Hence, time course of induction is dose dependent (Patsalos & Perucca, 2003a). Using the population PK approach, the possibility to examine the influence of various PB doses on CBZ metabolism (CL/F) was shown, and the results indicate a linear relationship (Table 2).

Clinical significance in population modelling converts the estimated values of population PK models into potential benefits for an individual patient. In modelling, clinical relevance of the covariate effect usually assumes reduction in the interindividual variability of the specific PK parameter while adding a covariate/factor to a model. On the other hand, clinical relevance can also be evaluated by estimating the change in the predicted individual parameter values. For example, if predicted CL/F of a CBZ in a patient increases by 20% after adding PB (as a covariate) in the model, PB co-therapy may be regarded as a clinically relevant predictor of CBZ CL/F. In order to make the effect of a covariate on PK parameter robust, 95% CI of the value of parameter explaining covariate effect should be addressed. Finally, what is regarded as clinically relevant varies between investigators, physicians and regulators (EMEA, 2007).

Knowledge of population PK models can assist in choosing initial dosing regimen of a drug, modifying dosing regimens according to observed drug levels, and they can elucidate certain clinical questions. Identification of the factors which contribute to PK variability of AEDs provides a foundation for individualization of the therapy. An adjustment of drug therapy is directed by individual values of PK parameters which depend on patient and disease characteristics.

In order to optimize dosing regimen for a specific patient, individual PK parameters are needed. Hence, patient's CL/F represents fundamental PK parameter for individualization of therapy (given by equation (3)). Bayes approach is used to determine individual PK parameters using mutually the data from individual patient and population PK models of a drug defined via population typical values of PK parameters and their variability (Bonate, 2006; Jelliffe et al., 1993; Sheiner et al., 1979). This prediction is possible to perform using different PK softwares. Though, in Bayes regression approach it is of a great importance to use population PK model that represents individual patients. Furthermore, if population PK behaviour of AEDs is integrated with pharmacological and clinical effects, it would provide a better rationale for the proper selection of optimal dose, type and duration of administration of AED therapy in different patient populations.

5. Conclusion

Clinical experience demonstrated the need of therapeutic drug monitoring in optimizing therapy of epilepsy. Identification of sources of intra- and interindividual variability among patients is essential for individualization of drug therapy, and it can be accomplished by population approach to data analysis. The major strength of the population pharmacokinetics approach is that useful information can be extracted from sparse data collected during routine clinical care. Therefore, population approach serves as a natural and expected extension of therapeutic drug monitoring and it can significantly contribute to more rational pharmacotherapy of antiepileptic drugs. Knowledge of population pharmacokinetic models can assist in selecting an initial dosing regimen, and modifying dosing regimen appropriately according to the observed drug level and patients' characteristics. In order to truly individualize dosing regimen, patient's individual PK parameters are required, and they can be estimated as a function of significant covariates by Bayes analysis and the population pharmacokinetic model.

6. Acknowledgment

The work is prepared as a part of the project *Experimental and Clinical-Pharmacological Investigations of Mechanisms of Drug Action and Interactions in Nervous and Cardiovascular System* (N° 175023) funded by Ministry of Science and Technological Development, Belgrade, Republic of Serbia. The authors of this manuscript do not have any conflict of interests.

7. References

Barrett, J.S. (2002). Population Pharmacokinetics, In: *Pharmacokinetics in drug discovery and development*, R.D. Schoenwald (Ed.), pp. 315-356, CRC Press, ISBN 1-56676-973-6, London

Bauer, L.A. (2008). *Applied Clinical Pharmacokinetics* (2nd ed.), McGrawHill, ISBN 0-07-159372-1, New York

Beal, S.L. & Sheiner, L.B. (Eds.). (1989-2006). *NONMEM User's Guides*, Icon Development Solutions, ISBN Ellicott City, Maryland, USA

Beal, S.L. (2002). Commentary on Significance Levels for Covariate Effects in NONMEM. *Journal of Pharmacokinetics and Pharmacodynamics*, Vol. 29, No. 4, pp. 403-410, ISSN 1567-567X

Blanco-Serrano, B.; Otero, M.J.; Santos-Buelga, D.; Garcia-Sanchez, M.J.; Serrano, J. & Dominguez-Gil, A. (1999). Population Estimation of Valproic Acid Clearance in Adult Patients Using Routine Clinical Pharmacokinetic Data. *Biopharmaceutics & Drug Disposition*, Vol. 20, No. 5, pp. 233-240, ISSN 1099-081X

Bonate, L.B. (2006). *Pharmacokinetic-Pharmacodynamic Modeling and Simulation* (1st ed.), Springer, ISBN 0-387-27197-X, New York

Bonate, P.L. (2005). Covariate Detection in Population Pharmacokinetics Using Partially Linear Mixed Effects Models. *Pharmaceutical Research*, Vol.22, No.4, pp. 541-549, ISSN 1573-904X

Booth, B.P. & Gobburu, J.V.S. (2003). Considerations in Analysing Single-trough Concentrations Using Mixed-Effects Modeling. *The Journal of Clinical Pharmacology*, Vol.43, No.12, pp. 1307-1315, ISSN 1552-4604

Buchthal, F.; Svensmark, O. & Schiller P.J. (1960). Clinical and Electroencephalographic Correlations with Serum Levels of Diphenylhydantin. *Archives of Neurology*, Vol.2, No.6, pp. 624-630, ISSN 0003-9942

Chan, E.; Lee, H.S. & Hue, S.S. (2001). Population Pharmacokinetics of Carbamazepine in Singapore Epileptic Patients. *British Journal of Clinical Pharmacology*, Vol.51, No.6, pp. 567-576, ISSN 1365-2125

Commission on Antiepileptic Drugs. International League against Epilepsy. (1993). Guidelines for therapeutic monitoring on antiepileptic drugs. *Epilepsia*, Vol. 34, No.4, pp. 585-587, ISSN 1528-1167

Dhillon, S. & Kostrzewski, A. (Eds.). (2006). *Clinical Pharmacokinetics* (1st ed.), Pharmaceutical Press, ISBN 10-0-853695717, London

El Desoky, E.S.; Fuseau, E.; El Din Amry, S. & Cosson, V. (2004). Pharmacokinetic Modelling of Valproic Acid from Routine Clinical Data in Egyptian Epileptic Patients. *European Journal of Clinical Pharmacology*, Vol. 59, No.11, pp. 783-790, ISSN 0031-6970

Ette, E.I. & Williams, P.J. (2004a). Population Pharmacokinetics I: Background, Concepts, and Models. *The Annals of Pharmacotherapy*, Vol. 38, No. 10, pp. 1702-1706, ISSN 1060-0280

Ette, E.I. & Williams, P.J. (2004b). Population Pharmacokinetics II: Estimation Methods. *The Annals of Pharmacotherapy*, Vol. 38, No. 11, pp. 1907-1915, ISSN 1060-0280

European Medicines Agency (EMEA). Committee for Medicinal Products for Human Use. (2007). Guideline on Reporting the Results of Population Pharmacokinetic Analyses, 20.09.2008, Available from: http://www.ema.europa.eu/

Food and Drug Administration (FDA). (1999). Guidance for Industry, Population Pharmacokinetics, 15.08.2008, Available from: http://www.fda.gov

Gidal, B.E. & Garnett, W.R. (2005). Epilepsy. In: *Pharmacotherapy: a Pathophysiologic Approach,* J.T. DiPiro, R.L. Talbert, G.C. Yee, G.R. Matzke, B.G. Wells & L.M. Posey (Eds.), pp. 1023-1048, McGraw-Hill, ISBN 0071363610, New York

Grasela, T.H.; Antal, E.J.; Ereshefski, L.; Wells, B.G.; Evans, R.L. & Smith, R.B. (1987). An Evaluation of Population Pharmacokinetics in Therapeutic Trials. Part II. Detection of a Drug-Drug Interaction. *Clinical Pharmacology & Therapeutics*, Vol. 42, No. 4, pp. 433-441, ISSN 0009-9236

Graves, N.M.; Brundage, R.C.; Wen, Y.; Cascino, G. & So Leppik, I.E. (1988). Population Pharmacokinetics of Carbamazepine in Adults with Epilepsy. *Pharmacotherapy*, Vol. 18, No. 2, pp. 273-281, ISSN 0277-0008

Jelliffe, R.W.; Schumitzky, A.; Guilder, M.V.; Liu, M.; Hu, L.; Maire, P.; Gomis, P.; Barbaut, X. & Tahani, B. (1993). Individualizing Drug Dosage Regimens: Roles of Population Pharmacokinetic and Dynamic Models, Bayesian Fitting, and Adaptive Control. *Therapeutic Drug Monitoring,* Vol. 15, No. 5, pp. 380-393, ISSN 0163-4356

Jiao, Z.; Shi, X.J.; Zhao, Z.G. & Zhong, M.K. (2004). Population Pharmacokinetic Modeling of Steady State Clearance of Carbamazepine and its Epoxide Metabolite from Sparse Routine Clinical Data. *Journal of Clinical Pharmacy and Therapeutics*, Vol. 29, No. 3, pp. 247-256, ISSN 1365-2710

Jiao, Z.; Zhong, M.K.; Shi, X.J.; Hu, M. & Zhang, J.H. (2003). Population Pharmacokinetics of Carbamazepine in Chinese Epilepsy Patients. *Therapeutic Drug Monitoring*, Vol. 25, No. 3, pp. 279-86, ISSN 0163-4356

Jonsson, E.N. & Karlsson, M.O. (1998). Automated Covariate Model Building within NONMEM. *Pharmaceutical Research*, Vol. 15, No. 9, pp. 1463-1468, ISSN 0724-8741

Kutt, H. & Penry, J.K. (1974). Usefulness of Blood Levels of Antiepileptic Drugs. *Archives of Neurology*, Vol. 31, No. 5, pp. 283-288, ISSN 0003-9942

Mentre, F. & Mallet, A. (1994). Handling Covariates in Population Pharmacokinetics. *International Journal of Bio-Medical Computing*, Vol. 36, No. 1-2, pp. 25-33, ISSN 0020-7101

Miljković, B.; Pokrajac, M.; Varagić, V. & Lević Z. (1991). Single Dose and Steady State Pharmacokinetics of Valproic Acid in Adult Epileptic Patients. *International Journal of Clinical Pharmacology Research,* Vol. 11, No. 3, pp. 137-141, ISSN 0251-1649

Patsalos, P.N. & Perucca, E. (2003a). Clinically important drug interactions in epilepsy: general features and interactions between antiepileptic drugs. *The Lancet Neurology*, Vol. 2, No. 6, pp. 347-356, ISSN 1474-4422

Patsalos, P.N. & Perucca, E. (2003b). Clinically important drug interactions in epilepsy: interactions between antiepileptic drugs and other drugs. *The Lancet Neurology*, Vol. 2, No. 8, pp. 473-481, ISSN 1474-4422

Patsalos, P.N.; Berry, D.J.; Bourgeois, F.D., Cloyd J.C.; Glauser, T.A.; Johannessen, S.I.; Leppik, I.E.; Tomson, T. & Perucca, E. (2008). Antiepileptic Drugs - Best practice Guidelines for Therapeutic Drug Monitoring: A Position Paper by the Subcommission on Therapeutic Drug Monitoring, ILAE Commission on Therapeutic Strategies. *Epilepsia*, Vol. 49, No. , pp. 1239-1276, ISSN 1528-1167

Perucca, E. (2006). Clinically relevant drug interactions with antiepileptic drugs. *British Journal of Clinical Pharmacology*, Vol. 61, No. 3, pp. 246-255, ISSN 1365-2125

Pokrajac, M. (2008). *Pharmacokinetics-handbook.* (3rd ed.), BiroGraf, ISBN 978-86-907323-2-6, Belgrade

Sheiner, L.B. & Beal, S.L. (1981). Evaluation of Methods for Estimating Population Pharmacokinetic Parameters. III. Monoexponential Model: Routine Clinical Pharmacokinetic Data. *Journal of Pharmacokinetics and Biopharmaceutics*, Vol. 11, No. 3, pp. 303-319, ISSN 0090-466X

Sheiner, L.B. & Beal, S.L. (1981). Some Suggestions for Measuring Predictive Performance. *Journal of Pharmacokinetics and Biopharmaceutics*, Vol. 9, No. 4, pp. 503-512, ISSN 0090-466X

Sheiner, L.B.; Beal, S.L.; Rosenberg, B. & Marathe, V.V. (1979). Forecasting Individual Pharmacokinetics. *Clinical Pharmacology & Therapeutics*, Vol. 26, No. 3, pp. 294-305, ISSN 0009-9236

Sheiner, L.B.; Rosenberg, B. & Marathe, V.V. (1977). Estimation of Population Characteristics of Pharmacokinetic Parameters from Routine Clinical Data. *Journal of Pharmacokinetics and Biopharmaceutics*, Vol. 5, No. 5, pp. 445-479, ISSN 0090-466X

Sun, H.; Fadiran, E.O.; Jones, C.D.; Lesko, L.; Huang, S.M.; Higgins, K.; Hu, C.; Machado, S.; Maldonado, S.; Williams, R.; Hossain, M. & Ette, E.I. (1999). Population Pharmacokinetics. A Regulatory Perspective. *Clinical Pharmacokinetics*, Vol. 37, No. 1, pp. 41-58, ISSN 0312-5963

Vučićević, K.; Miljković, B.; Petronijević, M.; Pokrajac, M.; Mrhar, A. & Grabnar, I. (2008). Effect of Co-treatment with Valproic Acid on Carbamazepine Elimination in

Epileptic Patients - A Population Pharmacokinetic Study. Pharmacy World & Science, Vol. 30, No. 5, pp. 673-674, ISSN 1573-739X

Vučićević, K.; Miljković, B.; Petronijević, M.; Pokrajac, M.; Veličković, R. & Grabnar, I. (2007a). Induction of Carbamazepine Metabolism During Co-treatment with Phenobarbitone - A Population Pharmacokinetic Study. *European Neuropsychopharmacology*, Vol. 17, No. S4, pp. S261-262, ISSN 0924-977X

Vučićević, K.; Miljković, B.; Pokrajac, M. & Grabnar, I. (2009). Effect of Topiramate on Valproic Acid Clearance in Adult Patients with Epilepsy: A Population Pharmacokinetic Study. *European Neuropsychopharmacology*, Vol. 19, No. S3, pp. S271, ISSN 0924-977X

Vučićević, K.; Miljković, B.; Pokrajac, M. & Petronijević, M. (2005). Population Pharmacokinetic Approach to Data Analysis. *Arhiv za farmaciju*, Vol. 55, No. 5-6, pp. 483-496, ISSN 0004-1963

Vučićević, K.; Miljković, B.; Pokrajac, M.; Prostran, M.; Martinović, Ž. & Grabnar, I. (2009b). The Influence of Drug-Drug Interaction and Patients' Characteristics on Valproic Acid's Clearance in Adults with Epilepsy using Nonlinear Mixed Effects Modeling. *European Journal of Pharmaceutical Sciences*, Vol. 38, No. 5, pp. 512-518, ISSN 0928-0987

Vučićević, K.; Miljković, B.; Veličković, R.; Pokrajac, M.; Mrhar, A. & Grabnar, I. (2007b). Population Pharmacokinetic Model of Carbamazepine Derived from Routine Therapeutic Drug Monitoring Data. *Therapeutic Drug Monitoring*, Vol. 29, No. , pp. 781-788, ISSN 01634356

Wade, J.R.; Kelman, A.W.; Howie, C.A. & Whiting, B. (1993). Effect of Misspecification of the Absorption Process on Subsequent Parameter Estimation in Population Analysis. *Journal of Pharmacokinetics and Biopharmaceutics*, Vol. 21, No. 2, pp. 209-222, ISSN 0090-466X

Wählby, U.E.; Jonsson, N. & Karlsson, M.O. (2001). Assessment of Actual Significance Levels for Covariate Effects in NONMEM. *Journal of Pharmacokinetics and Pharmacodynamics*, Vol. 28, No. 3, pp. 231-252, ISSN 1567-567X

Wu, G. (1995). Calculating Predictive Performance: A User's Note. *Pharmacological Reseach*, Vol. 31, No. 6, pp. 393-399, ISSN 1043-6618

Yukawa, E. & Aoyama, T. (1996). Detection of Carbamazepine Drug Interaction by Multi Peak Approach Screening using Routine Clinical Pharmacokinetic Data. *The Journal of Clinical Pharmacology*, Vol. 36, No. 8, pp. 752-759, ISSN 1552-4604

Yukawa, E. (1999). Population-based Investigations of Drug Relative Clearance using Nonlinear Mixed-Effect Modeling from Information Generated during the Routine Clinical Care of Patients. *Journal of Clinical Pharmacy and Therapeutics*, Vol. 24, No. 2, pp. 103-113, ISSN 1365-2710

Yukawa, E.; Nonaka, T.; Yukawa, M.; Higuchi, S.; Kuroda, T. & Goto, Y. (2003). Pharmacoepidemiologic Investigation of a Clonazepam-Valproic Acid Interaction by Mixed Effect Modeling using Routine Clinical Pharmacokinetic Data in Japanese Patients. *Journal of Clinical Pharmacy and Therapeutics*, Vol. 28, No. 6, pp. 497-504, ISSN 1365-2710

Zhou, H. (2006). Population-based Assessments of Clinical Drug-Drug Interactions: Qualitative Indices or Quantitative Measures? *The Journal of Clinical Pharmacology,* Vol. 46, No. 11, pp. 1268-1289, ISSN 1552-4604

7

Antiepileptic Drugs Targeting Cerebral Presynaptic Ion Channels Reduce Cerebral Excitability Decreasing Glutamate Release

María Sitges
Instituto de Investigaciones Biomédicas, Universidad Nacional Autónoma de México, México

1. Introduction

Ion channel dysfunction has been implicated in several neurological diseases including epilepsy. Cerebral ion channels, and particularly presynaptic channels controlling neurotransmitter release, are among the most important targets of various antiepileptic drugs. In comparison with other parts of the neuron, in presynaptic nerve endings Na^+ and Ca^{2+} channels controlling neurotransmitter release are particularly abundant. However, most studies directed to test the effect of antiepileptic drugs on ion channels are done in preparations suitable for electrophysiological approaches. Because using those approaches in the small sized cerebral nerve endings is almost impossible.

In the present chapter I describe the strategies that we have used for investigating the effects of several compounds known for their anticonvulsant properties, including several of the most commonly used antiepileptic drugs of the first and second generations, as well as of the new potential antiepileptic drug, vinpocetine on cerebral presynaptic ionic channels. For discriminating the effects of those compounds on presynaptic Na^+ and Ca^{2+} channels, we first used depolarizing strategies, such as veratridine that triggers the entrance of Na^+ by activation of cerebral presynaptic Na^+ channels even when the participation of Ca^{2+} channels is eliminated, or such as a high external concentration of K^+, that activates cerebral pre-synaptic Ca^{2+} channels even when the participation of Na^+ channels is eliminated (Sitges & Galindo, 2005; Sitges et al., 2007a; 2007b). More recently, we also test the effects of antiepileptic drugs in the cerebral nerve endings *in vitro* using 4-aminopyridine as depolarizing strategy. Because 4-aminopyridine exposure may more closely mimic some of the changes that may take place in the epileptic tissue, since in cerebral nerve endings 4-aminopyridine besides increasing the permeability of Na^+ and Ca^{2+} channels, also decreases the permeability of some K^+ channels, and by this mean arrests indirectly the Na^+/K^+ ATPase (Galván & Sitges, 2004), making even more difficult the limitation of neuronal excitability.

2. Effects of antiepileptic drugs on cerebral presynaptic Na^+ channel mediated responses induced with veratridine

Voltage sensitive Na^+ channels are responsible for the initiation and conduction of neuronal action potentials. Therefore, the pharmacological down-modulation of those channels in situations in which all neurons are firing, such as during epileptic seizures, is likely to be particularly beneficial.

Several of the most effective antiepileptic drugs are believed to stop the paroxysmal neuronal activity acting as Na^+ channel blockers. In comparison with other parts of the neuron, Na^+ channels in presynaptic boutons are particularly abundant (Engel & Jonas, 2005). Nonetheless since the small size of cerebral presynaptic boutons (< 0.3 μm) make electrophysiological approaches very difficult, most of the pioneer as well as the sophisticated and important actual studies directed to test the effect of antiepileptic drugs on Na^+ channels were done in preparations suitable for electrophysiological approaches. These preparations include molluscan giant axons, kidney cells and Chinese hamster ovary cells transfect with the alpha subunit (the pore moiety) of the channel, and cells in culture among others (Lipicky et al.,1972; Fohlmeister et al., 1984; Xie et al., 1995; Sun & Lin, 2000; Xie et al., 2001; Huang et al., 2006; Lenkey et al., 2010; Karoly et al., 2010); and there are only few studies in which the effect of antiepileptic drugs on presynaptic ion channels controlling neurotransmitter release in the brain were investigated.

Among the first evidences suggesting an involvement of brain presynaptic Na^+ channel blockade in the mechanism of action of some antiepileptic drugs, was the displacement of ^{3}H-batrachotoxin binding to Na^+ channels in cerebral membranes and brain isolated nerve endings by the antiepileptic drugs carbamazepine, phenytoin and lamotrigine (Willow & Catterall, 1982; Cheung et al., 1992; Deffois et al., 1996; Bonifacio et al., 2001; Santangeli et al., 2002; Lingamaneni & Hemmings, 2003). Batrachotoxin, like veratridine, is a toxin of natural origin that binds to the site 2 (voltage sensor) of the Na^+ channel impeding its inactivation and by this mean increases the rate of Na^+ entry and depolarizes the plasma membrane of cerebral isolated nerve endings (Krueger et al., 1980). With the aid of: SBFI, fura-2 and PBFI, that are selective indicator dyes which change their emission fluorescence in response to the changes in Na^+, Ca^{2+} or K^+ in its vicinity, respectively, the changes in those ion channel permeability can be monitored in cerebral isolated nerve endings. Using cerebral isolated nerve endings preloaded with the Na^+ selective indicator dye, SBFI, we found that veratridine was able to increase the internal concentration of Na^+ independently of the presence of external Ca^{2+} (Sitges et al., 1998). Figure 1 adapted from our previous work (Sitges & Galindo, 2005) shows that in hippocampus isolated nerve endings veratridine is still increasing Na^+ when presynaptic Ca^{2+} channels are blocked by ω-agatoxin-TK but not when Na^+ channels are blocked by tetrodotoxin, a toxin of natural origin that binds irreversible to the external pore of the Na^+ channel (*i.e.* site 1) and by this mean blocks Na^+ entrance into the cytoplasm. The hippocampus is a brain structure particularly involved in seizures.

Cerebral isolated nerve endings (commonly referred to as synaptosomes) preserve many physiological properties of intact nerve terminals, including a tight coupling of neurotransmitter release to ion fluxes during depolarization (Turner et al., 1992; Sitges & Chiu, 1995a; 1995b; Sitges et al., 1998; Galván & Sitges, 2004). Depolarization-evoked neurotransmitter release, including the release of the excitatory amino acid neurotransmitter glutamate, the most abundant neurotransmitter in cerebral isolated nerve endings (Sitges et al., 2000), is composed by two fractions: a Ca^{2+} dependent fraction released by exocytosis and a Na^+ dependent fraction released from the cytoplasm by reversal of the neurotransmitter transporters.

When the internal concentration of Na^+ is substantially elevated with toxins such as veratridine in the absence of external Ca^{2+} brain neurotransmitters can be released from the cytoplasm (Nicholls, 1989; Sitges 1989; Adam-Vizi, 1992; Sitges et al., 1993; 1994; Sitges & Chiu, 1995a; Sitges et al., 1998; Sitges & Galindo 2005). In hippocampus synaptosomes the release of glutamate induced by veratridine in the absence of external Ca^{2+} was sensitive to the EAAT (excitatory amino acid transporter) inhibitor, TBOA (Fig. 2), indicating that the release of glutamate induced by veratridine originates from the cytoplasm by reversal of the neurotransmitter transporters located at the level of the presynaptic nerve endings.

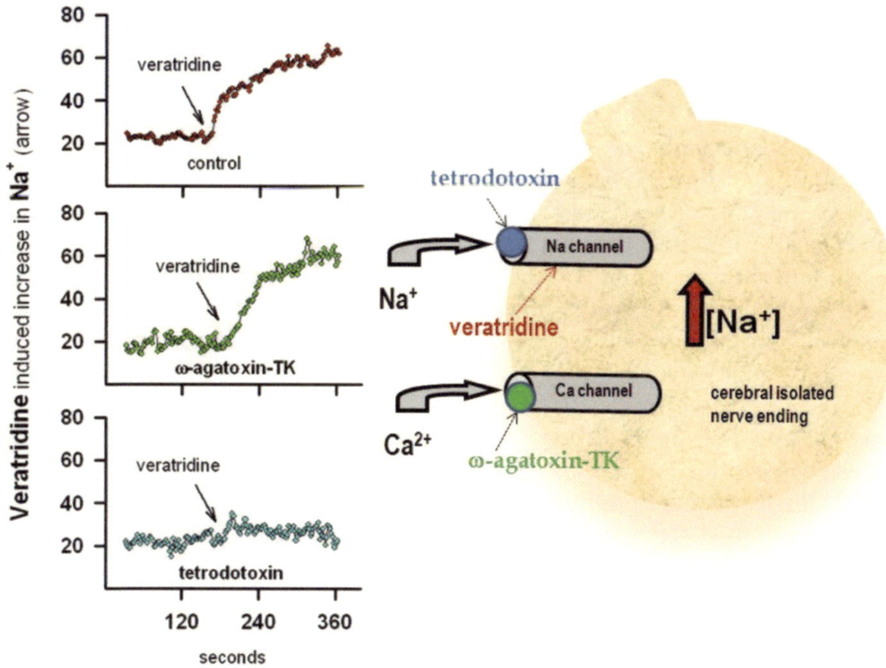

Fig. 1. The elevation of Na^+ (in mM) induced by veratridine is insensitive to ω-agatoxin-TK and completely blocked by tetrodotoxin. In this and the following cartoons channels are represented like tubes, although they are trans-membrane proteins well characterized.

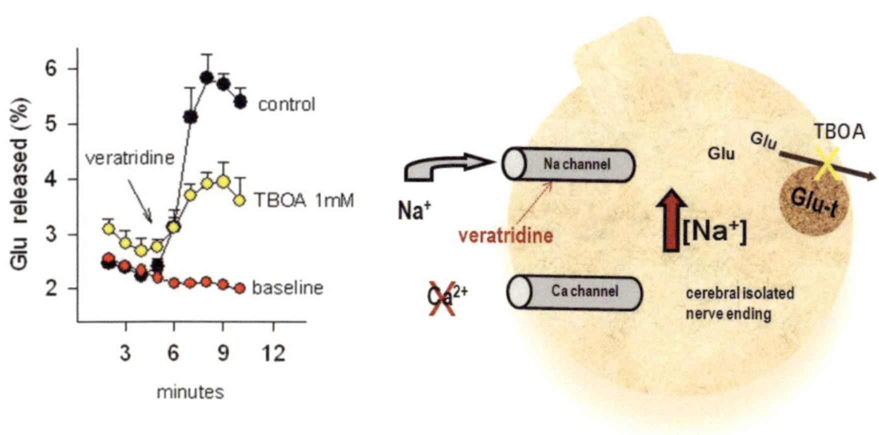

Fig. 2. Inhibition exerted by the EAAT inhibitor, TBOA, on glutamate (Glu) release induced by the Na^+ channel opener veratridine (arrow) via reversal of the glutamate transporter (Glu-t) in hippocampal synaptosomes.

Neurotransmitter release evoked by veratridine in synaptosomes isolated from the whole brain or different brain regions is also highly sensitive to the blockade of Na^+ channels with tetrodotoxin and absolutely dependent on the presence of external Na^+, but is independent of external Ca^{2+} (Sitges, 1989; Sitges & Chiu, 1995a; Galindo & Sitges, 2004; Sitges & Galindo, 2005). This Ca^{2+} independence of veratridine induced responses is particularly valuable as it allows testing the inhibitory effect of compounds on responses selectively mediated by activation of presynaptic voltage sensitive sodium channels in the cerebral isolated nerve endings.

The action of carbamazepine as a brain presynaptic Na^+ channel blocker was first indicated by the sensitivity of the veratridine-induced release of glutamate to that antiepileptic drug (Ambrosio et al., 2001). In a previous study in cerebral nerve endings isolated from the hippocampus we compared the effect of increasing concentrations of several antiepileptic drugs, including carbamazepine, on the release of glutamate induced by veratridine in the absence of external Ca^{2+}. Figure 3, adapted from our previous work (Sitges et al., 2007a; 2007b), shows that the antiepileptic drugs: carbamazepine, phenytoin, lamotrigine and oxcarbazepine, progressively inhibit glutamate release induced by veratridine in a range from 150 to 1500 μM, whereas the antiepileptic drug topiramate only exerted a modest inhibition (20%) at the highest concentration tested (1500 μM). Interestingly, valproate which mechanism of action has been related to the increase in GABAergic transmission (Loscher 2002) was unable to inhibit glutamate release to veratridine at all, although a very large range of valproate concentrations was tested.

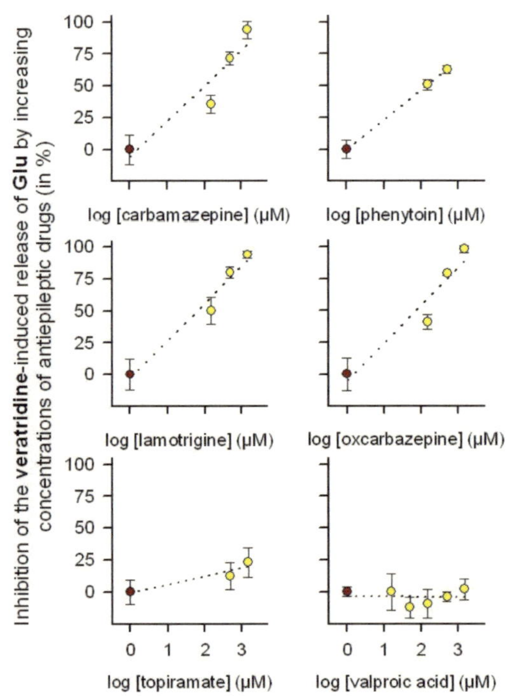

Fig. 3. Inhibition (in percentage of control) exerted by several antiepileptic drugs at increasing concentrations on glutamate (Glu) release induced by veratridine in hippocampus synaptosomes.

Results in figure 3 indicate that blockade of presynaptic Na^+ channels permeability contributes to the anticonvulsive action of carbamazepine, phenytoin, lamotrigine and oxcarbazepine, but not to the anticonvulsive action of topiramate or valproate.

3. Effects of antiepileptic drugs on high K^+ induced responses

On the basis of electrophysiological studies in dissociated cells, neurons in culture or brain slices also a reduction of Ca^{2+} channels permeability by several of the most effective antiepileptic drugs was suggested (Schirrmacher et al., 1993; Lees & Leach, 1993; Wang et al., 1996; Stefani et al., 1996; 1997; Kuzmiski et al., 2005). However, Ca^{2+} currents obtained in those preparations not necessarily reflect the effect of anticpileptic drugs on brain presynaptic Ca^{2+} channels controlling neurotransmitter release. Because in cell bodies, dendrites and nerve endings different types of calcium channels were localized (Timmerman et al., 2001), and Ca^{2+} currents obtained in the above preparations must be mainly somatic.
Again, as for the case of cerebral presynaptic ion Na^+ channels, cerebral presynaptic Ca^{2+} channels cannot be easily approached with electrophysiological techniques because of the small size of cerebral nerve endings. Nevertheless, with the selective Ca^{2+} indicator dye, fura-2, the changes in the internal concentration of Ca^{2+} concomitant to the changes in cerebral presynaptic Ca^{2+} channels permeability can be monitored directly in the cerebral isolated nerve endings. Using this technique it has been shown that among the several types of Ca^{2+} channels present in neurons, those sensitive to ω-agatoxin-IVA and to ω-agatoxin-TK, two peptides isolated from the venom of the spider Agelenopsis aperta, were particularly implicated in neurotransmitter release from cerebral nerve endings (Turner et al., 1992; Sitges & Chiu, 1995a; 1995b; Carvalho et al., 1995; Sitges & Galindo, 2005). P/Q type Ca^{2+} channels are pharmacologically characterized by their sensitivity to the above mentioned ω-agatoxins. In line, the cloned neuronal Ca^{2+} channel α_{1A}subunit encoding Ca^{2+} channels of the P/Q type was localized at a high density in presynaptic nerve terminals of many neurons (Westenbroek et al., 1995).

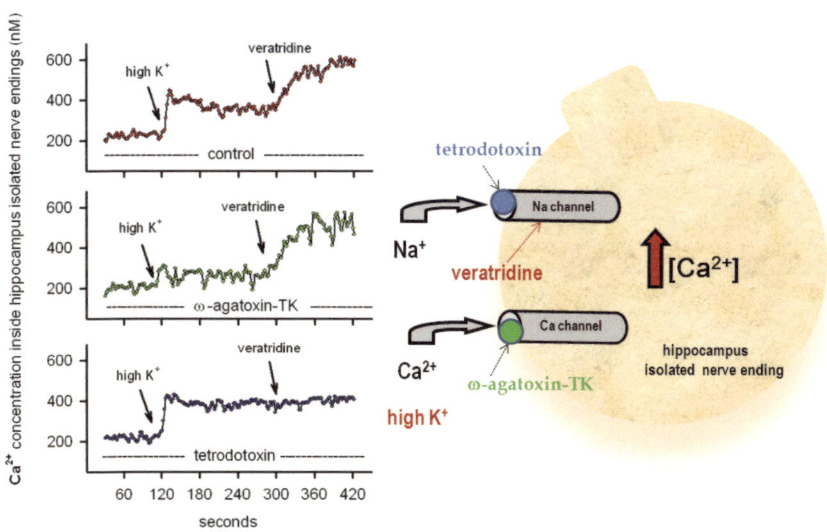

Fig. 4. The rise in Ca^{2+} induced by high K^+ depends on presynaptic Ca^{2+} channels availability and the rise in Ca^{2+} induced by veratridine depends on Na^+ channels availability (this figure was adapted from Sitges & Galindo (2005)

The top graph in figure 4 shows the increase in Ca^{2+} induced by high K^+ depolarization followed by the increase in Ca^{2+} induced by veratridine depolarization in hippocampal synaptosomes under control conditions. The middle graph shows the failure of high K^+ depolarization to increase Ca^{2+} when Ca^{2+} channels are blocked by ω-agatoxin-TK and the failure of this blockade to prevent the veratridine induced increase in Ca^{2+}. Oppositely, the bottom graph shows that when Na^+ channels are blocked by tetrodotoxin, high K^+ depolarization is still increasing Ca^{2+}, but veratridine does not.

It is important to mention that in the presence of external Ca^{2+}, veratridine depolarization also can increase the internal concentration of Ca^{2+} like high K^+ depolarization. Nonetheless, the underlying mechanisms are different. Because while the entrance of external Na^+ via tetrodotoxin sensitive Na^+ channels is strictly required for the increase in Ca^{2+} and the increase in neurotransmitter release induced by veratridine, the increase in Ca^{2+} induced by high K^+ is insensitive to the absence of external Na^+ or to the presence of tetrodotoxin (Sitges & Chiu, 1995a; Sitges et al., 1998; Sitges & Galindo 2005).

In the absence of Na^+ or in the presence of tetrodotoxin, high K^+ depolarization also is still increasing neurotransmitter release. In hippocampus isolated nerve endings the fraction of glutamate release induced by high K^+ depolarization in the absence of external Na^+, however, is completely dependent on external Ca^{2+} and is highly sensitive to nanomolar concentrations of ω-agatoxin-IVA and ω-agatoxin-TK, as shown in figure 5 adapted from Sitges & Galindo (2005). This figure shows that high K^+ depolarization induced responses in the absence of external Na^+ are directly linked to the inhibition of cerebral presynaptic Ca^{2+} channels permeability.

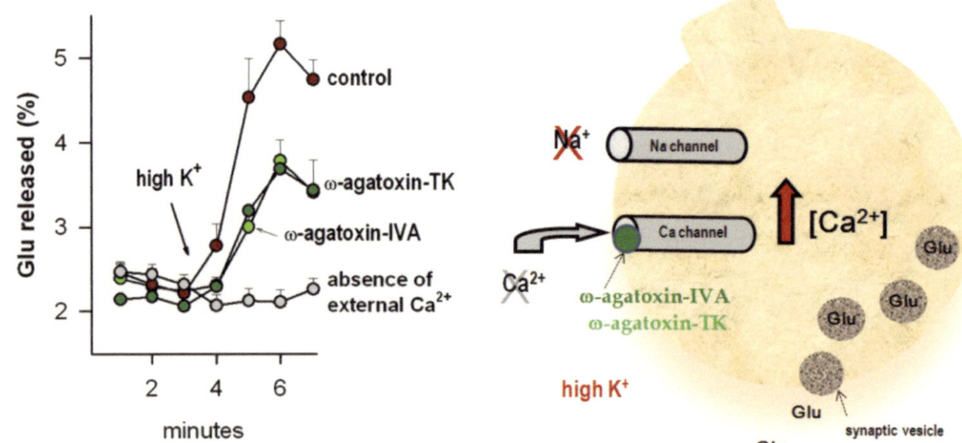

Fig. 5. Glutamate (Glu) release induced by high K^+ depends on the presence of external Ca^{2+} and is sensitive to the P/Q type Ca^{2+} channel blocker toxins. This figure was adapted from Sitges & Galindo (2005).

Since high K^+ can selectively release the Ca^{2+} dependent fraction of neurotransmitter release by exocytosis, for investigating the action of antiepileptic drugs on cerebral presynaptic Ca^{2+} channels permeability, we tested their effects at increasing concentrations on the Ca^{2+} channel-mediated release of glutamate evoked by high K^+ in the absence of external Na^+ in hippocampus isolated nerve endings. Figure 6, adapted from Sitges et al. (2007b), shows that carbamazepine, phenytoin and oxcarbazepine only reduced in about 30% and 55% glutamate release to high K^+ at concentrations of 500 μM and 1500 μM, respectively; that lamotrigine and topiramate were even less effective, as at the highest concentration tested (1500 μM) they only exerted a mild reduction (about 25%) of glutamate release to high K^+, and that valproate failed to modify the K^+ response at all. These results indicate that only some of the antiepileptic drugs tested, namely carbamazepine, phenytoin and oxcarbazepine, are able to reduce cerebral presynaptic Ca^{2+} channels permeability in some degree at high doses.

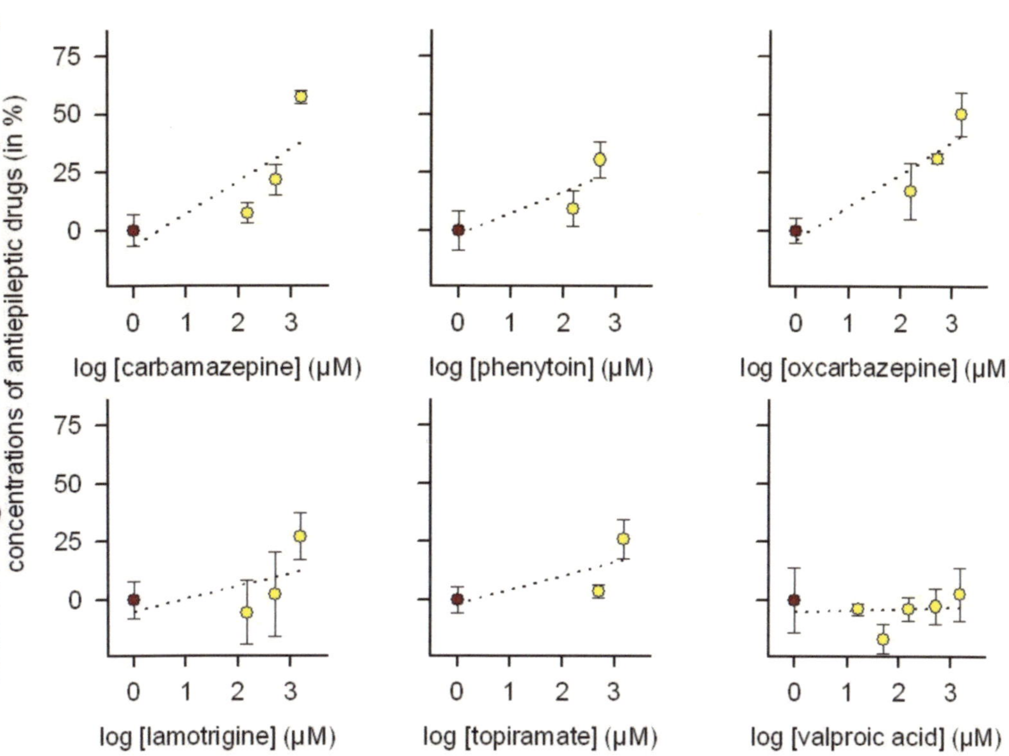

Fig. 6. Inhibition (in percentage of control) exerted by the indicated antiepileptic drug at increasing concentrations on glutamate (Glu) release induced by high K^+ in hippocampus synaptosomes.

4. Effects of antiepileptic drugs on 4-aminopyridine induced responses

4-aminopyridine is a convulsing agent that induces epileptiform activity in brain slices *in vitro* as in animal models of epilepsy *in vivo* (Ives & Jefferys, 1990; Perreault & Avoli, 1991; Yamaguchi & Rogawski, 1992; Psarropoulou & Avoli, 1996; Armand et al., 1999; Nekrassov & Sitges, 2003). 4-aminopyridine increases neurotransmitters release, including glutamate, the most important excitatory amino acid neurotransmitter in the brain, that is by far the most concentrated neurotransmitter in cerebral isolated nerve endings (Sitges et al., 2000).

The action of 4-aminopyridine at the brain presynaptic level is amply documented. Although the rise in the internal concentration of Ca^{2+} induced by 4-aminopyridine was not resolved using $^{45}Ca^{2+}$ (Tapia et al., 1985), it became evident when the more sensitive fura-2 technique was used in cerebral isolated nerve endings. The role of voltage sensitive sodium channels in the mode of action of 4-aminopyridine, first suggested by the sensitivity of the Ca^{2+} response induced by 4-aminopyridine to the Na^{+} channel blocker, tetrodotoxin (Tibbs et al., 1989; Heemskerk et al., 1991) was later demonstrated in cerebral isolated nerve endings using the Na^{+} selective indicator dye, SBFI (Galván & Sitges 2004). The involvement of K^{+} channels in the mode of action of 4-aminopyridine at the presynaptic brain level, first suggested by the changes on $^{86}Rb^{+}$ fluxes in brain nerve endings (Sitges et al., 1986), was confirmed later using the K^{+} selective indicator dye, PBFI (Galindo & Sitges 2004). In summary, in cerebral isolated nerve endings 4-aminopyridine increases Na^{+} channels permeability (Galván and Sitges, 2004), Ca^{2+} channels permeability (Tibbs et al., 1989; Heemskerk et al., 1991; Galván & Sitges, 2004; Sitges et al., 2005), and decreases K^{+} channels permeability (Sitges et al., 1986; Galván & Sitges, 2004). Therefore, the changes that may occur in cerebral nerve endings under the excitatory conditions that take place during seizures seem to be more closely resembled by 4-aminopyridine; although its mechanism of action is complicated. For instance, in contrast to veratridine, that can increase Na^{+} and glutamate release independently of Ca^{2+} channels activation, or in contrast to high K^{+} that can increase Ca^{2+} and glutamate release independently of Na^{+} channels activation (Sitges & Galindo, 2005; Sitges et al., 2007a; 2007b), 4-aminopyridine is unable to increase Ca^{2+} and to induce glutamate exocytosis, when Na^{+} channels are blocked by tetrodotoxin (Tibbs et al., 1989; Heemskerk et al., 1991; Galván & Sitges, 2004; Sitges et al., 2005). Thus, as the tetrodotoxin-sensitive fraction of glutamate release induced by 4-aminopyridine requires the presence of external Ca^{2+} and is sensitive to presynaptic Ca^{2+} channel blockade, the tetrodotoxin-sensitive fraction of glutamate release induced by 4-aminopyridine is expected to be the fraction released from the vesicular pool by exocytosis. This also contrasts with veratridine depolarization, that increases glutamate release in a tetrodotoxin sensitive manner via reversal of the neurotransmitter transporter independently of presynaptic Ca^{2+} channels, and with high K^{+} depolarization that increases Ca^{2+} and glutamate exocytosis from the vesicular pool in a tetrodotoxin insensitive manner independently of presynaptic Na^{+} channels (Sitges & Galindo, 2005; Sitges et al. 2007a; 2007b). Moreover, in addition to the tetrodotoxin-sensitive increases in Na^{+}, Ca^{2+} and glutamate exocytosis, 4-aminopyridine also produces an accumulation of Na^{+} that is tetrodotoxin insensitive and is accompanied by a decrease in the internal concentration of K^{+}, due to inhibition of the Na/K-ATPase that restores K^{+} (Galván & Sitges, 2004). This tetrodotoxin insensitive accumulation of Na^{+}, that is independent of presynaptic Na^{+} or Ca^{2+} channels activation, is likely to also release the cytoplasm fraction of glutamate by reversal of the glutamate transporter in a tetrodotoxin insensitive manner.

Figure 7 shows that the maximal inhibitory effect on glutamate release to 4-aminopyridine exerted by the antiepileptic drugs: carbamazepine, phenytoin, lamotrigine and oxcarbazepine in a range from 75 to 750 μM in hippocampus isolated nerve endings, that is almost reached with the concentration of 250 μM, is not larger than 50-60%. Similarly 1 μM tetrodotoxin also inhibited glutamate released to 4-aminopyridine only in about 50%; and at that concentration tetrodotoxin completely abolished the veratridine-induced responses in synaptosomes, indicating that the decrease in glutamate release to 4-aminopyridine exerted by the above antiepileptic drugs, is linked to the blockade of presynaptic Na^+ channels. Figure 7 also shows that topiramate at the highest concentration tested (750 μM) only exerted a modest inhibition of 4-aminopyridine induced glutamate release; further indicating that the anticonvulsant mechanism of action of that antiepileptic drug is unrelated with a reduction in cerebral presynaptic Na^+ channels permeability. In line with this last interpretation previous studies showed that neuronal Na^+ currents were only slightly reduced by topiramate at high doses (Zona et al., 1997; Taverna et al., 1999; Mc. Lean et al., 2000).

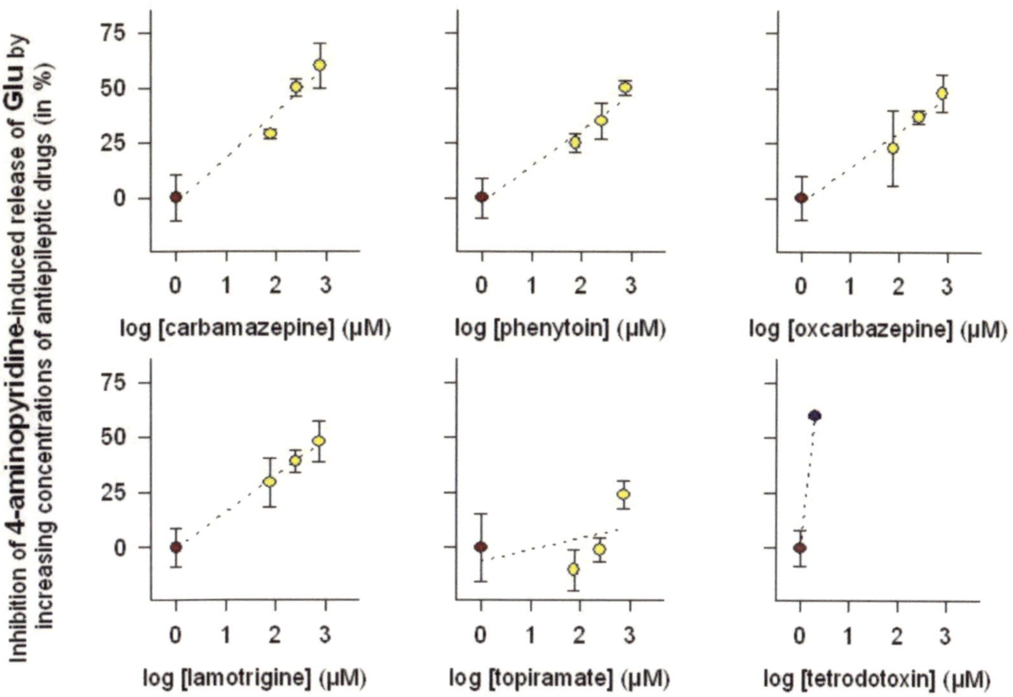

Fig. 7. Inhibition (in percentage of control) exerted by the indicated compounds at increasing concentrations on glutamate (Glu) release induced by 4-aminopyridine in hippocampus synaptosomes.

Figure 8 shows that similarly to glutamate release induced by 4-aminopyridine, the rise in Ca^{2+} induced by 4-aminopyridine also was partially sensitive to the blockade of Na^+ channels with 1 μM tetrodotoxin or with 250μM carbamazepine, phenytoin, lamotrigine and oxcarbazepine, and insensitive to topiramate at that concentration.

The antiepileptic drugs valproate and levetiracetam, even at a very high (1000 μM) concentration were unable to inhibit the rise in Ca^{2+} induced by 4-aminopyridine in hippocampus isolated nerve endings. In line, levetiracetam, like valproate, also was unable to inhibit glutamate release induced by the Na^+ channel opener, veratridine or by high K^+ (data not shown), suggesting that levetiracetam mechanism of action does not involve inhibition of cerebral presynaptic Na^+ or Ca^{2+} channels permeability as well.

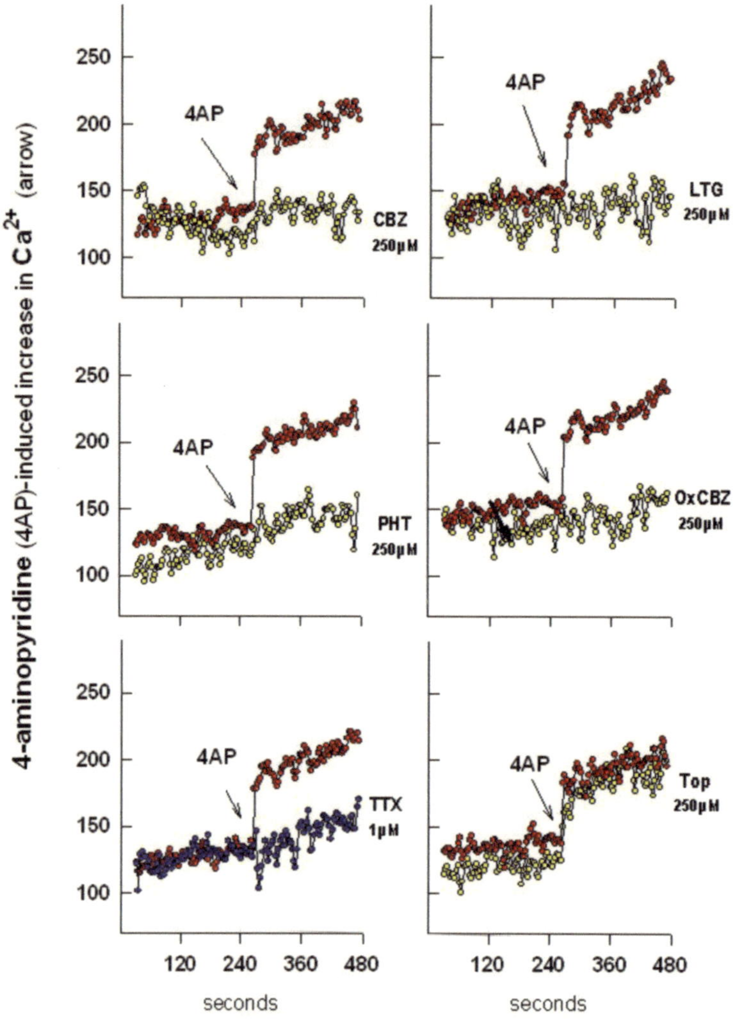

Fig. 8. The elevation of Ca^{2+} (in mM) induced by 4-aminopyridine in hippocampus isolated nerve endings is sensitive to carbamazepine (CBZ), lamotrigine (LTG), phenytoin (PHT), oxcarbazepine (OxCBZ) and tetrodotoxin (TTX), and insensitive to topiramate (Top).

5. Presynaptic Na^+ channels are better targets of antiepileptic drugs than presynaptic Ca^{2+} channels

Comparison of the inhibition exerted by the antiepileptic drugs on glutamate release triggered by the selective activation of Ca^{2+} channels with high K^+ with the inhibition exerted by the antiepileptic drugs on glutamate release evoked by the activation of Na^+ channels induced by veratridine, clearly shows that antiepileptic drugs targeting cerebral presynaptic channels are in general more effective blockers of presynaptic Na^+ than of presynaptic Ca^{2+} channel mediated responses.

Moreover, it is likely that all the compounds that inhibited the increase in Ca^{2+} and the release of glutamate induced by 4-aminopyridine were reducing presynaptic Na^+ channels permeability, and by this mean the entrance of Ca^{2+}. In agreement with this conclusion, lamotrigine that barely reduced the Ca^{2+} dependent release of glutamate induced by high K^+ (Fig. 6), markedly inhibited glutamate release induced by veratridine (Fig. 3). Thus, the inhibition exerted by lamotrigine on the rise in Ca^{2+} induced by 4-aminopyridine may also result from a blockade of tetrodotoxin sensitive Na^+ channels. In line with an indirect effect of lamotrigine, as well as of carbamazepine, on the rise in Ca^{2+} induced by 4-aminopyridine, a detailed model of the binding sites for carbamazepine, lamotrigine and phenytoin in the inner pore of voltage-gated Na^+ channels was recently provided by Lipkind and Fozzard (2010).

6. Effect of the new potential antiepileptic drug vinpocetine on presynaptic ion channels

Although there is an uncovered medical need for the treatment of epilepsies, neurologists are with reasons reluctant to believe in new antiepileptic drugs. Because also new antiepileptic drugs produce several secondary effects that in some cases are severe. In addition to the fact that as antiepileptic drugs control seizures but do not cure the illness, they have to be taken for all the life span.

Vinpocetine (ethyl apovincamine-22-oate) is a nootropic drug with neuroprotective capabilities discovered during the late 1960s that in animal models of hypoxia and ischemia exerts beneficial effects against neuronal damage and has been used in the treatment of central nervous system disorders of cerebral-vascular origin for decades. In brain isolated nerve endings vinpocetine inhibited the rise in the internal concentration of Na^+ and neurotransmitter release induced by veratridine (Tretter & Adam-Vizi, 1998; Sitges & Nekrassov, 1999; Trejo et al., 2001; Sitges et al., 2006), as well as the tetrodotoxin sensitive fraction of the rise in Na^+ and Ca^{2+} induced by 4-aminopyridine (Sitges et al., 2005). In hippocampus isolated nerve endings, vinpocetine inhibited glutamate release induced by increasing presynaptic Na^+ channels permeability with veratridine and by increasing presynaptic Ca^{2+} channels permeability with high K^+ in a much lower range of concentrations than carbamazepine, phenytoin, lamotrigine and oxcarbazepine (Sitges et al., 2007a; 2007b).

Moreover, in contrast to carbamazepine, phenytoin, lamotrigine and oxcarbazepine, which that at the highest dose tested (750 μM) only inhibited glutamate release to 4-aminopyridine between 50-60%, vinpocetine completely abolished glutamate release to 4-aminopyridine at a concentration of 25 μM, which is a much lower concentration. Since in molluscan neurons, 30 μM vinpocetine, but not other antiepileptic drugs, increases the fast inactivating 4-aminopyridine-sensitive K^+ current (IA) (Bukanova et al., 2002), one possible explanation of the higher efficacy of vinpocetine to inhibit glutamate release induced by 4-aminopyridine in the hippocampus nerve endings could be that, in addition to its action on Na^+ and Ca^{2+} channels, vinpocetine is capable to overcome the blockade of the IA current produced by 4-aminopyridine. Also at a tenfold lower concentration than of carbamazepine, phenytoin, lamotrigine and oxcarbazepine, vinpocetine reduced the Ca^{2+} response to 4-aminopyridine in hippocampus isolated nerve endings. Figure 9 summarizes some of the above findings.

Combination of antiepileptic drugs is a common practice in refractory epileptics not responding to mono-therapy. Interestingly, in striatum isolated nerve endings vinpocetine facilitated the inhibition exerted by carbamazepine on the rise in Na^+ and glutamate release induced by veratridine activation of Na^+ channels (Sitges et al., 2006).

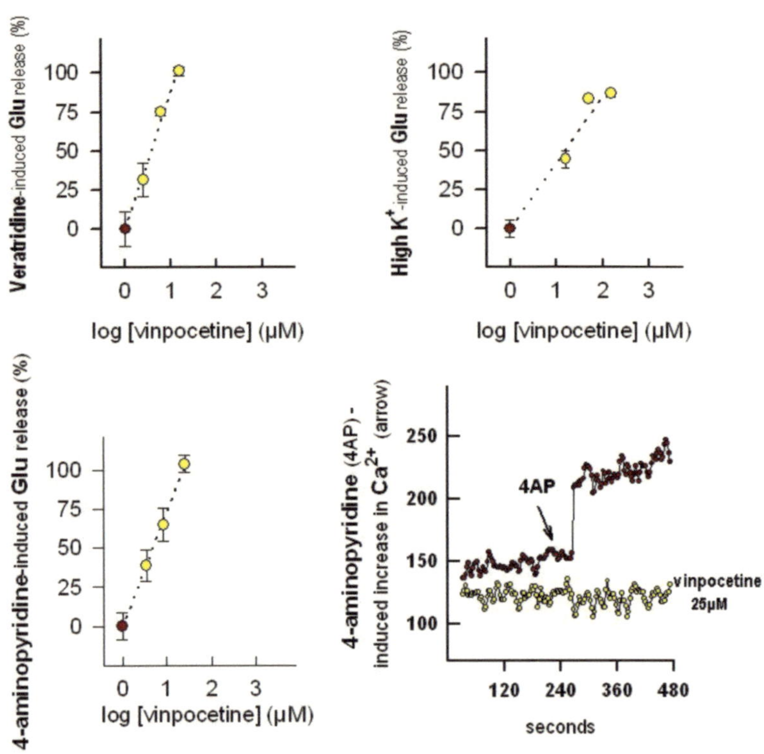

Fig. 9. Inhibition (in percentage of control) exerted by vinpocetine at increasing concentrations on the release of glutamate (Glu) induced by: veratridine, high K^+ and 4-aminopyridine, and on the elevation of Ca^{2+} induced by 4-aminopyridine in hippocampus synaptosomes.

7. Comparison of vinpocetine and some antiepileptic drugs effects on seizures and hearing in the animal *in vivo*

The high antiepileptic potential of vinpocetine also was evidenced in the guinea pig *in vivo;* where vinpocetine completely prevented seizures and the epileptic-like cortical activity induced by 4-aminopyridine at a convulsive dose (Sitges & Nekrassov, 2004).

The top traces in figures 10a and 10b show that the EEG recordings under control conditions (i.e. before the injection of the convulsive agent, 4-aminopyridine) in an animal administered with vehicle and an animal administered with vinpocetine are similar. In contrast, the abnormal EEG changes accompanying seizures observed 20, 30, 60 and 80 min after 4-aminopyridine administration in the control animal administered with vehicle are not observed in the animal pre-administered with 2 mg/kg vinpocetine.

Also seizures and the epileptiform activity induced by the convulsive agent pentylenetetrazole were vinpocetine sensitive (Nekrassov & Sitges, 2004). Representative EEG recordings before and 10, 20, 30 and 50 min after pentylenetetrazole administration are shown in figure 11a, and representative EEG recordings before and at the same periods of time after pentylenetetrazole administration in an animal pre-administered with vinpocetine are in figure 11b.

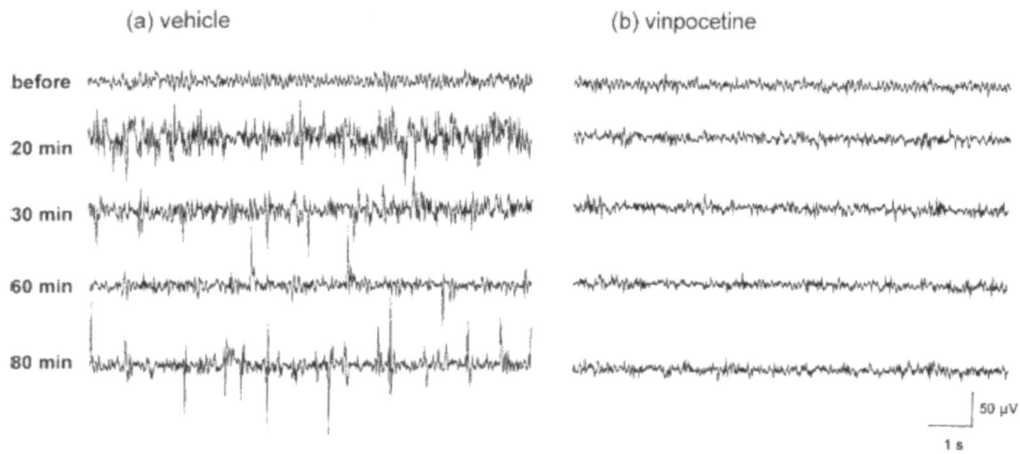

Fig. 10. Representative EEG recordings of the cortical activity before and at the indicated times after 4-aminopyridine in: (a) a control animal and (b) an animal pre-administered with vinpocetine.

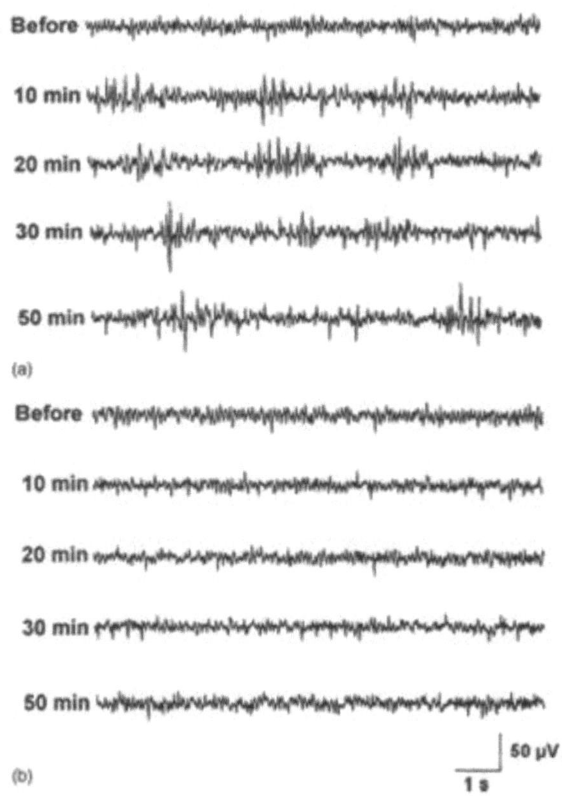

Fig. 11. Vinpocetine prevents pentylenetetrazole-induced epileptiform activity accompanying seizures.

Moreover, the epileptiform activity accompanying seizures induced by pentilenetetrazole was inhibited by vinpocetine at a lower dose than the classical antiepileptic drugs: carbamazepine, phenytoin and valproate (Nekrassov & Sitges, 2006), and a higher potency of vinpocetine than carbamazepine to inhibit seizures induced by 4-aminopyridine was observed too (Nekrassov & Sitges, 2008).

In a previous study, in which the acute, chronic and post-treatment effects of carbamazepine and vinpocetine were investigated on seizures induced by 4-aminopyridine in the guinea pig *in vivo* (Nekrassov & Sitges 2008) we found that: all the control animals developed seizures upon 4-aminopyridine exposure regardless on the time of vehicle administration; namely vehicle injection one hour before 4-aminopyridine (acute), 13 days of vehicle injections before 4-aminopyridine (chronic) or 4-aminopyridine one month after the end of the vehicle injections (post-treatment), as illustrated in figure 12a adapted from Nekrassov & Sitges, 2008. We also found that in the carbamazepine animal group, the acute carbamazepine treatment failed to prevent 4-aminopyridine-induced seizures in all the animals, whereas the chronic carbamazepine treatment, protected about half of the animals from developing seizures after 4-aminopyridine. However, one month after the end of treatment, all the animals of the carbamazepine group developed seizures again after 4-aminopyridine (Fig. 12b). In the vinpocetine animal group, the acute vinpocetine treatment already protected 43% of the animals from developing seizures and the chronic vinpocetine treatment 70% of the animals. Interestingly, 40% of the animals in the vinpocetine group did not developed seizures upon 4-aminopyridine administration one month after the end of treatment (Fig. 12c).

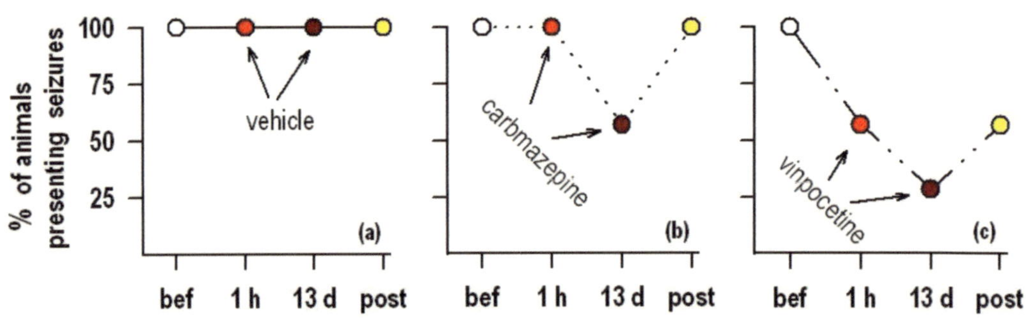

Fig. 12. Acute, chronic and post-treatment effects of carbamazepine and vinpocetine on seizures induced by 4-aminopyridine at a highly convulsive dose. Guinea pigs presenting seizures (in percentage) after the injection of 4-aminopyridine before any treatment was started (bef.), one hour after the first (1h) or of the last (13 d) injection of: (a) vehicle, (b) 17 mg/kg carbamazepine or (c) 3 mg/kg vinpocetine, and one month after the end of the above treatments (post).

Since the available antiepileptic drugs control seizures but do not cure the illness, the finding that vinpocetine even after post-treatment was able to prevent 4-aminopyridine-induced seizures is very hopefulness.

In another study, (Nekrassov & Sitges, 2006) we also investigated the auditory sensitivity, as indicated by brainstem auditory evoked potential thresholds at two tone frequencies (4 and 8 kHz) in guinea pigs daily injected with vehicle (control), 20 mg/kg carbamazepine, 6 mg/kg phenytoin, 30 mg/kg valproate or 2 mg/kg vinpocetine for 28 days before and after the administration of pentylenetetrazole at a convulsing dose (100 mg/kg). In that study we found that the long term treatment with carbamazepine, phenytoin or valproate increased the auditory threshold to a similar extent as the convulsing agent, pentylenetetrazole. In contrast, the 28 days treatment with vinpocetine even decreased the auditory threshold. Moreover, the increases exerted by the antiepileptic drugs and by pentylenetetrazole on the auditory thresholds were additive, indicating that the hearing loss produced by the long term treatment with the most commonly used antiepileptic drugs could be aggravated by the illness. On the contrary, vinpocetine at the anticonvulsive dose prevented the hearing decline accompanying seizures. In other words, oppositely to the classical antiepileptic drugs carbamazepine, phenytoin and valproate, vinpocetine was able to improve hearing loss by itself and to prevent hearing loss accompanying seizures (Nekrassov & Sitges, 2006). Figure 13 adapted from data reported in : (a) Nekrassov & Sitges, 2004 and (b) Sitges & Nekrassov, 2004 shows that vinpocetine pre-administered at a dose of 2 mg/kg (i.p.) prevents the hearing loss induced by pentylenetetrazole and 4-aminopyridine at convulsive doses in the guinea pig *in vivo*. Hearing loss was assessed by recording the auditory threshold at 8 kHz before, 30 and 60 min after administration of the convulsive agents.

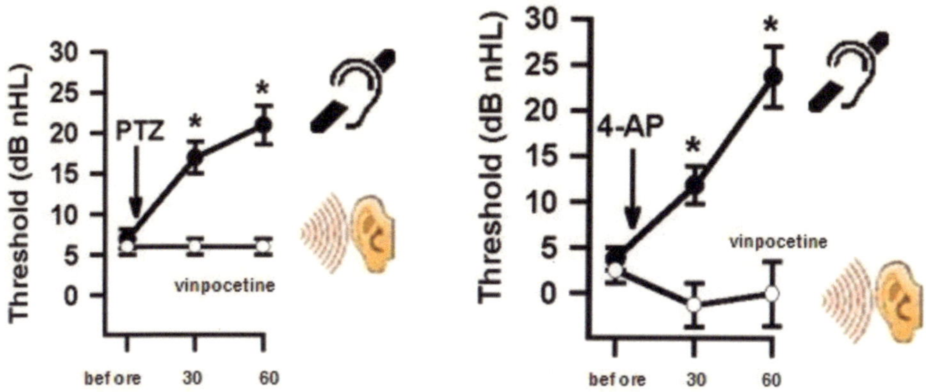

Fig. 13. Vinpocetine inhibits the rise in the auditory threshold induced by pentylenetetrazole (PTZ) and 4-aminopyridine (4-AP) at convulsive doses.

The high doses of antiepileptic drugs required to control seizures are frequently accompanied by adverse secondary effects. A great number of epileptic patients suffer from memory disturbances which are consequence of both, the disease (Prevey et al., 1998; Theodore et al., 1999; Meador, 2001; Elger et al., 2004) and the antiepileptic medication; as several studies show that antiepileptic drugs of either the "old and new generations" are also a causal factor (Vermeulen & Aldenkamp, 1995; Gates, 2000; Kwan & Brodie, 2001; Brunbech & Sabers, 2002; Schmidt, 2002). For instance, the classic antiepileptic drug carbamazepine deteriorates cognitive function particularly when administered at high doses or after a long term treatment (O´Dougherty et al., 1987; Gallassi et al., 1988; Forsythe et al., 1991; van der Meyden et al., 1992; Seidel & Mitchell, 1999). Fascinatingly previous studies in animals and humans show that vinpocetine is also a memory enhancer (Subhan & Hindmarch, 1985; Bhatti & Hindmarch, 1987; DeNoble, 1987: Lendvai et al., 2003).
The higher potency of vinpocetine not necessarily has to indicate a best side-effect profile than the conventional antiepileptic drugs. Nevertheless, vinpocetine has shown to be well tolerated and without contraindications (Hindmarch et al., 1991). Therefore, the higher

potency and efficacy of vinpocetine to reduce the permeability of presynaptic ionic channels controlling the release of the most important excitatory neurotransmitter in the brain must be advantageous in seizures control and epilepsy treatment. In line with this assumption it is worthy to mention that an unpublished investigation in course in epileptic children resistant to classic antiepileptic drugs the add-on-therapy of vinpocetine effectively controlled seizures at a dose more than tenfold lower than the dose of the classical antiepileptic drugs.

8. Conclusion

The findings summarized in the present chapter show that cerebral presynaptic ion channels, and particularly presynaptic Na^+ channels controlling glutamate release, are among the most important targets of various anticonvulsant drugs. Therefore, the pharmacological down-modulation of those channels in situations in which all neurons are firing is likely to be particularly beneficial in the control of epileptic seizures. In addition, since there is an uncovered medical need for the treatment of epilepsies and cerebral presynaptic channels are targets of the most effective antiepileptic drugs, the *in vitro* techniques presented in this chapter may represent powerful tools for the future screening and discover of anticonvulsive drugs controlling excitation by targeting brain presynaptic channels. The findings presented also show that the higher potency and efficacy of vinpocetine than the most effective antiepileptic drugs to inhibit presynaptic Na^+ and Ca^{2+} channels permeability is extensive to the control of seizures in experimental animal models of epilepsy. Current unpublished studies carried out in epileptic inpatients refractory to the classic antiepileptic drugs also show the high efficacy of this third generation antiepileptic drug in seizures control.

9. References

Adam-Vizi, V. (1992). External Ca(2+)-independent release of neurotransmitters, *Journal of Neurochemistry* 58 (2): 395-405.

Ambrosio, A.F., Silva, A.P., Araujo, I., Malva, J.O., Soares-da-Silva, P., Carvalho, A.P. & Carvalho, C.M. (2001). Inhibition of glutamate release by BIA 2-093 and BIA 2-024, two novel derivatives of carbamazepine, due to blockade of sodium but not calcium channels, *Biochemical Pharmacology* 61 (10): 1271-1275.

Armand, V., Hoffmann, P., Vergnes, M. & Heinemann, U. (1999). Epileptiform activity induced by 4-aminopyridine in entorhinal cortex hippocampal slices of rats with a genetically determined absence epilepsy (GAERS) 580, *Brain Research* 841(1-2): 62-69.

Bhatti, J.Z. & Hindmarch, I. (1987). Vinpocetine effects on cognitive impairments produced by flunitrazepam, *International Clinical Psychopharmacology* 2(4): 325-331.

Bonifacio, M.J., Sheridan, R.D., Parada, A., Cunha, R.A., Patmore, L. & Soares da Silva, P. (2001). Interaction of the novel anticonvulsant, BIA 2-093, with voltage-gated sodium channels: comparison with carbamazepine, *Epilepsia* 42(5): 600-608.

Brunbech, L. & Sabers, A. (2002). Effect of antiepileptic drugs on cognitive function in individuals with epilepsy: a comparative review of newer versus older agents, *Drugs* 62(4): 593-604.

Bukanova, J., Solntseva, E. & Skrebitsky, V. (2002). Selective suppression of the slow-inactivating potassium currents by nootropics in molluscan neurons, *International Journal of Neuropsychopharmacology* 5 (3): 229-237.

Carvalho, C.M., Ferreira, I.L., Duarte, C.V., Malva, J.O., Tretter, L., Adam-Vizi, V. & Carvalho, A.P. (1995). Relation of $[Ca^{2+}]_i$ to dopamine release in striatal synaptosomes: role of Ca2+ channels, *Brain Research* 669(2): 234-244.

Cheung, H., Kamp, D. & Harris, E. (1992). An in vitro investigation of the action of lamotrigine on neuronal voltage-activated sodium channels, *Epilepsy Research* 13(2): 107-112.

Deffois, A., Fage, D. & Carter, C. (1996). Inhibition of synaptosomal veratridine-induced sodium influx by antidepressants and neuroleptics used in chronic pain, *Neuroscience Letters* 220(2): 117-120.

DeNoble, V.J. (1987). Vinpocetine enhances retrieval of a step-through passive avoidance response in rats, *Pharmacology Biochem Behav* 26(1): 183-186.

Elger, C.E., Helmstaedter, C. & Kurthen, M. (2004). Chronic epilepsy and cognition, *Lancet Neurology* 3(11): 663-672.

Engel, D. & Jonas, P. (2005). Presynaptic action potential amplification by voltage-gated Na+ channels in hippocampal mossy fiber boutons, *Neuron* 45(3): 405-417.

Fohlmeister, J.F., Adelman, W. Jr. & Brennan, J.J. (1984). Excitable channel currents and gating times in the presence of anticonvulsants ethosuximide and valproate, *Journal of Pharmacology and Experimental Therapeutics* 230(1): 75-81.

Forsythe, I., Butler, R., Berg, I. & McGuire, R. (1991). Cognitive impairment in new cases of epilepsy randomly assigned to carbamazepine, phenytoin and sodium valproate, *Developmental Medicine and Child Neurology* 33(6): 524-534.

Galindo, C. & Sitges, M. (2004). Dihydropiridines mechanism of action in striatal isolated nerve endings. Comparison with -agatoxin IVA, *Neurochemical Research* 29 (4): 659-669.

Gallassi, R., Morreale, A., Lorusso, S., Procaccianti, G., Lugaresi, E. & Baruzzi, A. (1988). Carbamazepine and phenytoin. Comparison of cognitive effects in epileptic patients during monotherapy and withdrawal, *Archives of Neurology* 45(8): 892-894.

Galván, E. & Sitges, M. (2004). Characterization of the participation of sodium channels on the rise in Na+ induced by 4-aminopyridine (4-AP) in synaptosomes, *Neurochemical Research* 29(2): 347-355.

Gates, J.R. (2000). Side effect profiles and behavioral consequences of antiepileptic medications, *Epilepsy and Behavior* 1(3): 153-159.

Heemskerk, F.M., Schrama, L.H., Ghijsen, W.E., De Graan, P.N., Lopes da Silva, F.H. & Gispen, W.H. (1991). Presynaptic mechanism of action of 4-aminopyridine: changes in intracellular free Ca2+ concentration and its relationship to B-50 (GAP-43) phosphorylation, *Journal of Neurochemistry* 56(6): 1827-1835.

Hindmarch, I., Fuchs, H.H. & Erzigkeit, H. (1991). Efficacy and tolerance of vinpocetine in ambulant patients suffering from mild to moderate organic psychosyndromes, *International Clinical Psychopharmacology* 6(1): 31-43.

Huang, C.J., Harootunian, A., Maher, M.P., Quan, C., Raj, C.D., McCormack, K., Numann, R., Negulescu, P.A. & González, J.E. (2006). Characterization of voltage-gated sodium-channel blockers by electrical stimulation and fluorescence detection of membrane potential, *Nature Biotechnology* 24(4): 439-446.

Ives, A.E. & Jefferys, J.G. (1990). Synchronization of epileptiform bursts induced by 4-aminopyridine in the in vitro hippocampal slice preparation, *Neuroscience Letters* 112(2-3): 239-245.

Karoly, F., Lenkey, N., Juhasz, A.O., Vizi, E.S. & Mike, A. (2010). Fast- or slow-inactivated state preference of Na+ channel inhibitors: a simulation and experimental study, *PLoS Computational Biology* 6(6): e1000818.

Krueger, B.K., Blaustein, M.P. & Ratzlaff, R.W. (1980). Sodium channels in presynaptic nerve terminals, Regulation by neurotoxins, *Journal of General Physiology* 76(3): 287-313.

Kuzmiski, J.B., Barr, W., Zamponi, G.W. & MacVicar, B.A. (2005). Topiramate inhibits the initiation of plateau potentials in CA1 neurons by depressing R-type calcium channels, *Epilepsia* 46(4): 481-489.

Kwan, P. & Brodie, M.J. (2001). Neuropsychological effects of epilepsy and antiepileptic drugs, *Lancet* 357(9251): 216-222.

Lees, G. & Leach, M.J. (1993). Studies on the mechanism of action of the novel anticonvulsant lamotrigine (Lamictal) using primary neurological cultures from rat cortex, *Brain Research* 612(1-2): 190-199.

Lendvai, B., Zelles, T., Rozsa, B. & Vizi, E.S. (2003). A vinca alkaloid enhances morphological dynamics of dendritic spines of neocortical layer 2/3 pyramidal cells, *Brain Research Bulletin* 59(4): 257-260.

Lenkey, N., Karoly, R., Lukacs, P., Vizi, E.S., Sunesen, M., Fodor, L. & Mike, A. (2010). Classification of drugs based on properties of sodium channel inhibition: a comparative automated patch-clamp study, *PLoS One* 5(12): e15568.

Lingamaneni, R. & Hemmings, H.C.J. (2003). Differential interaction of anaesthetics and antiepileptic drugs with neuronal Na+ channels, Ca2+ channels, and GABA(A) receptors, *British Journal of Anaesthesiology* 90(2): 199-211.

Lipicky, R.J., Gilbert, D.L. & Stillman, I.M. (1972). Diphenylhydantoin inhibition of sodium conductance in squid giant axon, *Proceedings of the National Academy of Sciences* 69(7): 1758-1760.

Lipkind, G.M. & Fozzard, H.A. (2010). Molecular model of anticonvulsant drug binding to the voltage-gated sodium channel inner pore, *Molecular Pharmacology* 78(4): 631-638.

Loscher, W. (2002). Animal models of epilepsy for the development of antiepileptogenic and disease-modifying drugs. A comparison of the pharmacology of kindling and post-status epilepticus models of temporal lobe epilepsy, *Epilepsy Research* 50(1-2): 105-123.

McLean, M.J., Bukhari, A.A. & Wamil, A.W. (2000). Effects of topiramate on sodium-dependent action-potential firing by mouse spinal cord neurons in cell culture, *Epilepsia* 41(Suppl 1): S21-4

Meador, K.J. (2001). Can we treat cognitive deficits in patients with epilepsy?, *Epilepsy and Behavior* 2(4): 307-308.

Nekrassov, V. & Sitges, M. (2003). Effects of pentylenetetrazole and 4-aminopyridine on the auditory brainstem response (ABR) and on the hearing sensitivity in the guinea pig in vivo, *Epilepsy Research* 53(3): 245-254.

Nekrassov, V. & Sitges, M. (2004). Vinpocetine inhibits the epileptic cortical activity and auditory alterations induced by pentylenetetrazole in the guinea pig in vivo, *Epilepsy Research* 60(1): 63-71.

Nekrassov, V. & Sitges, M. (2006). Additive effects of antiepileptic drugs and pentylenetetrazole on hearing, *Neuroscience Letters* 406(3): 276-280.

Nekrassov, V. & Sitges, M. (2008). Comparison of acute, chronic and post-treatment effects of carbamazepine and vinpocetine on hearing loss and seizures induced by 4-aminopyridine, *Clinical Neurophysiology* 119(11): 2608-2614.

Nicholls, D.G. (1989). Release of glutamate, aspartate, and gamma-aminobutyric acid from isolated nerve terminals, *Journal of Neurochemistry* 52(2): 331-341.

O'Dougherty, M., Wright, F.S., Cox, S., & Walson, P. (1987). Carbamazepine plasma concentration. Relationship to cognitive impairment, *Archives of Neurology* 44(8): 863-867.

Perreault, P. & Avoli, M. (1991). Physiology and pharmacology of epileptiform activity induced by 4-aminopyridine in rat hippocampal slices, *Journal of Neurophysiology* 65(4): 771-785.

Prevey, M.L., Delaney, R.C., Cramer, J.A. & Mattson, R.H. (1998). Complex partial and secondarily generalized seizure patients: cognitive functioning prior to treatment with antiepileptic medication. VA Epilepsy Cooperative Study 264 Group, *Epilepsy Research* 30(1): 1-9.

Psarropoulou, C. & Avoli, M. (1996). Developmental features of 4-aminopyridine induced epileptogenesis, *Brain Research Development* 94(1): 52-59.

Santangeli, S., Sills, G.J., Thompson, G.G. & Brodie, M.J. (2002). Na^+ channel effects of remacemide and desglycinyl-remacemide in rat cortical synaptosomes, *European Journal of Pharmacology* 438(1-2): 63-68.

Schirrmacher, K., Mayer, A., Walden, J., Dusing, R. & Bingmann, D. (1993). Effects of carbamazepine on action potentials and calcium currents in rat spinal ganglion cells in vitro, *Neuropsychobiology* 27(3): 176-179.

Schmidt, D. (2002). The clinical impact of new antiepileptic drugs after a decade of use in epilepsy, *Epilepsy Research* 50(1-2): 21-32.

Seidel, W.T. & Mitchell, W.G. (1999). Cognitive and behavioral effects of carbamazepine in children: data from benign rolandic epilepsy, *Journal of Child Neurology* 14(11): 716-723.

Sitges, M. & Chiu, L.M. (1995a). w-Aga IVA selectively inhibits the calcium dependent fraction of the evoked release of [^{3}H]GABA from synaptosomes, *Neurochemical Research* 20(9): 1065-1071.

Sitges, M. & Chiu, L.M. (1995b). Characterization of the type of calcium channel primarily regulating GABA exocytosis from brain nerve endings, *Neurochemical Research* 20(9): 1073-1080.

Sitges, M. & Galindo, C.A. (2005). Omega-agatoxin-TK is a useful tool to study P-type Ca^{2+} channel-mediated changes in internal Ca^{2+} and glutamate release in depolarised brain nerve terminals, *Neurochemistry International* 46(1): 53-60.

Sitges, M. & Nekrassov, V. (1999). Vinpocetine selectively inhibits neurotransmitter release triggered by sodium channel activation, *Neurochemical Research* 24(12): 1585-1591.

Sitges, M. & Nekrassov, V. (2004). Vinpocetine prevents 4-aminopyridine-induced changes in the EEG, the auditory brainstem responses and hearing, *Clinical Neurophysiology* 115(12): 2711-2717.

Sitges, M. (1989). Effect of organic and inorganic calcium channel blockers on s-amino-n-butyric acid release induced by monensin and veratrine in the absence of external calcium, *Journal of Neurochemistry* 53(2): 436-441.

Sitges, M., Chiu, L.M. & Gonzalez, L. (1993). Vesicular and carrier-mediated depolarization-induced release of [3H]GABA: inhibition by amiloride and verapamil, *Neurochemical Research* 18(10): 1081-1087.

Sitges, M., Chiu L.M. & Nekrassov, V. (2006). Single and combined effects of carbamazepine and vinpocetine on depolarization-induced changes in Na(+), Ca(2+) and glutamate release in hippocampal isolated nerve endings, *Neurochemistry International* 49(1): 55-61.

Sitges, M., Chiu, L.M., Guarneros, A. & Nekrassov, V. (2007a). Effects of carbamazepine, phenytoin, lamotrigine, oxcarbazepine, topiramate and vinpocetine on Na+ channel-mediated release of [3H]glutamate in hippocampal nerve endings, *Neuropharmacology* 52(2): 598-605.

Sitges, M., Galvan, E. & Nekrassov, V. (2005). Vinpocetine blockade of sodium channels inhibits the rise in sodium and calcium induced by 4-aminopyridine in synaptosomes, *Neurochemistry International* 46(7): 533-540.

Sitges, M., Guarneros, A. & Nekrassov, V. (2007b). Effects of carbamazepine, phenytoin, valproic acid, oxcarbazepine, lamotrigine, topiramate and vinpocetine on the presynaptic Ca2+ channel-mediated release of [3H]glutamate: comparison with the Na+ channel-mediated release, *Neuropharmacology* 53(7): 854-862.

Sitges, M., Nekrassov, V. & Guarneros, A. (2000). Simultaneous action of MK-801 (dizclopine) on dopamine, glutamate, aspartate and GABA release from striatum isolated nerve endings, *Brain Research* 854(1-2): 48-56.

Sitges, M., Peña, F., Chiu, L.M. & Guarneros, A. (1998). Study on the possible involvement of protein kinases in the modulation of brain presynaptic sodium channels; comparison with calcium channels, *Neurochemistry International* 32(2): 177-190.

Sitges, M., Possani, L.D. & Bayon, A. (1986). Noxiustoxin, a short-chain toxin from the Mexican scorpion Centruroides noxius, induces transmitter release by blocking K+ permeability, *Journal of Neuroscience* 6(6): 1570-1574.

Sitges, M., Reyes, A. & Chiu, L.M. (1994). Dopamine transporter mediated release of dopamine: role of chloride, *Journal of Neuroscience Research* 39(1): 11-22.

Stefani, A., Spadoni, F. & Bernardi, G. (1997). Voltage-activated calcium channels: targets of antiepileptic drug therapy?, *Epilepsia* 38(9): 959-965.

Stefani, A., Spadoni, F., Siniscalchi, A. & Bernardi, G. (1996). Lamotrigine inhibits Ca2+ currents in cortical neurons: functional implications, *European Journal of Pharmacology* 307(1): 113-116.

Subhan, Z. & Hindmarch, I. (1985). Psychopharmacological effects of vinpocetine in normal healthy volunteers, *European Journal of Clinical Pharmacology* 28(5): 567-571.

Sun, L. & Lin, S.S. (2000). The anticonvulsant SGB-017 (ADCI) blocks voltage-gated sodium channels in rat and human neurons: comparison with carbamazepine, *Epilepsia* 41(3): 263-270.

Tapia, R., Sitges, M. & Morales, E. (1985). Mechanism of the calcium-dependent stimulation of transmitter release by 4-aminopyridine in synaptosomes, *Brain Research* 361(1-2): 373-382.

Taverna, S., Sancini, G., Mantegazza, M., Franceschetti, S. & Avanzini, G. (1999). Inhibition of transient and persistent Na+ current fractions by the new anticonvulsant topiramate, *Journal of Pharmacology and Experimental Therapeutics* 288(3): 960-968.

Theodore, W.H., Bhatia, S., Hatta, B.S., Fazilat, S., DeCarli, C., Bookheimer, S.Y. & Gaillard, W.D. (1999). Hippocampal atrophy, epilepsy duration and febrile seizures in patients with partial seizures, *Neurology* 52(1): 132-136.

Tibbs, G.R., Barrie, A.P., Van, Mieghem, F.J.E., McMahon, H.T. & Nicholls, D.G. (1989). Repetitive action potentials in isolated nerve terminals in the presence of 4-aminopyridine: Effects on cytosolic free Ca^{2+} and glutamate release, *Journal of Neurochemistry* 53(6): 1693-1699.

Timmermann, D.B., Lund, T.M., Belhage, B. & Schousboe, A. (2001). Localization and pharmacological characterization of voltage dependent calcium channels in cultured neocortical neurons, *International Journal of Developmental Neuroscience* 19(1): 1-10.

Trejo, F., Nekrassov, V., & Sitges, M. (2001). Characterization of vinpocetine effects on DA and DOPAC release in striatal isolated nerve endings, *Brain Research* 909(1-2): 59-67.

Tretter, L. & Adam-Vizi, V. (1998). The neuroprotective drug vinpocetine prevents veratridine-induced [Na+]i and [Ca2+]i rise in synaptosomes, *Neuroreport* 9(8): 1849-1853.

Turner, T.J., Adams, M.E. & Dunlap, K. (1992). Calcium channels coupled to glutamate release identified by w-Aga-IVA, *Science* 258(5080): 310-313.

van der Meyden, C.H., Bartel, P.R., Sommers, D.K., Blom, M., Becker, P., Erasmus, S. & Griesel, D. (1992). Effect of acute doses of controlled-release carbamazepine on clinical, psychomotor, electrophysiological, and cognitive parameters of brain function, *Epilepsia* 33(2): 335-342.

Vermeulen, J. & Aldenkamp, A.P. (1995). Cognitive side-effects of chronic antiepileptic drug treatment: a review of 25 years of research, *Epilepsy Research* 22(2): 65-95.

Wang, S.J., Huang, C.C., Hsu, K.S., Tsai, J.J. & Gean, P.W. (1996). Inhibition of N-type calcium currents by lamotrigine in rat amygdalar neurons, *Neuroreport* 7(18): 3037-3040.

Westenbroek, R.E., Sakurai, T., Elliott, E.M., Hell, J.W., Starr, T.V., Snutch, T.P. & Catterall, W.A. (1995). Immunochemical identification and subcellular distribution of the alpha 1A subunits of brain calcium channels, *Journal of Neuroscience* 15(10): 6403-6418.

Willow, M. & Catterall, W.A. (1982). Inhibition of binding of [3H]batrachotoxinin A 20-alpha-benzoate to sodium channels by the anticonvulsant drugs diphenylhydantoin and carbamazepine, *Molecular Pharmacology* 22(3): 627-635.

Xie, X., Dale, T.J., John, V.H., Cetr, H.L., Peakman, T.C. & Clare, J.J. (2001). Electrophysiological and pharmacological properties of the human brain type IIA Na+ channel expressed in a stable mammalian cell line, *Pflugers Archives* 441(4): 425-433.

Xie, X., Lancaster, B., Peakman, T. & Garthwaite, J. (1995). Interaction of the antiepileptic drug lamotrigine with recombinant rat brain type IIA Na+ channels and with native Na+ channels in rat hippocampal neurons, *Pflugers Archives* 430(3): 437-446.

Yamaguchi, S. & Rogawski, M.A. (1992). Effects of anticonvulsant drugs on 4-aminopyridine-induced seizures in mice, *Epilepsy Research* 11(1): 9-16.

Zona, C., Ciotti, M.T. & Avoli, M. (1997). Topiramate attenuates voltage-gated sodium currents in rat cerebellar granule cells, *Neuroscience Letters* 231(3): 123-126.

8

Therapeutic Drug Monitoring of Antiepileptic Medications

Matthew D. Krasowski
University of Iowa Hospitals and Clinics, United States

1. Introduction

Medications used to treat and prevent seizures (antiepileptic medications, AEMs) have been commonly managed by therapeutic drug monitoring (TDM) to optimize efficacy and avoid toxicity (Neels et al., 2004; Patsalos et al., 2008). TDM has been applied mostly to the first-generation AEMs that have been used clinically in the United States and Europe for several decades, namely carbamazepine, ethosuximide, phenobarbital, phenytoin, primidone, and valproic acid. First-generation AEMs generally have significant inter-individual variability in their pharmacokinetics (absorption, distribution, metabolism, and excretion) and low therapeutic indices. Two randomized, controlled studies of AEM TDM showed that practitioners often apply information from TDM incorrectly (Fröscher et al., 1981; Januzzi et al., 2000). Consequently, improved education of medical practitioners on TDM is important for the future.

In the last twenty-five years, 14 new AEMs have entered the market in the United States and/or Europe (LaRoche & Helmers, 2004a,b; Patsalos, 1999). These drugs are sometimes characterized as second- or third-generation AEMs and include the following drugs: eslicarbazepine acetate, felbamate, gabapentin, lacosamide, lamotrigine, levetiracetam, oxcarbazepine, pregabalin, rufinamide, stiripentol, tiagabine, topiramate, vigabatrin and zonisamide. Eslicarbazepine acetate, lacosamide, rufinamide, and stiripentol have not yet been approved in the United States. In contrast to the first-generation AEMs, the newer agents generally (although not always) have wider therapeutic ranges and less adverse effects. This chapter focuses on TDM of AEMs in treatment of epilepsy, emphasizing whether the pharmacokinetics and clinical profile of the drug make TDM useful. AEMs are sometimes used to treat disorders other than epilepsy such as trigeminal neuralgia, fibromyalgia, and migraine headaches (Johannessen Landmark, 2008; LaRoche & Helmers, 2004a).

There are several main challenges in TDM of AEMs (Patsalos et al., 2008). First, there are no simple diagnostic or laboratory tests for seizure disorders. The electroencephalogram (EEG) is useful for diagnosis of seizure disorders but is too labor-intensive for long-term patient observation. Second, seizures often occur unpredictably, sometimes with long periods of time between episodes. Lastly, the toxicity of AEMs can resemble neurologic disease, sometimes leading to inappropriate escalations of medication therapy even when the dose is actually too high.

One of the most basic assumptions of TDM is that the concentration of drug being measured correlates with the concentration at the target site of action (e.g., brain tissue). TDM of AEMs is usually performed on plasma or serum, or occasionally on some other body fluid such as saliva. TDM is difficult to apply when there are factors (e.g., irreversibility of action, drug tolerance) that lessen the correlation between clinical effect and serum/plasma concentration. AEMs with active metabolites also present a special challenge for TDM. For drugs with active metabolites (e.g., oxcarbazepine, primidone), TDM can include measurement of the concentrations of both parent drug and its metabolite(s) or just of the metabolite(s).

TDM of AEMs in saliva has not yet been widely applied (Liu & Delgado, 1999), but has been studied for ten drugs: carbamazepine (Ruiz et al., 2010; Tennison et al., 2004), gabapentin (Benetello et al., 1997; Berry et al., 2003), lamotrigine (Incecayir et al., 2007; Malone et al., 2006; Ryan et al., 2003), levetiracetam (Grim et al., 2003; Guo et al., 2007; Mecarelli et al., 2007), oxcarbazepine (Cardot et al., 1995), phenobarbital (Tennison et al., 2004), phenytoin (Tennison et al., 2004), topiramate (Miles et al., 2003), valproic acid (al Za'abi et al., 2003), and zonisamide (Kumagai et al., 1993). Of these ten drugs, gabapentin and valproic acid are clearly unsuited for salivary concentration analysis. Gabapentin shows low concentration in saliva versus plasma (salivary concentrations are only ~5-10% that of serum or plasma) and valproic acid has poor correlation between serum and salivary concentrations. Monitoring of salivary concentrations of AEMs has clear appeal in some patient populations, especially in the pediatric and geriatric populations. One study showed that salivary samples can be collected by the patient and mailed to a clinical laboratory without loss of sample integrity (Jones et al., 2005).

2. Application of TDM to AEMs

The most common reason to employ TDM for AEM therapy is that the drug shows unpredictable and/or variable pharmacokinetics, often related to differences in drug metabolism (Bialer, 2005; Perucca, 2006). Variability in pharmacokinetics may also occur due to alterations in drug absorption or distribution. Metabolism of AEMs may vary due to impaired organ function (typically kidney or liver), genetic factors, or drug-drug interactions. Many of the AEMs are metabolized by hepatic enzymes including cytochrome P450 (CYP) enzymes such as CYP3A4 and CYP2C9. A number of drugs are known to increase (induce) the expression of hepatic drug-metabolizing enzymes. Well-known inducers include carbamazepine, phenobarbital, phenytoin, rifampin (tuberculosis drug) and St. John's wort (herbal antidepressant) (Komoroski et al., 2004; Skolnick et al., 1976; Van Buren et al., 1984). In patients taking AEMs, the co-ingestion of liver enzyme inducers can lead to inappropriately low serum/plasma concentrations of the AEM if dose adjustments are not made. Some drugs may inhibit metabolism of AEMs, often by acting as antagonists of CYP enzyme activity, potentially leading to excessively high concentrations of drug unless the dose is reduced appropriately. Valproic acid inhibits multiple liver enzymes and has been well-documented to cause drug-drug interactions with other AEMs, which often requires careful TDM when valproic acid is used in multi-drug regimens to treat epilepsy (Neels et al., 2004). AEMs may be used in patients with some degree of renal impairment which can affect AEM pharmacokinetics by decreased clearance, or by removal of drug during dialysis procedures. In general, AEMs with low degrees of plasma protein binding are cleared more effectively by dialysis than AEMs that are highly protein bound (Lacerda et al., 2006).

Special considerations apply to TDM of AEMs that are highly (> 90%) bound to serum proteins. For these AEMs, monitoring of unbound (free) concentrations may be clinically useful (Dasgupta, 2007). Serum protein concentrations of drug can vary due to factors such as drug interactions, liver disease, pregnancy and old age. Co-administered medications (e.g., valproic acid) or endogenous substances can displace drugs from serum protein binding sites, increasing free drug concentrations. Uremia, typically secondary to renal failure, can also displace AEMs from serum protein binding sites. Free drug concentrations can be measured by preparing an ultrafiltrate of plasma (e.g., by centrifugation through a membrane) and then analyzing the concentration of drug. The main technical challenge is that free drug concentrations may be substantially lower than total drug concentrations in drugs that are highly bound to plasma proteins. Therefore, analytical methods to measure free drug concentrations need to have lower limits of quantitation than methods to measure total drug concentrations. Analytical methods used to measure total drug concentrations may have insufficient analytical sensitivity for free drug analysis (Dasgupta, 2007). A further practical challenge is that the ultrafiltration process needed for free drug analysis is not easily automated and adds processing time and effort to the clinical laboratory analysis.

The last common reason for TDM of AEMs is to assess compliance (adherence) to therapy such as in a patient who shows a lack of clinical response or the loss of efficacy in a therapy that was previously effective (Patsalos et al., 2008). Epilepsy therapy can occur over long periods of time even in the absence of seizures. Similar to other medications that may be taken chronically (e.g., anti-depressants, anti-hypertensives), patients may skip doses or stop taking the medication due to side effects, medication expense, or other factors.

3. Reference ranges for AEMs

Reference ranges for AEMs are challenging to establish. Ideally, TDM would guide physicians towards serum/plasma concentrations that optimally control seizures while avoiding or minimizing adverse effects. The 'reference range' of an AEM can be defined by a lower limit below which therapeutic effect is unlikely and an upper limit above which toxicity is likely (Patsalos et al., 2008). Reference ranges may vary with different types of seizures, or when AEMs are used for other purposes such as treatment of bipolar disorder or chronic pain. A special challenge occurs with defining reference ranges for the newer generation AEMs, which were generally studied in clinical trials as adjunctive therapy and not as monotherapy. Perucca has advocated the concept of 'individual therapeutic concentrations' (Perucca, 2000) wherein a patient is treated until good seizure control is achieved. The serum/plasma concentration at which good seizure control occurs serves as the patient's individual therapeutic concentration that can be used as the target concentration to maintain during chronic therapy. TDM for AEMs is especially important when there are factors that can alter AEM pharmacokinetics, e.g., pregnancy, impaired kidney or liver function, or concomitant therapy with hepatic enzyme-inducing or -inhibiting drugs.

With the background and theory on TDM above, each of the AEMs will be discussed in turn with regard to TDM. Table 1 summarizes the pharmacokinetic properties of the AEMs, while Table 2 presents a summary of the justifications of TDM for the AEMs. References for reference ranges used in Table 1 are as follows: carbamazepine, clonazepam, phenobarbital, phenytoin, primodone, valproic acid (Hardman et al., 1996), felbamate (Faught et al., 1993; Sachdeo et al., 1992), gabapentin (Lindberger et al., 2003), lacosamide (Kellinghaus, 2009), lamotrigine (Bartoli et al., 1997), levetiracetam (Leppik et al., 2002), oxcarbazepine (10-hydroxycarbazepine metabolite) (Friis et al., 1993), pregabalin (Patsalos et al., 2008), stiripentol (Farwell et al., 1993), tiagabine (Uthman et al., 1998), topiramate (Johannessen et al., 2003), vigabatrin (Patsalos, 1999), and zonisamide (Glauser & Pippenger, 2000; Mimaki, 1998).

4. TDM of the first generation AEMs

The first generation AEMs are commonly managed by TDM, in large part due to complex and variable pharmacokinetics. In general, the first generation agents have narrow therapeutic indices, with high plasma concentrations frequently associated with central nervous system (CNS) and other adverse effects. Several of the first generation AEMs, especially phenytoin, have high degrees of binding to plasma proteins; consequently, free drug concentrations in plasma can be clinically useful in some patients (Dasgupta, 2007). Three of the first generation AEMs (carbamazepine, phenobarbital, and phenytoin) are strong inducers of liver drug-metabolizing enzymes, particularly of CYP3A4. CYP3A4 has very wide substrate specificity including for cyclosporine, tacrolimus, and theophylline, as well as endogenous compounds such as estradiol and vitamin D (Luo et al., 2004). The accelerated metabolism of ethinyl estradiol that can occur during therapy with CYP3A4 inducers can lead to ineffectiveness of estrogen-containing oral contraceptives and unintended pregnancy (Crawford, 2002). Chronic therapy with carbamazepine, phenobarbital, and phenytoin is also well-known to have the potential risk of osteomalacia secondary to vitamin D deficiency (Zhou et al., 2006).

4.1 Carbamazepine

Carbamazepine has complicated pharmacokinetics that favors use of TDM (Neels et al., 2004; Warner et al., 1998). Carbamazepine is generally well-absorbed following oral administration; however, absorption may be delayed considerably by large doses. The metabolism of carbamazepine is quite complex, with the main metabolite being carbmazepine 10,11-epoxide, a compound that shows similar anticonvulsant activity to carbamazepine. In chronic therapy, concentrations of the epoxide metabolite may reach plasma concentrations 50% that of the parent drug. As described above, carbamazepine is a strong inducer of liver drug-metabolizing enzymes, including the CYP3A4 enzyme that metabolizes carbamazepine itself. Thus, carbamazepine represents an example of a drug that shows 'autoinduction', namely that the metabolism of carbamazepine increases as the drug is used chronically (Pitlick & Levy, 1977). Auto-induction is usually complete by 2-3 weeks, although it can take longer in some individuals.

Like other first generation AEMs, neurological side effects are common with high doses of carbamazepine, particularly when the plasma concentration exceeds 9 mg/L. Carbamazepine can also produce rare idiosyncratic adverse effects including severe dermatologic reactions such as Steven-Johnson Syndrome or toxic epidermal necrolysis. There is an association with severe skin reactions during carbamazepine therapy with the human leukocyte antigen (HLA) allele HLA-B*1502 which is common in patients with South Asian ancestry, particularly India (Alfirevic et al., 2006; Lonjou et al., 2006). Pharmacogenetic testing for this allele may be useful in patients of South Asian descent who are being considered for therapy with carbamazepine.

Drug	Oral bioavailability	Serum protein binding	Time to peak conc. (hrs)	Serum half-life (hrs)	Reference range in serum (mg/L)
Carbamazepine	>70	75	4-8	10-20	4-10
Clonazepam	>95	85	1-2	20-26	0.005-0.07
Eslicarbazepine acetate	≥80	30	1-4	20-24	Not established
Ethosuximide	>90	0	2-4	30-50	40-100
Felbamate	>90	25	2-6	16-22[a]	30-60
Gabapentin	<60	0	2-3	5-9	2-20
Lacosamide	≥95	15	0.5-4	12-13	5-10
Lamotrigine	≥95	55	1-3	15-35[a, b]	3-14
Levetiracetam	≥95	0	1	6-8	12-46
Oxcarbazepine	90	40	3-6	8-15[a]	3-35
Phenobarbital	>95	50	4-12	90-110	10-25
Phenytoin	90	>95	4-12	6-24	10-20
Primidone	>90	20	2-4	10-20	8-12
Pregabalin	≥90	0	1-2	5-7	2.8-8.3
Rufinamide	85	30	5-6	8-12[a]	Not established
Stiripentol	≥90	99	1-2	Variable	4-22
Tiagabine	≥90	96	1-2	5-9[a]	0.02-0.2
Topiramate	≥80	15	2-4	20-30	5-20
Valproic acid	>95	>90	1-4	11-17	30-100
Vigabatrin	≥60	0	1-2	5-8	0.8-36
Zonisamide	≥65	50	2-5	50-70[a]	10-40

[a] Serum half-life significant decreased with concomitant therapy with liver enzyme inducers (rifampin, carbamazepine, phenobarbital, phenytoin, St. John's wort)
[b] Serum half-life significantly increased with concomitant therapy with valproic acid.

Table 1. Pharmacokinetic Parameters and Reference Ranges for the AEMs

TDM is frequently used in carbamazepine therapy due to the challenging pharmacokinetics. Monitoring of carbamazepine is usually achieved by a variety of marketed immunoassays that have high specificity for the parent drug and limited cross-reactivity with the metabolites (Warner et al., 1998). TDM sometimes also includes monitoring of the epoxide metabolite, which can contribute a substantial amount of the therapeutic effect. One challenge of monitoring the epoxide metabolite is that commercial immunoassays specific for this metabolite are not available, and thus a technology such as high-performance liquid chromatography (HPLC) is generally needed, which usually means the analysis is performed at reference laboratories.

4.2 Clonazepam

Clonazepam is a benzodiazepine used in treatment of epilepsy, as well as in a variety of other conditions such as anxiety or panic disorders, restless legs syndrome, and mania (Riss et al., 2008). Other benzodiazepines such as diazepam and lorazepam are used commonly for acute management of seizures but not as often for long-term management. In general, benzodiazepines are limited by tolerance during chronic therapy. Clonazepam is extensively metabolized, with less than 1% of the administered dose recovered as parent drug. The main metabolite is 7-aminoclonazepam, which is therapeutically inactive.

TDM has a relatively limited role in clonazepam therapy (Warner et al., 1998). Plasma concentrations do not correlate all that tightly with therapeutic effect, with a wide range of concentations (5 to 70 ng/mL) associated with effective management of seizures. Higher plasma concentrations are associated with increased frequency of CNS side effects such as drowsiness or lethargy. Other than to establish an individual therapeutic concentration or to assess compliance with therapy or evaluate possible toxic effects, monitoring of clonazepam is generally of limited value.

4.3 Ethosuximide

Ethosuximide has excellent bioavailability and is not bound to any appreciable degree to plasma proteins (Brodie & Dichter, 1997; Perucca, 1996). Approximately 25% of the ingested drug is excreted unchanged. The remainder of the excretion is mostly to a hydroxyethyl metabolite, which is inactive with respect to anticonvulsant effect. Ethosuximide has a fairly wide therapeutic range with effective antiseizure activity commonly occurring with plasma concentrations of 40-100 mg/L. CNS and gastrointestinal side effects are more common with plasma concentrations exceeding 100 mg/L. TDM is commonly applied to ethosuximide therapy, although not as commonly as first generation AEMs such as carbamazepine, phenobarbital, and phenytoin that have more challenging pharmacokinetics (Warner et al., 1998).

4.4 Phenobarbital and primidone

Phenobarbital and primidone are structurally related compounds used in the management of epilepsy (Brodie & Dichter, 1997; Perucca, 1996). Primidone is converted to phenobarbital and phenylethylmalonamide (PEMA) by metabolism, with both metabolites contributing significant anticonvulsant activity. Phenobarbital and primidone show excellent absorption following oral dosing, although absorption of phenobarbital can be slow, especially with high doses. One of the striking pharmacokinetic features of phenobarbital is a long half-life, up to 100 hrs or more in adults and somewhat shorter (~80 hrs) in neonates.

TDM is commonly use for both phenobarbital and primidone (Warner et al., 1998). Plasma concentrations of 10-35 mg/L are generally recommended for phenobarbital management of seizures. Above 35 mg/L, CNS-related adverse effects are more frequent. TDM of primidone is complicated to interpret due to the formation of two active metabolites (phenobarbital and PEMA). Monitoring of primidone therapy often involves measurement of both primidone and phenobarbital plasma concentrations, both of which can be done with commercial immunoassays.

4.5 Phenytoin

Phenytoin is likely the AEM for which TDM is applied most frequently (Warner et al., 1998). Phenytoin has very challenging pharmacokinetic properties. While absorption of the drug following ingestion is high, time to peak concentrations are variable (3-12 hrs) depending on dosage and intake relative to meals. Phenytoin is extensively bound to plasma proteins, and clinically significant increased free fractions are observed in neonates, patients with hypoalbuminemia, and in patients with uremia due to renal failure (Dasgupta, 2007). Phenytoin has complex metabolism, with saturation of hepatic enzymes at therapeutic plasma concentrations, leading to zero-order (saturation) elimination kinetics. Two of the enzymes that catalyze the metabolism of phenytoin, CYP2C9 and CYP2C19, show pharmacogenetic variation, with individuals with lower catalytic acvitity (poor metabolizers) at risk for developing supra-therapeutic concentrations (Ninomiya et al., 2000). Phenytoin's unusual pharmacokinetic profile makes maintaining patients at therapeutic plasma concentrations a tricky and time-consuming goal that depends on recurrent TDM. Unfortunately, TDM cannot currently predict some of the annoying and occasionally serious adverse effects of phenytoin such as dermatologic reactions, hirsutism, and gingival overgrowth (Perucca, 1996). The latter two reactions occur unpredictably with chronic phenytoin therapy.

4.6 Valproic acid

Valproic acid has overall excellent bioavailability, although absorption can be delayed considerably with higher doses or when the drug is ingested with meals (Brodie & Dichter, 1997; Perucca, 1996). Valproic acid is approximately 90% bound to plasma proteins. Although measurement of free valproic acid concentrations in plasma is usually not needed for TDM, patients with hypoalbuminemia are at higher risk of having supra-therapeutic free concentrations. Valproic acid is extensively metabolized, with some of the metabolites having some anticonvulsant activity. Valproic acid is an inhibitor of multiple CYP enzymes and as such can cause drug-drug interactions, including with other AEMs such as carbamazepine, felbamate, lamotrigine, phenobarbital, phenytoin, and stiripentol (Besag & Berry, 2006). Valproic acid can cause hepatitis (with elevations of enzymes such as alanine aminotransferase), in some cases manifesting as fulminant liver failure. Consequently, many physicians periodically monitor hepatic enzymes and also instruct patients to seek medical attention with any signs or symptoms of liver damage such as abdominal pain or jaundice.

Valproic acid has a therapeutic range of 30-100 mg/L. CNS side effects are more common when plasma concentrations exceed 100 mg/L although some patients may have plasma concentrations of 150 mg/L or higher without adverse effects. Given the wide range of plasma concentrations associated with successful therapy, TDM can be especially valuable in valproic acid therapy in establishing an individual therapeutic concentration (Warner et al., 1998).

5. TDM of the new generation AEMs

5.1 Eslicarbazepine

Eslicarbazepine acetate [(S)-licarbazepine acetate] is a pro-drug that is rapidly and nearly completely metabolized to eslicarbazepine by liver esterases (Falcao et al., 2007; Maia et al., 2005). TDM focuses on eslicarbazepine and not on the minor metabolites oxcarbazepine (also used as an AEM) and (R)-licarbazepine. Unlike carbamazepine, eslicarbazepine does not exhibit auto-induction in metabolism, has low (~30%) binding to serum proteins, and overall has a low potential for drug-drug interactions (Almeida et al., 2010; Bialer et al., 2009). Eslicarbazepine has an elimination half-life of 20-24 hr during chronic administration

(Almeida et al., 2005). Mild to moderation hepatic failure has minimal impact on the pharmacokinetics of eslicarbazepine (Almeida et al., 2008). The main route of elimination of eslicarbazepine and other minor metabolites of eslicarbazepine acetate is via the kidneys, with moderate or severe renal failure significantly reducing the clearance of eslicarbazepine. Hemodialysis effectively removes eslicarbazepine and other metabolites of eslicarbazepine acetate (Maia et al., 2008).

Overall, TDM has a minor role in the therapeutic use of eslicarbazepine given the relatively predictable pharmacokinetics of the drug. TDM for eslicarbazepine may be useful in patients with renal failure. An enantioselective high-performance liquid chromatography-ultraviolet (HPLC-UV) method has been developed for the specific monitoring of eslicarbazepine and its metabolites (Alves et al., 2007).

5.2 Felbamate

Felbamate is approved in the United States for the treatment of partial seizures in adults and for Lennox-Gastaut Syndrome, a type of childhood epilepsy that is often refractory to AEM therapy (Bourgeois, 1997; Pellock et al., 2006). The use of felbamate has been limited due to the risks of aplastic anemia and severe liver failure, which led to revised labeling and restricted use of felbamate (Pellock et al., 2006). It is suspected that one or more metabolites of felbamate mediate the rare but serious adverse effects (Shumaker et al., 1990). Approximately 50% of the parent drug is metabolized by the liver to inactive metabolites (Shumaker et al., 1990; Thompson et al., 1999). Inducers of hepatic metabolism increase the metabolism of felbamate (Sachdeo et al., 1993; Wagner et al., 1991), while valproic acid inhibits the metabolism (Ward et al., 1991).

A clear reference range has not been established for felbamate, but seizure control usually occurs with serum/plasma concentrations of 30-60 mg/L (Faught et al., 1993; Sachdeo et al., 1992). Children clear felbamate approximately 20-65% faster than adults (Perucca, 2006). TDM may be helpful in felbamate therapy given the variable metabolism across individuals. Close monitoring of liver function and blood counts are advised during felbamate therapy, with the goal to discontinue therapy if any signs of bone marrow or liver damage appear.

5.3 Gabapentin

Gabapentin was originally approved in the United States for the treatment in epilepsy but is currently used more often for the management of chronic pain (LaRoche & Helmers, 2004b; McLean, 1995). Gabapentin is rapidly absorbed by the *L*-amino acid transport system (Vollmer et al., 1988), and a study published in 1998 showed possible saturability of this system, with a decrease in bioavailability at doses of 4,800 mg/day of gabapentin as compared to lower doses (Gidal et al., 1998). However, a later study showed linear absorption up to 4,800 mg/day (Berry et al., 2003). Gabapentin does not distribute much into saliva, precluding the utility of salivary gabapentin concentrations for TDM (Berry et al., 2003). Gabapentin is not metabolized to any appreciable degree and has low binding to serum proteins (Vollmer et al., 1988). The bulk of excretion is via the kidneys, with the half-life increasing in patients with renal failure. Hemodialysis effectively clears gabapentin (Hung et al., 2008; Wong et al., 1995).

Gabapentin does not have a clear reference range (Armijo et al., 2004), although effective control of seizures generally requires concentrations of 2 mg/L or higher (Sivenius et al.,

1991). An approximate reference range of 2-20 mg/L for management of seizure disorders has been proposed (Lindberger et al., 2003). TDM is not usually necessary for gabapentin therapy other than to adjust dosing in patients with impaired kidney function or to assess adherance to therapy (Patsalos et al., 2008)

5.4 Lacosamide

Lacosamide is a novel functionalized amino acid that enhances inactivation of voltage-gated sodium channels (Curia et al., 2009; Perucca et al., 2008b). Lacosamide was approved in Europe in 2008 for partial-onset seizures in patients 16 years and older (Chung et al., 2010). Lacosamide has high bioavailability (~100%) and serum protein binding (Ben-Menachem et al., 2007; Luszczki, 2009). Approximately 60% of the parent drug is metabolized, mainly by CYP2C19 to an inactive metabolite. The remaining 40% is excreted unchanged by the kidneys. The low plasma protein binding of lacosamide suggests that the drug should be cleared effectively by dialysis, although data on this has not yet been published (Lacerda et al., 2006). The half-life of lacosamide is approximately 12 hours. Drug-drug interactions involving lacosamide appear to be uncommon (Beydoun et al., 2009; Johannessen Landmark & Patsalos, 2010). The predictable pharmacokinetics of lacosamide, along with lack of clinically significant drug-drug interactions, suggests a limited role for TDM in managing lacosamide pharmacotherapy. Consequently, TDM of lacosamide has limited benefit except in patients with severe liver and/or kidney failure, or to assess compliance with therapy (Cross & Curran, 2009; Thomas et al., 2006).

5.5 Lamotrigine

Lamotrigine has been approved by the United States Food and Drug Administration (FDA) for treatment of partial seizures and bipolar disorder (Neels et al., 2004; Patsalos et al., 2008). The major adverse effect of lamotrigine is dermatologic reaction, including severe Stevens-Johnson and toxic epidermal necrolysis syndromes (Knowles et al., 1999). Harm from skin reactions have been reduced by the clinical practice of cautiously escalating dose and promptly ceasing therapy if potential skin reactions appear. One of the major advantages of lamotrigine is a solid safety record in pregnancy, which contrasts with the teratogenic effects of first-generation AEMs such as carbamazepine, phenytoin, and valproic acid (Sabers & Tomson, 2009; Tomson & Battino, 2007).

Lamotrigine is quickly and completely absorbed from the gastrointestinal tract and is only ~50% bound to serum proteins. Lamotrigine distributes into saliva, and salivary lamotrigine concentrations correlate well with those in serum, allowing for saliva to serve as an alternative sample for TDM (Ryan et al., 2003; Tsiropoulos et al., 2000). Lamotrigine is extensively metabolized, principally by glucuronidation to form an inactive metabolite (Hussein & Posner, 1997; Rambeck & Wolf, 1993). Similar to carbamazepine, lamotrigine shows the phenomenon of autoinduction during chronic therapy. Autoinduction is usually complete within two weeks, with a ~20% reduction in steady-state serum/plasma concentrations if the dose is not increased (Hussein & Posner, 1997). Classic liver enzyme inducers significantly increase the metabolism of lamotrigine, reducing the serum half-life from 15-35 hr to approximatley 8-20 hr (Hussein & Posner, 1997; Rambeck & Wolf, 1993). Ethinyl estradiol-containing oral contraceptives also significantly increase the clearance of lamotrigine (Reimers et al., 2007; Sabers et al., 2001; Sabers et al., 2003). Valproic acid inhibits the metabolism of lamotrigine and can increase the serum half-life to up to 60 hr (Biton,

2006; Ramsay et al., 1991). Severe renal failure increases the serum half-life to ~50 hr in patients. Hemodialysis effectively clears lamotrigine (Fillastre et al., 1993). The clearance of lamotrigine is higher in children (Bartoli et al., 1997; Perucca, 2006) and much higher (~300%) in pregnancy (Perucca, 2006). A reference range of 3-14 mg/L has been advocated for refractory epilepsy therapy (Morris et al., 1998). The risk of toxicity increases significantly when serum/plasma concentrations exceed 15 mg/L (Besag et al., 1998; Morris et al., 1998).

TDM of lamotrigine is useful for several main reasons. First, the drug shows significant interindividual variation in liver metabolism, which can be affected by concomitant medications. Second, the clearance of lamotrigine varies across development and particularly increases during pregnancy (Pennell et al., 2008). Lastly, there is a fairly clear concentration (> 15 mg/L) above which adverse effects become more frequent (Bartoli et al., 1997; Biton, 2006; Rambeck & Wolf, 1993).

5.6 Levetiracetam

Levetiracetam is a novel anticonvulsant structurally unrelated to other AEMs (Klitgaard, 2001; Leppik, 2001). Following oral administration, levetiracetam is rapidly and nearly completely absorbed, with the rate of oral absorption slowed by co-ingestion with food (Fay et al., 2005; Patsalos, 2000). Levetiracetam distribute extensively into saliva, with salivary concentrations usually being slightly higher than serum concentrations in patients receiving chronic therapy (Lins et al., 2007). Salivary and serum levetiracetam concentrations correlate well with one another, making saliva an alternative sample to perform TDM (Grim et al., 2003; Mecarelli et al., 2007).

Levetiracetam shows low binding to serum proteins and has linear pharmacokinetics. Nearly 100% of the absorbed drug is ultimately excreted by the kidneys (Patsalos, 2004), with approximately two-thirds as the parent drug and one-thirds as a metabolite that is formed by hydrolysis in the blood (Patsalos et al., 2006). There is very little, if any, metabolism of levetiracetam by the liver and, consequently low probability of significant drug-drug interactions (Johannessen Landmark and Patsalos, 2010). Given the low plasma protein binding, levetiracetam is likely efficiently cleared by hemodialysis (Lacerda et al., 2006). The serum half-life of levetiracetam is shorter in adult (6-8 hr) compared to neonates (16-18 hr) (Patsalos et al., 2008). Clearance of levetiracetam increases significantly in pregnancy, with an approximately 60% decrease in serum concentrations (Tomson and Battino, 2007).

A reference range of 12-46 mg/L has been proposed based on a study of 470 patients in a specialty epilepsy clinic (Leppik et al., 2002). Other than to assess compliance or investigate potential toxicity, the main value of TDM for levetiracetam is in adjusting dosage for renal insufficiency (Patsalos, 2000, 2004; Patsalos et al., 2008; Radtke, 2001). In collecting samples for drug monitoring, serum or plasma should be separated from whole blood rapidly, as *in vitro* hydrolysis of levetiracetam can occur in the blood tube and thus lead to artifactually low concentrations (Patsalos et al., 2006).

5.7 Oxcarbazepine

Oxcarbazepine has a chemical structure related to carbamazepine but causes less induction of liver enzymes. Oxcarbazepine is rapidly and completely absorbed and metabolized to its monohydroxy derivative 10-hydroxycarbazepine (Larkin et al., 1991; Lloyd et al., 1994; May et al., 2003). 10-Hydroxycarbazepine is further metabolized, primarily by glucuronidation. The clearance of 10-hydroxycarbazepine is reduced in renal insufficiency (Rouan et al., 1994) and in the elderly (Perucca, 2006). The clearance of 10-hydroxycarbazepine is increased in pregnancy (Christensen et al., 2006; Mazzucchelli et al., 2006) and in patients taking liver enzyme-inducing drugs (May et al., 2003). Children require higher doses of oxcarbazepine per body weight than adults (Battino et al., 1995). 10-Hydroxycarbazepine and oxcarbazepine have similar potencies for anticonvulsant activity; however, 10-hydroxycarbazepine generally accumulates to higher concentrations in serum and thus accounts for the majority of the antiseizure activity (Lloyd et al., 1994).

Consequently, TDM for oxcarbazepine generally focuses on measurement of serum/plasma concentrations of the monohydroxy metabolite (Patsalos et al., 2008). Although 10-hydroxycarbazepine distributes into saliva, there are dose-dependent variations in the correlation between 10-hydroxycarbazepine saliva and serum concentrations that limit the utility of saliva as an alternative specimen for TDM of oxcarbazepine (Cardot et al., 1995; Kristensen et al., 1983; Miles et al., 2004). In clinical research studies, a wide range of 10-hydroxycarbazepine serum concentrations (3-35 mg/L) were observed to be clinically effective in seizure treatment (Friis et al., 1993), with toxic side effects being more common at serum/plasma concentrations of 35 mg/L or higher (Striano et al., 2006). TDM for oxcarbazepine is justified when changes are expected that might alter 10-hydroxycarbazepine clearance including pregnancy, concomitant use of liver enzyme-inducing drugs, or renal insufficiency.

5.8 Pregabalin

Pregabalin was originally designed to be a more potent analog of gabapentin (Selak, 2001) and shares many clinical similarities to gabapentin, including widespread use to manage conditions other than epilepsy such as neuropathic pain and fibromyalgia (Acharya et al., 2005; LaRoche & Helmers, 2004a). Pregabalin has very advantageous pharmacokinetics including high bioavailability, low binding to plasma proteins, minimal metabolism, and no significant drug-drug interactions (Busch et al., 1998). The majority of the absorbed dose (~98%) is excreted unchanged in the urine. Clearance of pregabalin approximates glomerular filtration rate (Corrigan et al., 2001), and dosing of pregabalin may need adjustment in patients with impaired renal function (Randinitis et al., 2003). Pregabalin is effectively cleared by hemodialysis (Yoo et al., 2009). An approximate reference range of 2.8-8.3 mg/L has been proposed for the use of pregabalin in managing seizures (Patsalos et al., 2008). The favorable pharmacokinetics of pregabalin generally obviates the need for TDM, other than to adjust dosing during renal failure or to assess compliance. If monitoring is performed, the short half-life of pregabalin (4.6-5.8 hr) (Bockbrader et al., 2000) necessitates that care must be taken in the timing of blood draws for TDM.

5.9 Rufinamide

Rufinamide is a novel anticonvulsant approved for use in Europe in January 2007 and in the United States in December 2008 for Lennox-Gastaut syndrome (Hakimian et al., 2007; Heaney & Walker, 2007; Wheless & Vazquez, 2010; Wisniewski, 2010). Rufinamide is well-absorbed (80-90%) following oral administration (Perucca et al., 2008a). The peak exposure to rufinamide may increase significantly when taken with food as compared to an empty stomach. Consequently, patients are often counseled to take rufinamide in the same temporal relation to meals. Rufinamide is extensively metabolized, primarily by carboxyesterases, with only trace amounts of the parent drug excreted in feces or urine. The primary metabolite is inactive and mainly excreted by the kidneys.

Hepatic enzyme inducers such as carbamazepine and rifampin increase the excretion of rufinamide (Perucca et al., 2008a). Impaired renal function has minimal effect on clearance of rufinamde; however, increased doses of rufinamide are often needed in patients receiving hemodialysis due to removal of the drug by the dialysis procedure. Although reference ranges for rufinamide have not been well-defined yet, serum/plasma concentrations generally correlate with seizure control, allowing for determination of an individual therapeutic concentration that can be monitored over the course of chronic therapy (Luszczki, 2009; Perucca et al., 2008a; Wheless & Vazquez, 2010) TDM for rufinamide can be especially helpful in patients receiving hemodialysis or who are also taking liver enzyme inducers.

5.10 Stiripentol

Stiripentol is an AEM that was originally approved in Europe in 2001 but is currently infrequently used. Stiripentol is rapidly absorbed following oral administration but has overall low bioavailability, in large part due to extensive first-pass metabolism by the liver. The hepatic metabolism of stiripentol is very complex, with at least 5 different metabolic pathways generating over a dozen metabolites. The dosing of stiripentol is further complicated by zero-order (saturation) elimination kinetics, with a marked decrease in clearance with increased dosage (Levy et al., 1983). Stiripentol is also highly (>99%) protein bound and prone to drug interactions that can alter the free fraction (Lacerda et al., 2006). A well-defined reference range for stiripentol has not been established, although one study showed that serum concentrations of 4-22 mg/L correlate with control of absence seizures in children (Farwell et al., 1993).

The complex pharmacokinetics of stiripentol (extensive hepatic metabolism, high binding to plasma protein, and saturation kinetics) resemble that of phenytoin (Luszczki, 2009). Measurement of the free drug fraction of stiripentol may be clinically useful; however, methods to measure free fractions have not yet been reported. When used in combination AEM therapies, stiripentol may cause drug-drug interactions by inhibiting the metabolism of carbamazepine, clobazam, phenobarbital, phenytoin, and valproic (Levy et al., 1984; Tran et al., 1997; Tran et al., 1996).

5.11 Tiagabine

Tiagabine is currently approved in the United States and Europe but is used infrequently due to a propensity to cause non-convulsive status epilepticus (Eckardt & Steinhoff, 1998; Kellinghaus et al., 2002; Schapel & Chadwick, 1996). Tiagabine is rapidly absorbed with high bioavailability but, unlike many of the other newer AEMs, is highly bound to proteins (> 96%) (Gustavson & Mengel, 1995). Co-therapy with valproic acid can increase the free concentrations of tiagabine by displacing tiagabine from serum protein binding sites (Patsalos et al., 2002). The hepatic metabolism of tiagabine is complex and extensive with less than 1% of the absorbed parent drug excreted unchanged (Gustavson & Mengel, 1995). The metabolism of tiagabine can be altered by concomitant therapy with liver enzyme inhibitors or inducers. The serum half-life is typically 5-9 hr for patients on tiagabine monotherapy. The half-life is reduced to 2-4 hr in patients receiving enzyme inducers (So et al., 1995). The serum half-life increases to 12-16 h in severe liver failure (Lau et al., 1997). Children have higher clearance than adults (Gustavson et al., 1997). Renal dysfunction does not significantly impact the pharmacokinetics of tiagabine (Cato et al., 1998).

The inter-individual variation in hepatic metabolism makes tiagabine a candidate for TDM. Further, the extensive binding of tiagabine to plasma proteins further suggests that measurement of free drug concentrations may be clinically useful (Dasgupta, 2007). However, a clear relationship between tiagabine serum/plasma concentration and therapeutic efficacy has not yet been established, with a broad reference range of 20-200 ng/mL proposed (Patsalos et al., 2008; Uthman et al., 1998). For measurement of free drug concentrations, analytical sensitivity is an issue, with some assays having insufficiently low limits of sensitivity to measure clinically relevant free drug concentrations (Williams et al., 2003). Consequently, such analysis is only performed at specialized reference laboratories.

5.12 Topiramate

Topiramate has approval for treatment of epilepsy of children and adults, and also for the treatment of migraine headaches (LaRoche & Helmers, 2004a). Topiramate has high bioavailability (~80%) and low binding to serum proteins (Easterling et al., 1988). Salivary topiramate concentrations correlate well with those in serum (with salivary concentrations being roughly 0.9 that in serum), which makes saliva an alternative specimen type for TDM (Jones et al., 2005; Miles et al., 2003). Approximately 50% of the absorbed dose is metabolized by the liver. Hepatic enzyme inducers can decrease the serum half-life of topiramate from 20-30 hr to approximately 12 hr (Britzi et al., 2005; Sachdeo et al., 1996). Children generally eliminate topiramate faster than adults (Perucca, 2006; Rosenfeld et al., 1999). A reference range of 5-20 mg/L has been proposed for topiramate for epilepsy therapy (Johannessen et al., 2003). TDM of topiramate is most useful due to variability in metabolism.

5.13 Vigabatrin

Vigabatrin is an irreversible inhibitor of GABA transaminase, an enzyme that catalyzes the elimination of GABA (Rey et al., 1992; Schechter, 1989). Vigabatrin has high bioavailability (60-80%), low binding to serum proteins and is primarily excreted unchanged in the urine (Durham et al., 1993; Rey et al., 1992). Dose reductions of vigabatrin are generally needed in patients with renal failure (Rey et al., 1992). Clearance of vigabatrin increased during hemodialysis (Jacqz-Aigrain et al., 1997). The irreversible action of vigabatrin on its molecular target is likely the reason a wide range of serum/plasma concentrations (0.8-36 mg/L) of vigabatrin are associated with successful treatment with with vigabatrin. Other than to assess compliance or possible drug overdose, there is little value in monitoring vigabatrin plasma/serum concentrations (Patsalos, 1999).

Drug	Need for TDM	Factors Favoring TDM	Limitations of TDM
Carbamazepine	Frequent	Auto-induction of metabolism; drug-drug interactions; high serum protein binding	Free drug concentrations needed for some patients
Clonazepam	Uncommon	Distinguish tolerance from inadequate dosing	Wide reference range; low toxicity incidence
Eslicarbazepine acetate	Intermediate	Decreased clearance with chronic dosing and liver failure	Generally predictable pharmacokinetics
Ethosuximide	Intermediate	Complex metabolism	Wide reference range, variable toxicity range
Felbamate	Intermediate	Variable metabolism, potential for severe toxicity	Uncertain reference range
Gabapentin	Uncommon	Decreased clearance with renal failure	Wide reference range; low toxicity incidence
Lacosamide	Uncommon		Predictable dosing
Lamotrigine	Frequent	Variable metabolism; significant drug-drug interactions	
Levetiracetam	Intermediate	Decreased clearance with renal failure	Wide reference range, low toxicity incidence
Oxcarbazepine	Intermediate to Frequent	Variable metabolism, well-defined toxic range	
Phenobarbital	Frequent	Drug-drug interactions, long half-life	Tolerance to drug can complicate TDM
Phenytoin	Frequent	Variable absorption; high serum protein binding; drug-drug interactions; zero-order kinetics	Free drug concentrations needed in some populations
Primidone	Intermediate	Long half-life of metabolites, potential for toxicity	Need to monitor phenobarbital as well
Pregabalin	Uncommon	Decreased clearance with renal failure	Wide reference range, low toxicity incidence
Rufinamide	Intermediate to Frequent	Variable absorption; drug-drug interactions; decreased clearance with renal failure	Uncertain reference range
Stiripentol	Frequent	Extensive first-pass metabolism, high serum protein binding, zero-order kinetics	
Tiagabine	Intermediate	High serum protein binding	Uncertain reference range
Topiramate	Intermediate	Variable metabolism	
Valproic acid	Frequent	Well-established therapeutic range	Limited correlation of plasma concentration and efficacy
Vigabatrin	Uncommon		Irreversible action
Zonisamide	Frequent	Variable metabolism, well-define toxic range	

Table 2. Summary of Justifications of TDM of AEMs

5.14 Zonisamide

Zonisamide is approved in the United States for adjunctive treatment of partial seizures but is also used 'off-label' for bipolar disorder and migraine headaches (Leppik, 1999; Mimaki, 1998). After oral administration, zonisamide is rapidly absorbed and is only approximately 50% bound to serum proteins. Zonisamide is extensively metabolized by acetylation, oxidation, and other enzymatic pathways (Buchanan et al., 1996). CYP3A4 is responsible for some of the metabolism of zonisamide. Consequently, the metabolism of zonisamide can be significantly affected by CYP inducers and inhibitors. The elimination half-life of zonisamide is approximately 50-70 hr for patients receiving zonisamide as monotherapy but decreases to 25-35 hr in patients concomitantly taking enzyme inducers such as carbamazepine or phenobarbital. On the other hand, liver enzyme inhibitors such as ketoconazole and valproic acid may prolong zonisamide half-life (Perucca & Bialer, 1996). Zonisamide is cleared effectively by hemodialysis (Ijiri et al., 2004). In general, children require higher doses by weight than adults (Perucca, 2006). A serum/plasma reference range of 10-40 mg/L has been proposed for seizure management (Glauser & Pippenger, 2000; Mimaki, 1998). Toxic side effects are uncommon at serum concentrations below 30 mg/L (Miura, 1993). The main reason to perform TDM for zonisamde is inter-individual variability in metabolism, particularly in patients concomitantly taking CYP enzyme inducers or inhibitors.

6. Conclusion

TDM has traditionally been applied to the first generation AEMs such as carbamazepine, phenobarbital, phenytoin, and valproic acid, mainly due to the challenging pharmacokinetics of this group of drugs. The newer generation AEMs generally have more favorable pharmacokinetics and fewer adverse effects. The strongest evidence for routine TDM for the new generation AEMs are for lamotrigine, oxcarbazepine (10-hydroxycarbazepine metabolite), stiripentol, tiagabine, and zonisamide. For other AEMs, TDM may have value in adjusting dosing for organ failure or to assess compliance with therapy. Future research is needed to better delineate reference ranges and to establish the benefit of TDM in clinical practice.

7. References

Acharya, NV, Pickering, RM, Wilton, LW, Shakir, SA. (2005). The safety and effectiveness of newer antiepileptics: a comparative postmarketing cohort study. *Journal of Clinical Pharmacology*. Vol. 45, No. 4., (Apr 2005) 385-393. Print ISSN 0091-2700

al Za'abi, M, Deleu, D, Batchelor, C. (2003). Salivary free concentrations of anti-epileptic drugs: an evaluation in a routine clinical setting. *Acta Neurologica Belgica*. Vol. 103, No. 1. (Mar 2003) 19-23. Print ISSN 0300-9009

Alfirevic, A, Jorgensen, AL, Williamson, PR, Chadwick, DW, Park, BK, Pirmohamed, M. (2006). HLA-B locus in Caucasian patients with carbamazepine hypersensitivity. *Pharmacogenomics*. Vol. 7, No. 6. (Sep 2006) 813-818. Print ISSN 1462-2416

Almeida, L, Falcao, A, Maia, J, Mazur, D, Gellert, M, Soares-da-Silva, P. (2005). Single-dose and steady-state pharmacokinetics of eslicarbazepine acetate (BIA 2-093) in healthy elderly and young subjects. *Journal of Clinical Pharmacology*. Vol. 45, No. 9. (Sep 2005) 1062-1066. Print ISSN 0091-2700

Almeida, L, Nunes, T, Sicard, E, Rocha, JF, Falcao, A, Brunet, JS, Lefebvre, M, Soares-da-Silva, P. (2010). Pharmacokinetic interaction study between eslicarbazepine acetate and lamotrigine in healthy subjects. *Acta Neurologica Scandinavica*. Vol. 121, No. 4. (Dec 2010) 257-264. Print ISSN 1600-0404

Almeida, L, Potgieter, JH, Maia, J, Potgieter, MA, Mota, F, Soares-da-Silva, P. (2008). Pharmacokinetics of eslicarbazepine acetate in patients with moderate hepatic impairment. *European Journal of Clinical Pharmacology*. Vol. 64, No. 3. (Mar 2008) 267-273. Print ISSN 0031-6970

Alves, G, Figueiredo, I, Castel-Branco, M, Loureiro, A, Fortuna, A, Falcao, A, Caramona, M. (2007). Enantioselective HPLC-UV method for determination of eslicarbazepine acetate (BIA 2-093) and its metabolites in human plasma. *Biomedical Chromatography*. Vol. 21, No. 11. (Nov 2007) 1127-1134. Print ISSN 0269-3879

Armijo, JA, Perna, MA, Adin, J, Vega-Gil, N. (2004). Association between patient age and gabapentin serum concentration-to-dose ratio: a preliminary multivariate analysis. *Therapeutic Drug Monitoring*. Vol. 26, No. 6. 633-637. (Dec 2004) Print ISSN 0163-4356

Bartoli, A, Guerrini, R, Belmonte, A, Alessandri, MG, Gatti, G, Perucca, E. (1997). The influence of dosage, age, and comedication on steady state plasma lamotrigine concentrations in epileptic children: a prospective study with preliminary assessments of correlations with clinical response. *Therapeutic Drug Monitoring*. Vol. 19, No. 3. (Jun 1997) 252-260. Print ISSN 0163-4356

Battino, D, Estienne, M, Avanzini, G. (1995). Clinical pharmacokinetics of antiepileptic drugs in pediatric patients. Part II. Phenytoin, carbamazepine, sulthiame, lamotrigine, vigabatrin, oxcarbazepine and felbamate. *Clinical Pharmacokinetics* Vol. 29, No. 5. (Nov 1995) 341-369. Print ISSN 0312-5963

Ben-Menachem, E, Biton, V, Jatuzis, D, Abou-Khalil, B, Doty, P, Rudd, GD. (2007). Efficacy and safety of oral lacosamide as adjunctive therapy in adults with partial-onset seizures. *Epilepsia*. Vol. 48, No. 7. (Jul 2007) 1308-1317. Print ISSN 0013-9580

Benetello, P, Furlanut, M, Fortunato, M, Baraldo, M, Pea, F, Tognon, A, Testa, G. (1997). Oral gabapentin disposition in patients with epilepsy after a high-protein meal. *Epilepsia*. Vol. 38, No. 10. (Oct 1997) 1140-1142. Print ISSN 0013-9580

Berry, DJ, Beran, RG, Plunkeft, MJ, Clarke, LA, Hung, WT. (2003). The absorption of gabapentin following high dose escalation. *Seizure*. Vol. 12, No. 1. (Jan 2003) 28-36. Print ISSN 1059-1311

Besag, FM, Berry, D. (2006). Interactions between antiepileptic and antipsychotic drugs. *Drug Safety*. Vol. 29, No. 2. (2006) 95-118. Print ISSN 0114-5916

Besag, FM, Berry, DJ, Pool, F. (1998). Carbamazepine toxicity with lamotrigine: pharmacokinetic or pharmacodynamic interaction. *Epilepsia*. Vol. 39, No. 2. (Feb 1998) 183-187. Print ISSN 0013-9580

Beydoun, A, D'Souza, J, Hebert, D, Doty, P. (2009). Lacosamide: pharmacology, mechanisms of action and pooled efficacy and safety data in partial-onset seizures. *Expert Review of Neurotherapeutics*. Vol. 9, No. 1. (Jan 2009) 33-42. Print ISSN 1744-8360

Bialer, M. (2005). The pharmacokinetics and interactions of new antiepileptic drugs: an overview. *Therapeutic Drug Monitoring*. Vol. 27, No. 6. (Dec 2005) 722-726. Print ISSN 0163-4356

Bialer, M, Johannessen, SI, Levy, RH, Perucca, E, Tomson, T, White, HS. (2009). Progress report on new antiepileptic drugs: a summary of the Ninth Eilat Conference (EILAT IX). *Epilepsy Research*. Vol. 83, No. 1. (Jan 2009) 1-43. Print ISSN 1872-6844

Biton, V. (2006). Pharmacokinetics, toxicology and safety of lamotrigine in epilepsy. *Expert Opinion in Drug Metabolism and Toxicology*. Vol. 2, No. 6. (Dec 2006) 1009-1018. Print ISSN 1742-5255

Bockbrader, HN, Hunt, T, Strand, J, Posvar, EL, Sedman, A. (2000). Pregabalin pharmacokinetics and safety in health volunteers: results from two phase I studies. *Neurology*. Vol. 11, Suppl 3. (2000) 412. Electronic ISSN 1526-632X

Bourgeois, BF. (1997). Felbamate. *Seminars in Pediatric Neurology*. Vol. 4, No. 1. (Mar 1997) 3-8. Print ISSN 1071-9091

Britzi, MP, E., Soback, S, Levy, RH, Fattore, C, Crema, F, Gatti, G, Doose, DR, Maryanoff, BE, Bialer, M. (2005). Pharmacokinetic and metabolic investigation of topiramate disposition in healthy subjects in the absence and in the presence of enzyme induction by carbamazepine. *Epilepsia*. Vol. 46, No. 3. (Mar 2005) 378-384. Print ISSN 0013-9580

Brodie, MJ, Dichter, MA. (1997). Established antiepileptic drugs. *Seizure*. Vol. 6, No. 3. (Jun 1997) 159-174. Print ISSN 1059-1311

Buchanan, R, Bockbrader, HN, Chang, T, Sedman, AJ. (1996). Single- and multiple-dose pharmacokinetics of zonisamide. *Epilepsia*. Vol. 37, No. Suppl 5. (1996) 172. Print ISSN 0013-9580

Busch, JA, Strand, JC, Posvar, EL, Bockbrader, HN, Radulovic, LL. (1998). Pregabalin (CI-1008) single-dose pharmacokinetics and safety/tolerance in healthy subjects after oral administration of pregabalin solution or capsule doses. *Epilepsia*. Vol. 39, No. Suppl 6. (1998) 58. Print ISSN 0013-9580

Cardot, JM, Degen, P, Flesch, G, Menge, P, Dieterle, W. (1995). Comparison of plasma and saliva concentrations of the active monohydroxy metabolite of oxcarbazepine in patients at steady state. *Biopharmaceutics & Drug Disposition*. Vol. 16, No. 7. (Oct 1995) 603-614. Print ISSN 0142-2782

Cato, A, 3rd, Gustavson, LE, Qian, J, El-Shourbagy, T, Kelly, EA. (1998). Effect of renal impairment on the pharmacokinetics and tolerability of tiagabine. *Epilepsia*. Vol. 39, No. 1. (Jan 1998) 43-47. Print ISSN 0013-9580

Christensen, J, Sabers, A, Sidenius, P. (2006). Oxcarbazepine concentrations during pregnancy: a retrospective study in patients with epilepsy. *Neurology*. Vol. 24, No. 8. (Aug 2006) 1497-1499. Electronic ISSN 1526-632X

Chung, S, Sperling, MR, Biton, V, Krauss, G, Hebert, D, Rudd, GD, Doty, P. (2010). Lacosamide as adjunctive therapy for partial-onset seizures: A randomized controlled trial. *Epilepsia*. Vol. 51, No. 6 (June 2010) Print ISSN 0013-9580

Corrigan, BW, Poole, WF, Posvar, EL, Strand, JC, Alvey, CW, Radulovic, LL. (2001). Metabolic disposition of pregabalin in healthy volunteers. *Clinical Pharmacology and Therapeutics*. Vol. 69, Suppl. (2001) P18. Print ISSN 0009-9236

Crawford, P. (2002). Interactions between antiepileptic drugs and hormonal contraception. *CNS Drugs*. Vol. 16, No. 4. (Apr 2002) 263-272. Print ISSN 1172-7047

Cross, SA, Curran, MP. (2009). Lacosamide: in partial-onset seizures. *Drugs*. Vol. 69, No. 4. (Apr 2009) 449-459. Print ISSN 0012-6667

Curia, G, Biagini, G, Perucca, E, Avoli, M. (2009). Lacosamide: a new approach to target voltage-gated sodium currents in epileptic disorders. *CNS Drugs*. Vol. 23, No. 7. (Jul 2009) 555-568. Print ISSN 1172-7047

Dasgupta, A. (2007). Usefulness of monitoring free (unbound) concentrations of therapeutic drugs in patient management. *Clinica Chimca Acta*. Vol. 377, No. 1-2. (Feb 2007) 1-13. Print ISSN 009-8981

Durham, SL, Hoke, JF, Chen, TM. (1993). Pharmacokinetics and metabolism of vigabatrin following a single oral dose of [^{14}C]vigabatrin in healthy male volunteers. *Drug Metabolism and Disposition*. Vol. 21, No. 3. (May-Jun 1993) 480-484. Print ISSN 0090-9556

Easterling, DE, Zakszewski, T, Moyer, MD, Margul, BL, Marriott, TB, Nayak, RK. (1988). Plasma pharmacokinetics of topiramate, a new anticonvulsants in humans. *Epilepsia*. Vol. 29, Suppl. (1988) Print ISSN 0013-9580

Eckardt, KM, Steinhoff, BJ. (1998). Nonconvulsive status epilepticus in two patients receiving tiagabine treatment. *Epilepsia*. Vol. 39, No. 6. (Jun 1998) 671-674. Print ISSN 0013-9580

Falcao, A, Maia, J, Almeida, L, Mazur, D, Gellert, M, Soares-da-Silva, P. (2007). Effect of gender on the pharmacokinetics of eslicarbazepine acetate (BIA 2-093), a new voltage-gated sodium channel blocker. *Biopharmaceutics & Drug Disposition*. Vol. 28, No. 5. (Jul 2007) 249-256. Print ISSN 0142-2782

Farwell, JR, Anderson, GD, Kerr, BM, Tor, JA, Levy, RH. (1993). Stiripentol in atypical absence seizures in children: an open trial. *Epilepsia*. Vol. 34, No. 2. (Mar-Apr 1993) 305-311. Print ISSN 0013-9580

Faught, E, Sachdeo, RC, Remler, MP, Chayasirisobhon, S, Iragui-Madoz, VJ, Ramsay, RE, Sutula, TP, Kanner, A, Harner, RN, Kuzniecky, R, Kramer, LD, Karmin, M, Rosenberg, A. (1993). Felbamate monotherapy for partial-onset seizures: an active-controlled trial. *Neurology*. Vol. 43, No. 4. (Apr 1993) 688-692. Electronic ISSN 1526-632X

Fay, MA, Sheth, RD, Gidal, BE. (2005). Oral absorption kinetics of levetiracetam: the effect of mixing with food or enteral nutrition formulas. *Clinical Therapeutics*. Vol. 27, No. 5. (May 2005) 594-598. Print ISSN 0149-2918

Fillastre, JP, Taburet, AM, Fialaire, A, Etienne, I, Bidault, R, Singlas, E. (1993). Pharmacokinetics of lamotrigine in patients with renal impairment: influence of haemodialysis. *Drugs Under Experimental and Clinical Research*. Vol. 19, No. 1. (Jan 1993) 25-32. Print ISSN 0378-6501

Friis, ML, Kristensen, O, Boas, J, Dalby, M, Deth, SH, Gram, L, Mikkelsen, M, Pedersen, B, Sabers, A, Worm-Petersen, J. (1993). Therapeutic experiences with 947 epileptic out-patients in oxcarbazepine treatment. *Acta Neurologica Scandanavica*. Vol. 87, No. 3. (Mar 1993) 224-227. Print ISSN 0001-6314

Fröscher, W, Eichelbaum, M, Gugler, R, Hildebrand, G, Penin, H. (1981). A prospective randomized trial on the effect of monitoring plasma anticonvulsant levels in epilepsy. *Journal of Neurology*. Vol. 224, No. 3. (Mar 1981) 193-201. Print ISSN 0340-5354

Gidal, BE, DeCerce, J, Bockbrader, HN, Gonzalez, J, Kruger, S, Pitterle, ME, Rutecki, P, Ramsay, RE. (1998). Gabapentin bioavailability: effect of dose and frequency of administration in adult patients with epilepsy. *Epilepsy Research*. Vol. 31, No. 2. (Jul 1998) 91-99. Print ISSN 0920-1211

Glauser, TA, Pippenger, CE. (2000). Controversies in blood-level monitoring: re-examining its role in the treatment of epilepsy. *Epilepsia*. Vol. 41, Suppl 8. (2000) S6-S15. Print ISSN 0013-9580

Grim, SA, Ryan, M, Miles, MV, Tang, PH, Strawsburg, RH, de Grauw, TJ, Fakhoury, TA, Baumann, RJ. (2003). Correlation of levetiracetam concentrations between serum and plasma. *Therapeutic Drug Monitoring*. Vol. 25, No. 1. (Dec 2003) 61-66. Print ISSN 0277-0008

Guo, T, Oswald, LM, Mendu, DR, Soldin, SJ. (2007). Determination of levetiracetam in human plasma/serum/saliva by liquid chromatography-electrospray tandem mass spectrometry. *Clinica Chimica Acta*. Vol. 375, No. 1-2. (Jan 2007) 115-118. Print ISSN 0009-8981

Gustavson, LE, Boellner, SW, Granneman, GR, Qian, JX, Guenther, HJ, el-Shourbagy, T, Sommerville, KW. (1997). A single-dose study to define tiagabine pharmacokinetics in pediatric patients with complex partial seizures. *Neurology*. Vol. 48, No. 4. (Apr 1997) 1032-1037. Electronic ISSN 1526-632X

Gustavson, LE, Mengel, HB. (1995). Pharmacokinetics of tiagabine, a g-aminobutyric acid-uptake inhibitor, in healthy subjects after single and multiple doses. *Epilepsia*. Vol. 36, No. 6. (Jun 1995) 605-611. Print ISSN 0013-9580

Hakimian, S, Cheng-Hakimian, A, Anderson, GD, Miller, JW. (2007). Rufinamide: a new anti-epileptic medication. *Expert Opinion on Pharmacotherapy*. Vol. 8, No. 12. (Aug 2007) 1931-1940. Print ISSN 1744-7666

Hardman JG, Limbird LE, Molinoff PB, Ruddon RW, Gilman AG. (1996). Pharmacokinetic data, In: *Goodman & Gilman's The Pharmacological Basis of Therapeutics*, Hardman JG, Limbird LE, Molinoff PB, Ruddon RW, Gilman AG (eds), pp. 1712-1792, McGraw-Hill, ISBN 0-070-026266-7, New York.

Heaney, D, Walker, MC. (2007). Rufinamide. *Drugs Today (Barcelona)*. Vol. 43, No. 7. (Jul 2007) 455-460. Print ISSN 1699-3993

Hung, TY, Seow, VK, Chong, CF, Wang, TL, Chen, CC. (2008). Gabapentin toxicity: an important cause of altered consciousness in patients with uraemia. *Emergency Medicine Journal*. Vol. 25, No. 3. (Mar 2008) 178-179. Print ISSN 1472-0213

Hussein, Z, Posner, J. (1997). Population pharmacokinetics of lamotrigine monotherapy in patients with epilepsy: retrospective analysis of routine monitoring data. *British Journal of Clinical Pharmacology*. Vol. 43, No. 5. (May 1997) 457-464. Print ISSN 0306-5251

Ijiri, Y, Inoue, T, Fukuda, F, Suzuki, K, Kobayashi, T, Shibahara, N, Takenaka, H, Tanaka, K. (2004). Dialyzability of the antiepileptic drug zonisamide in patients undergoing hemodialysis. *Epilepsia*. Vol. 45, No. 8. (Aug 2004) 924-927. Print ISSN 0013-9580

Incecayir, T, Agabeyoglu, I, Gucuyener, K. (2007). Comparison of plasma and saliva concentrations of lamotrigine in healthy volunteers. *Arzneimittelforschung*. Vol. 57, No. 8. (Aug 2007) 517-521. Print ISSN 0004-4172

Jacqz-Aigrain, E, Guillonneau, M, Rey, E, Macher, MA, Montes, C, Chiron, C, Loirat, C. (1997). Pharmacokinetics of the S(+) and R(-) enantiomers of vigabatrin during chronic dosing in a patient with renal failure. *British Journal of Clinical Pharmacology*. Vol. 44, No. 2. (Aug 1997) 183-185. Print ISSN 0306-5251

Januzzi, G, Cian, P, Fattore, C, Gatti, G, Bartoli, A, Monaco, F, Perucca, E. (2000). A multicenter randomized controlled trial on the clinical impact of therapeutic drug monitoring in patients with newly diagnosed epilepsy. *Epilepsia*. Vol. 41, No. 2. (Feb 2000) 222-230. Print ISSN 0013-9580

Johannessen Landmark, C. (2008). Antiepileptic drugs in non-epilepsy disorders: relations between mechanisms of action and clinical efficacy. *CNS Drugs*. Vol. 22, No. 1. (Jan 2008) 27-47. Print ISSN 1172-7047

Johannessen Landmark, C, Patsalos, PN. (2010). Drug interactions involving the new second- and third-generation antiepileptic drugs. *Expert Review of Neurotherapeutics*. Vol. 10, No. 1. (Jan 2010) 119-140. Print ISSN 1744-8360

Johannessen, SI, Battino, D, Berry, DJ, Bialer, M, Kramer, G, Tomson, T, Patsalos, PN. (2003). Therapeutic drug monitoring of the newer antiepileptic drugs. *Therapeutic Drug Monitoring*. Vol. 25, No. 3. (Mar 2003) 347-363. Print ISSN 0277-0008

Jones, MD, Ryan, M, Miles, MV, Tang, PH, Fakhoury, TA, Degrauw, TJ, Baumann, RJ. (2005). Stability of salivary concentrations of the newer antiepileptic drugs in the postal system. *Therapeutic Drug Monitoring*. Vol. 27, No. 5. (Oct 2005) 576-579. Print 0163-4356

Kellinghaus, C. (2009). Lacosamide as treatment for partial epilepsy: mechanisms of action, pharmacology, effects, and safety. *Therapeutics and Clinical Risk Management*. Vol. 5, (2009) 757-766. Print ISSN 1176-6336

Kellinghaus, C, Dziewas, R, Ludemann, P. (2002). Tiagabine-related non-convulsive status epilepticus in partial epilepsy: three case reports and a review of the literature. *Seizure*. Vol. 11, No. 4. (Jun 2002) 243-249. Print ISSN 1059-1311

Klitgaard, H. (2001). Levetiracetam: the preclinical profile of a new class of antiseizure drugs? *Epilepsia*. Vol. 42, Suppl 4. (2001) S13-S18. Print ISSN 0013-9580

Knowles, SR, Shapiro, LE, Shear, NH. (1999). Anticonvulsant hypersensitivity syndrome: incidence, prevention and management. *Drug Safety*. Vol. 21, No. 6. (Dec 1999) 489-501. Print ISSN 0114-5916

Komoroski, BJ, Zhang, S, Cai, H, Hutzler, JM, Frye, R, Tracy, TS, Strom, SC, Lehmann, T, Ang, CYW, Cui, YY, Venkataramanan, R. (2004). Induction and inhibition of cytochromes P450 by the St. John's wort constituent hyperforin in human hepatocyte cultures. *Drug Metabolism and Disposition*. Vol. 32, No. 5. (May 2004) 512-518. Print ISSN 0090-9556

Kristensen, O, Klitgaard, NA, Jonsson, B, Sindrup, S. (1983). Pharmacokinetics of 10-OH-carbazepine, the main metabolite of the antiepileptic oxcarbazepine, from serum and saliva concentrations. *Acta Neurologica Scandinavica*. Vol. 68, No. 3. (Sep 1983) 145-150. Print ISSN 0001-6314

Kumagai, N, Seki, T, Yamada, T, Takuma, Y, Hirai, K. (1993). Concentrations of zonisamide in serum, free fraction, mixed saliva and cerebrospinal fluid in epileptic children treated with monotherapy. *The Japanese Journal of Psychiatry and Neurology*. Vol. 47, No. 2. (Jun 1993) 291-292. Print ISSN 0912-2036

Lacerda, G, Krummel, T, Sabourdy, C, Ryvlin, P, Hirsch, E. (2006). Optimizing therapy of seizures in patients with renal or hepatic dysfunction. *Neurology*. Vol. 67, No. 12 Suppl 4. (Dec 2006) S28-33. Electronic ISSN 1526-632X

Larkin, JG, McKee, PJ, Forrest, G, Beastall, GH, Park, BK, Lowrie, JI, Lloyd, P, Brodie, MJ. (1991). Lack of enzyme induction with oxcarbazepine (600 mg daily) in healthy subjects. *British Journal of Clinical Pharmacology*. Vol. 31, No. 1. (Jan 1991) 65-71. Print ISSN 0306-5251

LaRoche, SM, Helmers, SL. (2004a). The new antiepileptic drugs: clinical applications. *JAMA*. Vol. 291, No. 5. (Feb 2004) 615-620. Print ISSN 0098-7484

LaRoche, SM, Helmers, SL. (2004b). The new antiepileptic drugs: scientific review. *JAMA*. Vol. 291, No. 5. (Feb 2004) 605-614. Print ISSN 0098-7484

Lau, AH, Gustavson, LE, Sperelakis, R, Lam, NP, El-Shourbagy, T, Qian, JX, Layden, T. (1997). Pharmacokinetics and safety of tiagabine in subjects with various degrees of hepatic function. *Epilepsia*. Vol. 38, No. 4. (Apr 1997) 445-451. Print ISSN 0013-9580

Leppik, IE. (1999). Zonisamide. *Epilepsia*. Vol. 40, Suppl 5. (1999) S23-S29. Print ISSN 0013-9580

Leppik, IE. (2001). The place of levetiracetam in the treatment of epilepsy. *Epilepsia*. Vol. 42, No. Suppl 4. (2001) S44-S45. Print ISSN 0013-9580

Leppik, IE, Rarick, JO, Walczak, TS, Tran, TA, White, JR, Gumnit, RJ. (2002). Effective levetiracetam doses and serum concentrations: age effects. *Epilepsia*. Vol. 43, Suppl 7. (2002) 240. Print ISSN 0013-9580

Levy, RH, Lin, HS, Blehaut, HM, Tor, JA. (1983). Pharmacokinetics of stiripentol in normal man: evidence of nonlinearity. *Journal of Clinical Pharmacology*. Vol. 23, No. 11-12. (Nov-Dec 1983) 523-533. Print ISSN

Levy, RH, Loiseau, P, Guyot, M, Blehaut, HM, Tor, J, Moreland, TA. (1984). Stiripentol kinetics in epilepsy: nonlinearity and interactions. *Clinical Pharmacology and Therapeutics*. Vol. 36, No. 5. (Nov 1984) 661-669. Print ISSN 0009-9236

Lindberger, M, Luhr, O, Johannessen, SI, Larsson, S, Tomson, T. (2003). Serum concentrations and effects of gabapentin and vigabatrin: observations from a dose titration study. *Therapeutic Drug Monitoring*. Vol. 25, No. 4. (Apr 2003) 457-462. Print ISSN 0277-0008

Lins, RL, Otoul, C, De Smedt, F, Coupez, R, Stockis, A. (2007). Comparison of plasma and saliva concentrations of levetiracetam following administration orally as a tablet and as a solution in healthy adult volunteers. *International Journal of Clinical Pharmacology and Therapeutics*. Vol. 45, No. 1. (Jan 2007) 47-54. Print ISSN 0946-1965

Liu, H, Delgado, MR. (1999). Therapeutic drug concentration monitoring using saliva samples. Focus on anticonvulsants. *Clinical Pharmacokinetics*. Vol. 36, No. 6. (Jun 1999) 453-470. Print ISSN 0312-5963

Lloyd, P, Flesch, G, Dieterle, W. (1994). Clinical pharmacology and pharmacokinetics of oxcarbazepine. *Epilepsia*. Suppl 3 (1994) 10-13. Print ISSN 0013-9580

Lonjou, C, Thomas, L, Borot, N, Ledger, N, de Toma, C, LeLouet, H, Graf, E, Schumacher, M, Hovnanian, A, Mockenhaupt, M, Roujeau, JC. (2006). A marker for Stevens-Johnson syndrome ...: ethnicity matters. *Pharmacogenomics Journal*. Vol. 6, No. 4. (Jul-Aug 2006) 265-268. Print ISSN 1470-269X

Luo, G, Guenthner, T, Gan, L-S, Humphreys, WG. (2004). CYP3A4 induction by xenobiotics: biochemistry, experimental methods and impact on drug discovery and development. *Current Drug Metabolism*. Vol. 5, No. 6. (Dec 2004) 483-505. Print ISSN 1389-2002

Luszczki, JJ. (2009). Third-generation antiepileptic drugs: mechanisms of action, pharmacokinetics and interactions. *Pharmacological Reports*. Vol. 61, No. 2. (Mar-Apr 2009) 197-216. Print ISSN 1734-1140

Maia, J, Almeida, L, Falcao, A, Soares, E, Mota, F, Potgieter, MA, Potgieter, JH, Soares-da-Silva, P. (2008). Effect of renal impairment on the pharmacokinetics of eslicarbazepine acetate. *International Journal of Clinical Pharmacology and Therapeutics*. Vol. 46, No. 3. (Mar 2008) 119-130. Print ISSN 0946-1965

Maia, J, Vaz-da-Silva, M, Almeida, L, Falcao, A, Silveira, P, Guimaraes, S, Graziela, P, Soares-da-Silva, P. (2005). Effect of food on the pharmacokinetic profile of eslicarbazepine acetate (BIA 2-093). *Drugs R D*. Vol. 6, No. 4. (Apr 2005) 201-206. Print ISSN 1174-5886

Malone, SA, Eadie, MJ, Addison, RS, Wright, AW, Dickinson, RG. (2006). Monitoring salivary lamotrigine concentrations. *Journal of Clinical Neuroscience*. Vol. 13, No. 9. (Nov 2006) 902-907. Print ISSN 0967-5868

May, TW, Korn-Merker, E, Rambeck, B. (2003). Clinical pharmacokinetics of oxcarbazepine. *Clinical Pharmacokinetics*. Vol. 42, No. 12. (Dec 2003) 1023-1042. Print ISSN 0312-5963

Mazzucchelli, I, Onat, FY, Ozkara, C, Atakli, D, Specchio, LM, Neve, AL, Gatti, G, Perucca, E. (2006). Changes in the disposition of oxcarbazepine and its metabolites during pregnancy and the puerperium. *Epilepsia*. Vol. 47, No. 3. (Mar 2006) 504-509. Print ISSN 0013-9580

McLean, MJ. (1995). Gabapentin. *Epilepsia*. Vol. 36, Suppl 2. (1995) S57-S86. Print ISSN 0013-9580

Mecarelli, O, Li Voti, P, Pro, S, Romolo, FS, Rotolo, M, Pulitano, P, Accornero, N, Vanacore, N. (2007). Saliva and serum levetiracetam concentrations in patients with epilepsy. *Therapeutic Drug Monitoring*. Vol. 29, No. 3. (Jun 2007) 313-318. Print ISSN 0163-4356

Miles, MV, Tang, PH, Glauser, TA, Ryan, MA, Grim, SA, Strawsburg, RH, deGrauw, TJ, Baumann, RJ. (2003). Topiramate concentration in saliva: an alternative to serum monitoring. *Pediatric Neurology*. Vol. 29, No. 2. (Aug 2003) 143-147. Print ISSN 0887-8994

Miles, MV, Tang, PH, Ryan, MA, Grim, SA, Fakhoury, TA, Strawsburg, RH, DeGrauw, TJ, Baumann, RJ. (2004). Feasibility and limitations of oxcarbazepine monitoring using salivary monohydroxycarbamazepine (MHD). *Therapeutic Drug Monitoring*. Vol. 26, No. 3. (Jun 2004) 300-304. Print ISSN 0163-4356

Mimaki, T. (1998). Clinical pharmacology and therapeutic drug monitoring of zonisamide. *Therapeutic Drug Monitoring*. Vol. 20, No. 6. (Jun 1998) 593-597. Print ISSN 0277-0008

Miura, H. (1993). Developmental and therapeutic pharmacology of antiepileptic drugs. *The Japanese Journal of Psychiatry and Neurology*. Vol. 47, No. 2. (Feb 1993) 169-174. Print ISSN 0912-2036

Morris, RG, Black, AB, Harris, AL, Batty, AB, Sallustio, BC. (1998). Lamotrigine and therapeutic drug monitoring: retrospective survey following the introduction of a routine service. *British Journal of Clinical Pharmacology*. Vol. 46, No. 6. (Jun 1998) 547-551. Print ISSN 0306-5251

Neels, HM, Sierens, AC, Naelerts, K, Scharpé, SL, Hatfield, GM, Lambert, WE. (2004). Therapeutic drug monitoring of old and newer anti-epileptic drugs. *Clinical Chemstry and Laboratory Medicine*. Vol. 42, No. 11. (2004) 1228-1255. Print ISSN 1434-6621

Ninomiya, H, Mamiya, K, Matsuo, S, Ieiri, I, Higuchi, S, Tashiro, N. (2000). Genetic polymorphism of the CYP2C subfamily and excessive serum phenytoin concentration with central nervous system intoxication. *Therapeutic Drug Monitoring*. Vol. 22, No. 2. (Apr 2000) 230-232. Print 0163-4356

Patsalos, PN. (1999). New antiepileptic drugs. *Annals of Clinical Biochemistry*. Vol. 36, No. 1. (Jan 1999) 10-19. Print ISSN 0004-5632

Patsalos, PN. (2000). Pharmacokinetic profile of levetiracetam: toward ideal characteristics. *Pharmacology and Therapeutics*. Vol. 85, No. 2. (Feb 2000) 77-85. Print ISSN 0163-7258

Patsalos, PN. (2004). Clinical pharmacokinetics of levetiracetam. *Clinical Pharmacokinetics*. Vol. 43, No. 11. (Nov 2004) 707-724. Print ISSN 0312-5963

Patsalos, PN, Berry, DJ, Bourgeois, BFD, Cloyd, JC, Glauser, TA, Johannessen, SI, Tomson, T, Perucca, E. (2008). Antiepileptic drugs - best practice guidelines for therapeutic drug monitoring: a position paper by the subcommission on therapeutic drug monitoring, ILAE Commission on Therapeutic Strategies. *Epilepsia*. Vol. 49, No. 7. (Jun 2008) 1239-1276. Print ISSN 0013-9580

Patsalos, PN, Elyas, AA, Ratnaraj, N, Iley, J. (2002). Concentration-dependent displacement of tiagabine by valproic acid. *Epilepsia*. Vol. 43, Suppl 8. (2002) 143. Print ISSN 0013-9580

Patsalos, PN, Ghattaura, S, Ratnaraj, N, Sander, JW. (2006). In situ metabolism of levetiracetam in blood of patients with epilepsy. *Epilepsia*. Vol. 47, No. 11. (Nov 2006) 1818-1821. Print ISSN 0013-9580

Pellock, JM, Faught, E, Leppik, IE, Shinnar, S, Zupanc, ML. (2006). Felbamate: consensus of current clinical experience. *Epilepsy Research*. Vol. 71, No. 2-3. (Oct 2006) 89-101. Print ISSN 0920-1211

Pennell, PB, Peng, L, Newport, DJ, Ritchie, JC, Koganti, A, Holley, DK, Newman, M, Stowe, ZN. (2008). Lamotrigine in pregnancy: clearance, therapeutic drug monitoring, and seizure frequency. *Neurology*. Vol. 70, No. 22 Pt 2. (2008) 2130-2136. Electronic ISSN 1526-632X

Perucca, E. (1996). Established antiepileptic drugs. *Baillieres Clinical Neurology*. Vol. 5, No. 4. (Dec 1996) 693-722. Print ISSN 0961-0421

Perucca, E. (2000). Is there a role for therapeutic drug monitoring of new anticonvulsants? *Clinical Pharmacokinetics*. Vol. 38, No. 3. (Mar 2000) 191-204. Print ISSN 0312-5963

Perucca, E. (2006). Clinical pharmacokinetics of new-generation antiepileptic drugs at the extremes of age. *Clinical Pharmacokinetics* Vol. 45, No. 4. 351-364. Print ISSN 0312-5963

Perucca, E, Bialer, M. (1996). The clinical pharmacokinetics of the newer antiepileptic drugs. Focus on topiramate, zonisamide and tiagabine. *Clinical Pharmacokinetics* Vol. 31, No. 1. (Jan 1996) 29-46. Print ISSN 0312-5963

Perucca, E, Cloyd, J, Critchley, D, Fuseau, E. (2008a). Rufinamide: clinical pharmacokinetics and concentration-response relationships in patients with epilepsy. *Epilepsia*. Vol. 49, No. 7. (Jul 2008) 1123-1141. Print 0013-9580

Perucca, E, Yasothan, U, Clincke, G, Kirkpatrick, P. (2008b). Lacosamide. *Nature Reviews Drug Discovery*. Vol. 7, No. 12. (Dec 2008) 973-974. Print ISSN 1474-1784

Pitlick, WH, Levy, RH. (1977). Time-dependent kinetics I: Exponential autoinduction of carbamazepine in monkeys. *Journal of Pharmaceutical Sciences*. Vol. 66, No. 5. (May 1977) 647-649. Print ISSN 0022-3549

Radtke, RA. (2001). Pharmacokinetics of levetiracetam. *Epilepsia*. Vol. 42, Suppl. (2001) 24-27. Print ISSN 0013-9580

Rambeck, B, Wolf, P. (1993). Lamotrigine clinical pharmacokinetics. *Clinical Pharmacokinetics* Vol. 25, No. 6. (Jun 1993) 433-443. Print ISSN 0312-5963

Ramsay, RE, Pellock, JM, Garnett, WR, Sanchez, RM, Valakas, AM, Wargin, WA, Lai, AA, Hubbell, J, Chern, WH, Allsup, T, et al. (1991). Pharmacokinetics and safety of lamotrigine (Lamictal) in patients with epilepsy. *Epilepsy Research*. Vol. 10, No. 2-3. (Nov-Dec 1991) 191-200. Print ISSN 0920-1211

Randinitis, EJ, Posvar, EL, Alvey, CW, Sedman, AJ, Cook, JA, Bockbrader, HN. (2003). Pharmacokinetics of pregabalin in subjects with various degrees of renal functions. *Journal of Clinical Pharmacology*. Vol. 43, No. 3. (Mar 2003) 277-283. Print ISSN 0091-2700

Reimers, A, Skogvoll, E, Sund, JK, Spigset, O. (2007). Lamotrigine in children and adolescents: the impact of age on its serum concentrations and on the extent of drug interactions. *European Journal of Clinical Pharmacology*. Vol. 63, No. 7. (Jul 2007) 687-692. Print ISSN 0031-6970

Rey, E, Pons, G, Olive, G. (1992). Vigabatrin. Clinical pharmacokinetics. *Clinical Pharmacokinetics*. Vol. 23, No. 4. (Apr 1992) 267-278. Print ISSN 0312-5963

Riss, J, Cloyd, J, Gates, J, Collins, S. (2008). Benzodiazepines in epilepsy: pharmacology and pharmacokinetics. *Acta Neurologica Scandinavica*. Vol. 118, No. 2. (Aug 2008) 69-86. Print ISSN 1600-0404

Rosenfeld, WE, Doose, DR, Walker, SA, Baldassarre, JS, Reifer, RA. (1999). A study of topiramate pharmacokinetics and tolerability in children with epilepsy. *Pediatric Neurology*. Vol. 20, No. 5. (May 1999) 339-344. Print ISSN 0887-8994

Rouan, MC, Lecaillon, JB, Godbillon, J, Menard, F, Darragon, T, Meyer, P, Kourilsky, O, Hillion, D, Aldigier, JC, Jungers, P. (1994). The effect of renal impairment on the pharmacokinetics of oxcarbazepine and its metabolites. *European Journal of Clinical Pharmacology*. Vol. 47, No. 2. (Feb 1994) 161-167. Print ISSN 0031-6970

Ruiz, ME, Conforti, P, Fagiolino, P, Volonte, MG. (2010). The use of saliva as a biological fluid in relative bioavailability studies: comparison and correlation with plasma results. *Biopharmaceutics & Drug Disposition*. Vol. 31, No. 8-9. (Nov 2010) 476-485. Print ISSN 0142-2782

Ryan, M, Grim, SA, Miles, MV, Tang, PH, Fakhoury, TA, Strawsburg, RH, deGrauw, TJ, Baumann, RJ. (2003). Correlation of lamotrigine concentrations between serum and saliva. *Pharmacotherapy*. Vol. 23, No. 12. (Dec 2003) 1550-1557. Print ISSN 0277-0008

Sabers, A, Buchholt, JM, Uldall, P, Hansen, EL. (2001). Lamotrigine plasma levels reduced by oral contraceptives. *Epilepsy Research*. Vol. 47, No. 1-2. (Nov 2001) 151-154. Print ISSN 0920-1211

Sabers, A, Ohman, I, Christensen, J, Tomson, T. (2003). Oral contraceptives reduce lamotrigine plasma levels. *Neurology*. Vol. 61, No. 4. (Aug 26 2003) 570-571. Electronic ISSN 1526-632X

Sabers, A, Tomson, T. (2009). Managing antiepileptic drugs during pregnancy and lactation. *Current Opinion in Neurology*. Vol. 22, No. 2. (Apr 2009) 157-161. Print ISSN 1473-6551 (Electronic)

Sachdeo, RC, Kramer, LD, Rosenberg, A, Sachdeo, S. (1992). Felbamate monotherapy: controlled trial in patients with partial onset seizures. *Annals of Neurology*. Vol. 32, No. 3. (Sep 1992) 386-392. Print ISSN 0364-5134

Sachdeo, RC, Narang-Sachdeo, SKH, J.R., Dix, RK, Shumaker, RC, Perhach, JL, Rosenberg, A. (1993). Steady-state pharmacokinetics and dose-proportionality of felbamate after oral administration of 1200, 2400, and 3600 mg/day of felbamate. *Epilepsia*. Vol. 34, Suppl 6. (1993) 80. Print ISSN 0013-9580

Sachdeo, RC, Sachdeo, SK, Walker, SA, Kramer, LD, Nayak, RK, Doose, DR. (1996). Steady-state pharmacokinetics of topiramate and carbamazepine in patients with epilepsy during monotherapy and concomitant therapy. *Epilepsia*. Vol. 37, No. 8. (Aug 1996) 774-480. Print ISSN 0013-9580

Schapel, G, Chadwick, D. (1996). Tiagabine and non-convulsive status epilepticus. *Seizure*. Vol. 5, No. 2. (Jun 1996) 153-156. Print ISSN 1059-1311

Schechter, PJ. (1989). Clinical pharmacology of vigabatrin. *British Journal of Clinical Pharmacology*. Vol. 27, Suppl 1. (1989) 19S-22S. Print ISSN 0306-5251

Selak, I. (2001). Pregabalin (Pfizer). *Current Opinion in Investigational Drugs*. Vol. 2, No. 6. (Jun 2001) 828-834. Print ISSN 1472-4472

Shumaker, RC, Fantel, C, Kelton, E, Wong, K, Weliky, I. (1990). Evaluation of the elimination of (^{14}C) felbamate in healthy men. *Epilepsia*. Vol. 31, Suppl. (1990) 642. Print ISSN 0013-9580

Sivenius, J, Kälviäinen, R, Ylinen, A, Riekkinen, P. (1991). A double-blind study of gabapentin in the treatment of partial seizures. *Epilepsia*. Vol. 32, No. 4. (Apr 1991) 539-542. Print ISSN 0013-9580

Skolnick, JL, Stoler, BS, Katz, DB, Anderston, WH. (1976). Rifampin, oral contraceptives, and pregnancy. *JAMA*. Vol. 236, No. 12. (Sep 1976) 1382. Print ISSN 0098-7484

So, EL, Wolff, D, Graves, NM, Leppik, IE, Cascino, GD, Pixton, GC, Gustavson, LE. (1995). Pharmacokinetics of tiagabine as add-on therapy in patients taking enzyme-inducing antiepilepsy drugs. *Epilepsy Research*. Vol. 22, No. 3. (Nov 1995) 221-226. Print ISSN 0920-1211

Striano, S, Striano, P, Di Nocera, P, Italiano, D, Fasiello, C, Ruosi, P, Bilo, L, Pisani, F. (2006). Relationship between serum mono-hydroxy-carbazepine concentrations and adverse effects in patients with epilepsy on high-dose oxcabazepine therapy. *Epilepsy Research*. Vol. 69, No. 2. (Jun 2006) 170-176. Print ISSN 0920-1211

Tennison, M, Ali, I, Miles, MV, D'Cruz, O, Vaughn, B, Greenwood, R. (2004). Feasibility and acceptance of salivary monitoring of antiepileptic drugs via the US Postal Service. *Therapeutic Drug Monitoring*. Vol. 26, No. 3. (Jun 2004) 295-299. Print ISSN 0163-4356

Thomas, D, Schartenecker, U, Nickel, B, Doty, P, Cawello, W, Horstmann, R. (2006). Low potential for drug-drug interaction of lacosamide. *Epilepsia*. Vol. 47 Suppl, (2006) 200. Print ISSN 0013-9580

Thompson, CD, Barthen, MT, Hopper, DW, Miller, TA, Quigg, M, Hudspeth, C, Montouris, G, Marsh, L, Perhach, JL, Sofia, RD, Macdonald, TL. (1999). Quantification in patient urine samples of felbamate and three metabolites: acid carbamate and two mercapturic acids. *Epilepsia*. Vol. 40, No. 6. (Jun 1999) 769-776. Print ISSN 0013-9580

Tomson, T, Battino, D. (2007). Pharmacokinetics and therapeutic drug monitoring of newer antiepileptic drugs during pregnancy and the puerperium. *Clin Pharmacokinet*. Vol. 46, No. 3. (Mar 2007) 209-219. Print ISSN 0312-5963

Tran, A, Rey, E, Pons, G, Rousseau, M, d'Athis, P, Olive, G, Mather, GG, Bishop, FE, Wurden, CJ, Labroo, R, Trager, WF, Kunze, KL, Thummel, KE, Vincent, JC, Gillardin, JM, Lepage, F, Levy, RH. (1997). Influence of stiripentol on cytochrome P450-mediated metabolic pathways in humans: in vitro and in vivo comparison and calculation of in vivo inhibition constants. *Clinical Pharmacology and Therapeutics*. Vol. 62, No. 5. (Nov 1997) 490-504. Print ISSN 0009-9236

Tran, A, Vauzelle-Kervroedan, F, Rey, E, Pous, G, d'Athis, P, Chiron, C, Dulac, O, Renard, F, Olive, G. (1996). Effect of stiripentol on carbamazepine plasma concentration and metabolism in epileptic children. *European Journal of Clinical Pharmacology*. Vol. 50, No. 6. (Jun 1996) 497-500. Print ISSN 0031-6970

Tsiropoulos, I, Kristensen, O, Klitgaard, NA. (2000). Saliva and serum concentration of lamotrigine in patients with epilepsy. *Therapeutic Drug Monitoring*. Vol. 22, No. 5. (Oct 2000) 517-521. Print ISSN 0163-4356

Uthman, BM, Rowan, AJ, Ahmann, PA, Leppik, IE, Schachter, SC, Sommerville, KW, Shu, V. (1998). Tiagabine for complex partial seizures: a randomized, add-on, dose-response trial. *Archives of Neurology*. Vol. 55, No. 1. (Jan 1998) 56-62. Print ISSN 0003-9942

Van Buren, D, Wideman, CA, Ried, M, Gibbons, S, Van Buren, CT, Jarowenko, M, Flechner, SM, Frazier, OH, Cooley, DA, Kahan, BD. (1984). The antagonistic effect of rifampin upon cyclosporine bioavailability. *Transplantation Proceedings*. Vol. 16, No. 6. (Dec 1984) 1642-1645. Print ISSN 0041-1345

Vollmer, KO, von Hodenberg, A, Kölle, EU. (1988). Pharmacokinetics and metabolism of gabapentin in rat, dog and man. *Arzneimittelforschung*. Vol. 36, No. 5. (May 1988) 830-839. Print ISSN 0004-4172

Wagner, ML, Graves, NM, Marienau, K, Holmes, GB, Remmel, RP, Leppik, IE. (1991). Discontinuation of phenytoin and carbamazepine in patients receiving felbamate. *Epilepsia*. Vol. 32, No. 3. (May-Jun 1991) 398-406. Print ISSN 0013-9580

Ward, DL, Wagner, ML, Perhach, JL, Kramer, L, Graves, N, Leppik, I, Shumaker, RC. (1991). Felbamate steady-state pharmacokinetics during co-administration of valproate. *Epilepsia*. Vol. 32, Suppl 3. (1991) 8. Print ISSN 0013-9580

Warner, A, Privitera, M, Bates, D. (1998). Standards of laboratory practice: antiepileptic drug monitoring. National Academy of Clinical Biochemistry. *Clinical Chemistry*. Vol. 44, No. 5. (May 1998) 1085-1095. Print ISBN 0009-9147

Wheless, JW, Vazquez, B. (2010). Rufinamide: a novel broad-spectrum antiepileptic drug. *Epilepsy Currents*. Vol. 10, No. 1. (Jan 2010) 1-6. Print ISSN 1535-7511

Williams, J, Bialer, M, Johannessen, SI, Krämer, G, Levy, R, Mattson, RH, Perucca, E, Patsalos, PN, Wilson, JF. (2003). Interlaboratory variability in the quantification of new generation antiepileptic drugs based on external quality assessment data. *Epilepsia*. Vol. 44, No. 1. (Jan 2003) 40-45. Print ISSN 0013-9580

Wisniewski, CS. (2010). Rufinamide: a new antiepileptic medication for the treatment of seizures associated with lennox-gastaut syndrome. *Annals of Pharmacotherapy*. Vol. 44, No. 4. (Apr 2010) 658-667. Print ISSN 1542-6270

Wong, MO, Eldon, MA, Keane, WF, Turck, D, Bockbrader, HN, Underwood, BA, Sedman, AJ, Halstenson, CE. (1995). Disposition of gabapentin in anuric subjects on hemodialysis. *Journal of Clinical Pharmacology*. Vol. 35, No. 6. (Jun 1995) 622-626. Print ISBN 0091-2700

Yoo, L, Matalon, D, Hoffman, RS, Goldfarb, DS. (2009). Treatment of pregabalin toxicity by hemodialysis in a patient with kidney failure. *American Journal of Kidney Disease*. Vol. 54, No. 6. (Dec 2009) 1127-1130. Print ISSN 1523-6838

Zhou, C, Assem, M, Tay, JC, Watkins, PB, Blumberg, B, Schuetz, EG, Thummel, KE. (2006). Steroid and xenobiotic receptor and vitamin D receptor crosstalk mediates CYP24 expression and drug-induced osteomalacia. *Journal of Clinical Investigation*. Vol. 116, No. 6. (Jun 2006) 1703-1712. Print ISSN 0021-9738

9

Co-Morbidity and Medication Profiles of Patients with Epilepsy and Matched Controls in US and UK Electronic Health Records Systems

Lianna Ishihara and Michael Irizarry
GlaxoSmithKline PLC,
United Kingdom,
United States of America

1. Introduction

The global burden of epilepsy is substantial, especially in the developing regions of the world where treatments are less accessible (de Boer et al., 2008). One contribution to the overall disease burden is the higher prevalence of comorbidities among patients with epilepsy, compared to the general population. These include psychological comorbidities, such as depression, which have been associated with epilepsy, both before and after epilepsy diagnosis (Hesdorffer et al., 2005). Other neurological diseases such as migraine have also been associated with epilepsy (Ottman & Lipton, 1994).

Two database studies were utilised to assess the overall comorbidity profiles of patients with epilepsy and matched controls without epilepsy. The analyses allow for comparisons between the relative prevalence estimates of comorbidities within populations captured through electronic health data sources. The US Impact National Managed Care Benchmark Database (IHCIS) is an insurance claims database provided by Ingenix, Eden Prairie, MN, and the UK General Practice Research Database (GPRD) Gold contains electronic medical records and is managed by the Medicines and Healthcare products Regulatory Agency.

The IHCIS database contains medical (inpatient, outpatient, physician, and ancillary) and pharmacy claims from a national sample of 46 managed care health plans covering approximately 93 million lives over the period 1997 to 2009.

The GPRD Gold is the world's largest computerised database of anonymised longitudinal medical records from primary care (Jick et al., 2003). The data are drawn from the computer systems used by general practitioners (GPs) to maintain the clinical records within their practices, and contain all records that primary care deemed relevant to patient care. Currently, data are available from 561 "research standard" general practices throughout the UK, providing information from 4.0 million currently registered patients (c. 9.0 million in total).

The objectives of the current analyses were: (1) to calculate the prevalence of epilepsy diagnosis in a US and a UK electronic health record system, stratified by gender and age category; (2) to describe and compare the prevalence of co-morbidities, in epilepsy patients and matched controls without any record of epilepsy; and (3) to describe the prevalence of medication use by epilepsy patients during a one-year period of observation.

2. Methods

This study was a case-control study comparing comorbidities between patients with epilepsy and matched controls without epilepsy, and a descriptive study reporting medication use among patients with epilepsy.

2.1 Patient population

2.1.1 Case selection

The definitions of active epilepsy reflected the structure of the databases and how medical and pharmacy data are captured:

In IHCIS, epilepsy cases were identified based on at least two records of epilepsy on or before the index date and with 30 days or more between the first and last record of epilepsy. At least one of the records of epilepsy had to be recorded within the lead-in period to identify individuals with recently active epilepsy. Epilepsy was defined as the ICD-9 code 345*, with * indicating all terms under this hierarchy. AED treatment was not part of the case definition of epilepsy in the IHCIS in order to capture epilepsy patients in the claims database that may not have pharmacy benefits. Also, disease diagnoses are recorded on a regular basis in the insurance claims, therefore a repeat diagnosis could be used to confirm the epilepsy diagnosis.

In the GPRD, epilepsy cases were identified as those with one epilepsy diagnosis (READ) code on or before the index date. The relevant GPRD medical codes were identified and reviewed by a clinician. Within the GPRD, active epilepsy cases were required to have at least 2 anti-epileptic drug (AED) prescriptions within -3 and +6 months of any epilepsy diagnosis code AND at least 1 AED prescription within the lead-in or analysis period. In the GPRD, a diagnosis is often recorded only one time on the database therefore the medications were used as a proxy to confirm the diagnosis and that the diagnosis was still active near the time of the index date.

Full definitions of index date, analysis and lead-in periods are provided in Section Data Analysis.

2.1.2 Control selection

Controls were matched to cases at a ratio of 1:1 by: gender, exact year of birth, duration of prior continuous enrolment in the database (from index date) by the following categories (1-<2 years, 2-<3 years, 3-<4 years, 4 or more years).

For IHCIS specifically, controls were also matched on pharmacy benefits throughout the full analysis period (Yes/No), Mental Health benefits on the index date (Yes/No/Partial), and Provider/Plan Type (on the index date).

For GPRD specifically, the controls were also matched by General Practice site.

2.2 Data analysis

The analysis period was defined as the 12 month period from 01/Jan/2009 to 31/Dec/2009, inclusive. The first day of the analysis period (01/Jan/2009) was assigned as the "index date" for cases and their matched controls. The pre-analysis lead-in period was defined as the 12 month period from 01/Jan/2008 to 31/Dec/2008, inclusive. Thus, the study inclusion period contains all time from 01/Jan/2008 to 31/Dec/2009, inclusive.

A base population was defined containing all patients eligible for this study. This was the denominator for calculations of the population prevalence of epilepsy. All cases and controls were selected from this population.

For inclusion in the base population, a patient must have been:

- registered on the database for the full lead-in period to allow the identification of existing epilepsy patients.
- registered on the database for the full analysis period to allow the characterisation of patients' current medication and comorbidities.
- aged between 0 and 120 years inclusive, on the index date

For the IHCIS, the analyses of medication use were restricted to those cases with full pharmacy benefits throughout the analysis period and no gaps in pharmacy benefit greater than one day during the analysis period.

2.2.1 Analysis 1: prevalence of epilepsy

The prevalence of epilepsy on the index date was determined, by gender and age category, as appropriate. The denominator was taken as all patients within the base population. In IHCIS, the numerator was calculated as all patients (within the denominator population) with two or more records of epilepsy, and 30 days or more between the first and last record of epilepsy. In GPRD, the numerator was calculated as all patients (within the denominator population) with an epilepsy diagnosis prior to the index date, and at least 2 anti-epileptic drug (AED) prescriptions within -3 and +6 months of any epilepsy diagnosis code AND at least 1 AED prescription within the lead-in or analysis period. For both databases, at least one of the diagnoses must be on, or before, the index date.

2.2.2 Analysis 2: listing of comorbidities in epilepsy patients

The prevalence of comorbidities within the epilepsy and control populations was determined. A patient was considered to have a comorbidity if they had one or more records of this condition within the time period being considered. Prevalence of comorbid disease in the epilepsy population was calculated as the number of epilepsy cases with a record of the disease (within the time periods defined below) divided by the total number of epilepsy cases. Prevalence of comorbid diseases in the controls were similarly calculated. Analyses were repeated for two time periods, (1) the analysis period and (2) the analysis period, and any time before, within the period of continuous enrollment.

In GPRD, the comorbidities are listed as defined by disease headings which were based on the Meddra Dictionary and were reviewed by clinicians. A Read/MedDRA (version 13.0) mapping was created using the available Read/MedDRA (version 6) dictionary and the 2010-AB release of the Unified Medical Language System (UMLS). Approximately 41% of events were not mapped, but many of the events remaining unmapped were not of clinical significance. Some of these were mapped by further review of terms.

In IHCIS, comorbidities are reported by Clinical Classifications Software (CCS) level 4 (HCUP, 2011).

In addition, there were a number of conditions previously associated with epilepsy that were specifically explored including: depression, anxiety, bipolar disorder, suicidality, and migraine. These conditions were defined by clinician-reviewed coding lists using GPRD GOLD READ medical codes or ICD-9 codes for IHCIS.

In GPRD, medications are listed as defined by British National formulary (BNF) class, and in IHCIS by Universal System Classification (USC) Fourth Level. The USC is a categorization system, developed by IMS, to resolve a need for therapeutic classification of pharmaceutical products; the USC is widely accepted in North America as the standard for pharmaceutical product classification.

2.2.3 Analysis 3: comparative analyses of the occurrence co-morbidities

The relative prevalence of co-morbidities in epilepsy cases and matched controls was assessed. Unstratified matched analyses were conducted via conditional logistic regression using the SAS Proc PHREG procedure. Stratified analyses were conducted via the Fisher Exact tests using the SAS Proc FREQ procedure. Odds ratios (ORs) and 95% confidence intervals are presented (Note: p-values are not presented). Since these were exploratory (rather than hypothesis testing) analyses, and sample sizes are not based on statistical considerations, there was no adjustment for multiple testing. ORs are only presented where there were at least five patients in both the case and control populations with a record of the comorbidity within the time period being considered. Results are presented for the 25 most frequent comorbidities amongst cases, and for the 25 highest ORs comparing cases and controls.

2.2.4 Analysis 4: listing of prescribed medications used by epilepsy cases during a one-year period of observation

The prevalence of drug use within the analysis period is presented for the epilepsy population. A patient was considered to be using the drug of interest if they were issued a prescription during the analysis period. The prevalence of drug use was calculated as the number of eligible cases with a record of use within the analysis period divided by the total number of eligible cases. Results are presented for cases only, and reported at Universal System Classification Fourth Level.

3. Results

There were 27,328 active epilepsy cases and 27,328 matched controls identified in the UK GPRD, and 83,045 active epilepsy cases and 83,045 controls identified from the IHCIS. Active epilepsy in GPRD was defined if a patient diagnosed with epilepsy had at least one AED prescription within the one-year lead-in or one-year analysis period. Active epilepsy in the IHCIS was defined if the patient had at least one diagnosis code within the lead-in or analysis period. The overall prevalence of active epilepsy was 0.8% in GPRD and 0.5% in IHCIS. The prevalence in GPRD increased with age and was highest in the age group 65 years and older. The prevalence was similar across the age groups in IHCIS with a peak of 0.5% in the age group 45 to 64 years.

The studies within the US claims database (IHCIS) and UK general practice database (GPRD) compared the prevalence of a range of psychiatric conditions including anxiety, bipolar disorder, depression, schizophrenia/psychosis and suicidality (Table 1&Table 2). These psychiatric conditions were significantly more common in epilepsy cases than in controls (OR > 1.0, and lower bound of 95% CI excluding 1.0). The highest ORs were for suicidality, bipolar disorder and schizophrenia. Migraine was also included in the analyses, and it was significantly more common among cases than controls for the time period during or before analysis period. However, the association was not significant for the analysis period only in GPRD, and the associations were stronger in IHCIS than GPRD. Given the chronic nature of these conditions the prevalence was considered both during and prior to the analysis period (i.e. the latter period represented the patients' medical histories).

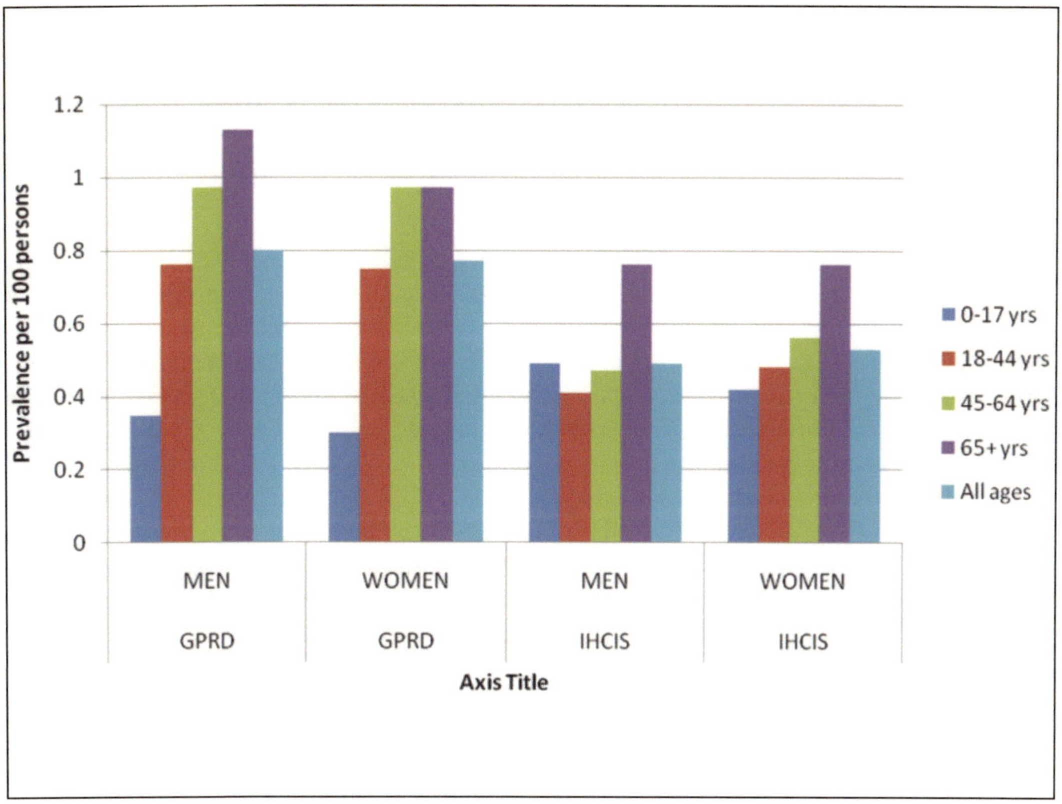

Fig. 1. The prevalence of active epilepsy per 100 persons on 1st January 2009 in the GPRD and IHCIS databases, stratified by age and sex

The top 25 most common diagnosed comorbidities among cases are reported for within the analysis period (Table 3 & Table 7) and within the analysis period or before (Table 4 & Table 8), for GPRD and IHCIS respectively. As expected, the medical condition headings related to epilepsy, seizures and convulsions were at the top of the lists. Other conditions included respiratory infections, skin conditions, and hypertension. The latter conditions were also common in controls.

The top 25 diagnosed comorbidities with the highest ORs comparing cases to controls were reported for the analysis period (Table 5 & Table 9) and within the analysis period or before (Table 6 & Table 10), for GPRD and IHCIS respectively. These listings can be considered for generating hypotheses about the associations between epilepsy and other conditions, though temporality cannot be established.

In the GPRD, mental retardation had a high OR of 24.9 (95%CI: 12.3-50.4) during the analysis period. During the GPRD analysis period, the conditions with the highest ORs included many neurological conditions and behaviour and socialisation disturbances (Table 5). In the GPRD analysis period or ever before, the conditions with the highest ORs also included neurological and developmental conditions, and the highest ORs were 50.7 (95%CI: 28.0-92.1) for "Cerebral disorders congenital", 38.1 (95%CI: 20.9-69.3) for "Congenital and peripartum cerebral disorders", and 33.9 (95%CI: 16.8-68.4) for "Neonatal neurological system disorders NEC" (Table 6).

The highest OR in the IHCIS was for intellectual disabilities, 143.1 (95%CI: 84.6-241.9) during the analysis period, and 79.8 (95%CI: 60.1-106.1) during the analysis period or ever before. The other conditions with high ORs included neurological disorders, cerebrovascular disease, developmental and learning disorders, and mental disorders (Table 9 & Table 10).

Medication use was reported for the analysis year, 2009, for epilepsy cases only (N=27,328 GPRD; N= 46,912 IHCIS). For IHCIS, only individuals with full pharmacy benefits throughout the year 2009 were included in medication analyses. The proportion of patients using anti-depressants and anti-epileptic drugs were reported using clinician-reviewed drug coding lists (Table 11 & Table 13). In the GPRD, 97% of the epilepsy cases had a prescription for an anti-epileptic drug in the analysis period, as expected since AED use either in the lead-in or analysis period was a requirement of the case definition (3% of cases only had AED use in the lead-in period). Eighteen percent of cases had a prescription for anti-depressants in the one-year analysis period. In the IHCIS, 76% of epilepsy patients had a prescription for an AED, and 22% for anti-depressants in 2009. The 24% of epilepsy cases who did not have an AED in the analysis period may either not have had pharmacy benefit, or they were not prescribed an AED in that time period. However, the relative proportions of patients using each type of AED are of interest, and there are differences in the AED use between the UK GPRD and US IHCIS. Two of the older AEDs, valproate (34%) and carbamazepine (32%) were the most frequently used AEDs among epilepsy patients in the GPRD, followed by lamotrigine (18%) and phenytoin (17%). Lamotrigine (15%) and phenytoin (15%) were the most commonly used AEDs in the IHCIS in 2009, followed by carbamazepine (12%) and topiramate (9%).

The top 25 most commonly prescribed medication categories in a one year time period, 2009, are reported for GPRD (Table 12) and IHCIS (Table 14). As in (Table 11), drugs classified as "Control of Epilepsy" were the most commonly prescribed in GPRD (97.3%). Other common medications were neuropathic pain (52.3%), non-opioid analgesics (39.7%), anti-manic drugs (32.4%), non-steroidal anti-inflammatory drugs (30.2%), opioid analgesics (23.8%), broad spectrum penicillins (21.1%), and statins (20.2%). In the IHCIS, 74% of epilepsy patients had a prescription in the "Seizure disorders" drug category during 2009. The other frequently prescribed medications were codeine (23%), extended spectrum macroli (19%), benzodiazepines (17%), and selective serotonin reuptake inhibitors (SSRI, 15%).

Comorbidity	GPRD					IHCIS				
	Number Cases	Percent Cases	Number Controls	Percent Controls	Odds Ratio (95% CI)	Number Cases	Percent Cases	Number Controls	Percent Controls	Odds Ratio (95% CI)
Anxiety	750	2.74	677	2.48	1.1 (1, 1.2)	9354	11.26	5062	6.1	2.0 (1.9, 2.1)
Bipolar Disorder	26	0.1	7	0.03	3.7 (1.6, 8.6)	2029	2.44	510	0.61	4.1 (3.7, 4.5)
Depression	1207	4.42	1034	3.78	1.2 (1.1, 1.3)	9696	11.68	4163	5.01	2.6 (2.5, 2.7)
Migraine	188	0.69	173	0.63	1.1 (0.9, 1.3)	5806	6.99	1556	1.87	4.1 (3.9, 4.4)
Schizophrenia (GPRD)/ Psychosis (IHCIS)	20	0.07	5	0.02	4.0 (1.5, 10.7)	2215	2.67	359	0.43	6.5 (5.8, 7.3)
Suicidality	76	0.28	20	0.07	3.8 (2.3, 6.2)	1389	1.67	252	0.3	5.6 (4.9, 6.4)

Suicidality = Suicide attempts, probable suicide attempts and suicidal ideation
CI= Confidence interval; GPRD= General Practice Research Database; IHCIS= Integrated Healthcare Information Services

Table 1. Prevalence and odds ratios for the comorbidities of interest comparing cases (N=27,328 GPRD; N=83,045 IHCIS) and controls (N=27,328 GPRD; N=83,045 IHCIS) during the analysis period

Comorbidity	GPRD					IHCIS				
	Number Cases	Percent Cases	Number Controls	Percent Controls	Odds Ratio (95% CI)	Number Cases	Percent Cases	Number Controls	Percent Controls	Odds Ratio (95% CI)
Anxiety	5858	21.44	4544	16.63	1.4 (1.3, 1.5)	21214	25.55	11965	14.41	2.1 (2.1, 2.2)
Bipolar Disorder	217	0.79	97	0.35	2.3 (1.8, 2.9)	3829	4.61	945	1.14	4.2 (3.9, 4.6)
Depression	7988	29.23	6196	22.67	1.5 (1.4, 1.5)	19762	23.8	9342	11.25	2.6 (2.5, 2.7)
Migraine	2378	8.70	1841	6.74	1.3 (1.3, 1.4)	13557	16.32	4490	5.41	3.7 (3.6, 3.8)
Schizophrenia (GPRD)/ Psychosis (IHCIS)	299	1.09	108	0.40	2.8 (2.3, 3.6)	7299	8.79	908	1.09	9.7 (9.0, 10.4)
Suicidality	1011	3.70	378	1.38	2.8 (2.5, 3.1)	4877	5.87	931	1.12	5.5 (5.2, 6.0)

Suicidality = Suicide attempts, probable suicide attempts and suicidal ideation
CI= Confidence interval; GPRD= General Practice Research Database; IHCIS= Integrated Healthcare Information Services

Table 2. Prevalence and odds ratios for the comorbidities of interest comparing cases (N=27,328 GPRD; N=83,045 IHCIS) and controls (N=27,328 GPRD; N=83,045 IHCIS) during or ever before the analysis period

Comorbidity	Number Cases	Percent Cases	Number Controls	Percent Controls	Odds Ratio (95% CI)
Social issues	4276	15.65	3527	12.91	1.29 (1.23, 1.36)
Musculoskeletal and connective tissue pain and discomfort	3751	13.73	3196	11.69	1.21 (1.15, 1.27)
Coughing and associated symptoms	3607	13.20	2728	9.98	1.39 (1.32, 1.47)
Upper respiratory tract infections NEC	3112	11.39	2693	9.85	1.18 (1.12, 1.25)
Upper respiratory tract infections	3111	11.38	2693	9.85	1.18 (1.12, 1.25)
Joint related signs and symptoms	2826	10.34	2405	8.80	1.20 (1.13, 1.28)
Seizures and seizure disorders NEC	2638	9.65	11	0.04	292.77 (152.18,563.22)
Dietary and nutritional therapies	2441	8.93	1977	7.23	1.32 (1.23, 1.41)
General signs and symptoms NEC	2313	8.46	1482	5.42	1.65 (1.54, 1.77)
Reproductive organ and breast histopathology procedures	2262	8.28	2499	9.14	0.87 (0.81, 0.93)
Lower respiratory tract and lung infections	1946	7.12	1138	4.16	1.80 (1.67, 1.95)
Lower respiratory tract infections NEC	1936	7.08	1125	4.12	1.82 (1.68, 1.96)
Non-site specific injuries NEC	1548	5.66	876	3.21	1.83 (1.68, 2.00)
Pain and discomfort NEC	1450	5.31	1116	4.08	1.32 (1.22, 1.44)
Bronchospasm and obstruction	1444	5.28	1128	4.13	1.30 (1.20, 1.41)
Neurological signs and symptoms NEC	1429	5.23	764	2.80	1.96 (1.79, 2.14)
Dermatitis and eczema	1400	5.12	1076	3.94	1.32 (1.22, 1.43)
Urinary tract infections	1349	4.94	754	2.76	1.88 (1.71, 2.07)
Asthenic conditions	1343	4.91	862	3.15	1.61 (1.47, 1.75)
Gastrointestinal and abdominal pains (excl oral and throat)	1318	4.82	1092	4,00	1.22 (1.12, 1.32)
Vascular hypertensive disorders NEC	1207	4.42	1381	5.05	0.86 (0.79, 0.93)
Oral soft tissue infections	1174	4.30	973	3.56	1.22 (1.12, 1.33)
Bladder and urethral symptoms	1135	4.15	683	2.50	1.70 (1.54, 1.88)
Gastrointestinal atonic and hypomotility disorders NEC	1128	4.13	598	2.19	1.95 (1.76, 2.16)
Headaches NEC	1079	3.95	751	2.75	1.46 (1.33, 1.61)

CI= Confidence Interval; GPRD= General Practice Research Database, NEC= Not elsewhere classified

Table 3. Prevalence and odds ratios for the top 25 most common comorbidities comparing cases and controls during the analysis period in the GPRD

Comorbidity	Number Cases	Percent Cases	Number Controls	Percent Controls	Odds Ratio (95% CI)
Seizures and seizure disorders NEC	26225	95.96	279	1.02	3707.51 (1767.33, 7777.61)
Social issues	17790	65.10	16830	61.59	1.23 (1.18, 1.28)
Upper respiratory tract infections NEC	16529	60.48	15504	56.73	1.20 (1.16, 1.24)
Upper respiratory tract infections	16529	60.48	15504	56.73	1.20 (1.16, 1.24)
Musculoskeletal and connective tissue pain and discomfort	15299	55.98	14339	52.47	1.18 (1.14, 1.22)
Coughing and associated symptoms	13657	49.97	11438	41.85	1.43 (1.38, 1.49)
General signs and symptoms NEC	12478	45.66	8900	32.57	1.96 (1.89, 2.04)
Joint related signs and symptoms	12153	44.47	10691	39.12	1.29 (1.24, 1.34)
Dietary and nutritional therapies	11088	40.57	10941	40.04	1.04 (0.99, 1.08)
Non-site specific injuries NEC	10949	40.07	7931	29.02	1.71 (1.64, 1.77)
Dermatitis and eczema	10442	38.21	8736	31.97	1.35 (1.30, 1.40)
Lower respiratory tract and lung infections	10357	37.90	7734	28.30	1.63 (1.57, 1.69)
Lower respiratory tract infections NEC	10326	37.79	7709	28.21	1.63 (1.57, 1.69)
Reproductive organ and breast histopathology procedures	9986	36.54	10502	38.43	0.66 (0.61, 0.72)
Pain and discomfort NEC	8849	32.38	7585	27.76	1.29 (1.24, 1.34)
Oral soft tissue infections	8693	31.81	8108	29.67	1.12 (1.08, 1.16)
Gastrointestinal and abdominal pains (excl oral and throat)	8637	31.60	7805	28.56	1.17 (1.13, 1.21)
Asthenic conditions	8219	30.08	5825	21.32	1.66 (1.59, 1.73)
Neurological signs and symptoms NEC	7933	29.03	4404	16.12	2.30 (2.19, 2.40)
Skin structures and soft tissue infections	7823	28.63	5654	20.69	1.58 (1.52, 1.64)
Headaches NEC	7733	28.30	5677	20.77	1.56 (1.49, 1.62)
Cardiac signs and symptoms NEC	7544	27.61	5307	19.42	1.67 (1.60, 1.74)
Allergies to foods, food additives, drugs and other chemicals	7499	27.44	6002	21.96	1.38 (1.33, 1.44)
Depressive disorders	7177	26.26	5660	20.71	1.41 (1.35, 1.47)
Urinary tract infections	7098	25.97	5133	18.78	1.63 (1.56, 1.70)

CI= Confidence Interval; GPRD= General Practice Research Database, NEC= Not elsewhere classified

Table 4. Prevalence and odds ratios for the top 25 most common comorbidities comparing cases and controls during or before the analysis period in the GPRD

Comorbidity	Number Cases	Percent Cases	Number Controls	Percent Controls	Odds Ratio (95% CI)
Seizures and seizure disorders NEC	2638	9.65	11	0.04	292.77 (152.18, 563.22)
Mental retardations	199	0.73	8	0.03	24.87 (12.27, 50.43)
Withdrawal and rebound effects	46	0.17	5	0.02	9.15 (3.64, 22.99)
Disability issues	277	1.01	33	0.12	9.13 (6.27, 13.31)
Abnormal behaviour NEC	47	0.17	6	0.02	7.81 (3.34, 18.26)
Sodium imbalance	156	0.57	20	0.07	7.78 (4.89, 12.39)
Pervasive developmental disorders NEC	44	0.16	6	0.02	7.32 (3.12, 17.17)
Behaviour and socialisation disturbances	197	0.72	29	0.11	6.79 (4.60, 10.02)
Calcium metabolism disorders	35	0.13	6	0.02	6.79 (2.66, 17.36)
Cerebellar coordination and balance disturbances	50	0.18	8	0.03	6.25 (2.96, 13.17)
Therapeutic bladder catheterisation	109	0.40	20	0.07	5.94 (3.61, 9.79)
Lower respiratory tract inflammatory and immunologic conditions	35	0.13	6	0.02	5.83 (2.45, 13.86)
Nervous system therapeutic procedures NEC	66	0.24	12	0.04	5.50 (2.97, 10.17)
Salivary gland disorders NEC	49	0.18	9	0.03	5.44 (2.67, 11.08)
Confusion and disorientation	179	0.66	38	0.14	4.81 (3.38, 6.85)
Cortical dysfunction NEC	199	0.73	43	0.16	4.80 (3.43, 6.73)
Thoracic cage fractures non-spinal (excl pathological)	32	0.12	7	0.03	4.57 (2.02, 10.36)
Thoracic cage fractures and dislocations	32	0.12	7	0.03	4.57 (2.02, 10.36)
Schizophrenia NEC	22	0.08	5	0.02	4.40 (1.67, 11.62)
Bipolar disorders	26	0.10	6	0.02	4.33 (1.78, 10.53)
Psychiatric elimination disorders	42	0.15	10	0.04	4.20 (2.11, 8.37)
Tremor (excl congenital)	223	0.82	57	0.21	3.91 (2.92, 5.23)
Nervous system haemorrhagic disorders	31	0.11	8	0.03	3.87 (1.78, 8.43)
Delusional symptoms	23	0.08	6	0.02	3.83 (1.56, 9.41)
Drug withdrawal therapies	33	0.12	9	0.03	3.67 (1.75, 7.66)

CI= Confidence Interval; GPRD= General Practice Research Database, NEC= Not elsewhere classified

Table 5. Prevalence and odds ratios for the 25 comorbidities with the highest odds ratios comparing cases and controls during the analysis period in the GPRD

Comorbidity	Number Cases	Percent Cases	Number Controls	Percent Controls	Odds Ratio (95% CI)
Seizures and seizure disorders NEC	26225	95.96	279	1.02	3707.51 (1767.33, 7777.61)
Cerebral disorders congenital	559	2.05	11	0.04	50.74 (27.95, 92.11)
Congenital and peripartum cerebral disorders	419	1.53	11	0.04	38.08 (20.93, 69.29)
Neonatal neurological system disorders NEC	271	0.99	8	0.03	33.87 (16.77, 68.42)
Nervous system neoplasms unspecified malignancy NEC	365	1.34	11	0.04	33.18 (18.21, 60.44)
Meningiomas benign	240	0.88	11	0.04	21.75 (11.90, 39.77)
Hydrocephalic conditions	345	1.26	18	0.07	20.19 (12.41, 32.85)
Mental retardations	1342	4.91	87	0.32	19.16 (15.04, 24.40)
Traumatic central nervous system haemorrhages	191	0.70	13	0.05	14.69 (8.38, 25.76)
Cerebrovascular embolism and thrombosis	59	0.22	5	0.02	14.50 (5.26, 39.92)
Developmental disorders cognitive	377	1.38	28	0.10	14.42 (9.69, 21.45)
Vascular anomalies congenital NEC	171	0.63	12	0.04	14.25 (7.93, 25.58)
Leukopenias NEC	69	0.25	5	0.02	13.80 (5.57, 34.19)
Paralysis and paresis (excl cranial nerve)	1458	5.34	114	0.42	13.80 (11.32, 16.82)
Encephalopathies NEC	154	0.56	12	0.04	12.83 (7.13, 23.09)
Congenital eye disorders NEC	137	0.50	11	0.04	12.45 (6.74, 23.02)
Disability issues	2277	8.33	212	0.78	12.28 (10.56, 14.28)
Pervasive developmental disorders NEC	495	1.81	44	0.16	12.27 (8.89, 16.94)
Nervous system haemorrhagic disorders	977	3.58	85	0.31	12.01 (9.58, 15.07)
Anterior pituitary hypofunction	86	0.31	8	0.03	10.75 (5.21, 22.18)
Cerebrovascular aneurysms and dissections	75	0.27	7	0.03	10.71 (4.94, 23.25)
Behaviour and socialisation disturbances	2575	9.42	308	1.13	9.52 (8.39, 10.80)
Inborn errors of amino acid metabolism	73	0.27	14	0.05	9.43 (4.33, 20.55)
Antidiuretic hormone related conditions	71	0.26	8	0.03	8.84 (4.26, 18.33)
Central nervous system aneurysms	61	0.22	7	0.03	8.68 (3.97, 18.95)

CI= Confidence Interval; GPRD= General Practice Research Database, NEC= Not elsewhere classified

Table 6. Prevalence and odds ratios for the 25 comorbidities with the highest odds ratios comparing cases and controls during or before the analysis period in the GPRD

Comorbidity	Number Cases	Percent Cases	Number Controls	Percent Controls	Odds Ratio (95% CI)
Epilepsy	45635	54.95	0	0	NA
Convulsions	41078	49.46	9	0.01	13688.40 (4415.0,42439.7)
Other connective tissue disease	25108	30.23	16519	19.89	1.80 (1.8,1.9)
Essential hypertension	24367	29.34	19961	24.04	1.50 (1.4,1.5)
Immunizations and screening for infectious disease	23827	28.69	20398	24.56	1.30 (1.2,1.3)
Disorders of lipid metabolism	23526	28.33	21045	25.34	1.20 (1.2,1.3)
Other and unspecified lower respiratory disease	20413	24.58	12854	15.48	1.80 (1.8,1.9)
Symptoms, signs and ill-defined conditions	20263	24.40	9946	11.98	2.50 (2.4,2.6)
Other non-traumatic joint disorders	18437	22.20	12774	15.38	1.60 (1.6,1.6)
Other skin disorders	18071	21.76	14957	18.01	1.30 (1.3,1.3)
Other and unspecified upper respiratory infections	17051	20.53	14692	17.69	1.20 (1.2,1.3)
Other nervous system symptoms and disorders	15474	18.63	4413	5.31	4.20 (4.1,4.4)
Malaise and fatigue	13586	16.36	7983	9.61	1.90 (1.8,1.9)
Other upper respiratory disease	12762	15.37	9794	11.79	1.40 (1.3,1.4)
Abdominal pain	11910	14.34	7637	9.20	1.70 (1.6,1.7)
Other eye disorders	11335	13.65	8142	9.80	1.50 (1.4,1.5)
Other injuries and conditions due to external causes	11228	13.52	4945	5.95	2.50 (2.4,2.6)
Depressive disorders	10907	13.13	4801	5.78	2.50 (2.4,2.6)
Other central nervous system disorders	10826	13.04	2403	2.89	5.10 (4.9,5.4)
Nonspecific chest pain	10769	12.97	6747	8.12	1.70 (1.7,1.8)
Acute upper respiratory infections of multiple or unspecified sites	10722	12.91	8206	9.88	1.40 (1.3,1.4)
Other headache	10462	12.60	4132	4.98	2.80 (2.7,2.9)
Other and unspecified gastrointestinal disorders	10127	12.19	5516	6.64	2.00 (1.9,2.0)
Other bone disease and musculoskeletal deformities	9909	11.93	7073	8.52	1.50 (1.4,1.5)
Other thyroid disorders	9886	11.90	6979	8.40	1.50 (1.5,1.6)

CI= Confidence interval; IHCIS= Integrated Healthcare Information Services

Table 7. Prevalence and odds ratios for the top 25 most common comorbidities comparing cases and controls during the analysis period in the IHCIS

Comorbidity	Number Cases	Percent Cases	Number Controls	Percent Controls	Odds Ratio (95% CI)
Convulsions	76929	92.64	58	0.07	76870.30 (10828.3,545702.2)
Epilepsy	69782	84.03	0	0	NA
Other connective tissue disease	50298	60.57	36898	44.43	2.10 (2.1,2.2)
Other and unspecified lower respiratory disease	46270	55.72	31447	37.87	2.20 (2.2,2.2)
Other non-traumatic joint disorders	42216	50.84	31641	38.10	1.80 (1.8,1.8)
Other skin disorders	41651	50.15	34760	41.86	1.40 (1.4,1.5)
Other and unspecified upper respiratory infections	41109	49.50	36734	44.23	1.30 (1.3,1.3)
Other nervous system symptoms and disorders	37912	45.65	11592	13.96	5.70 (5.5,5.9)
Disorders of lipid metabolism	37001	44.56	32157	38.72	1.40 (1.4,1.5)
Malaise and fatigue	35255	42.45	21419	25.79	2.30 (2.3,2.4)
Essential hypertension	33858	40.77	27249	32.81	1.70 (1.7,1.8)
Other upper respiratory disease	33727	40.61	26344	31.72	1.50(1.5,1.5)
Abdominal pain	32829	39.53	23175	27.91	1.70 (1.7,1.8)
Other injuries and conditions due to external causes	32800	39.50	16637	20.03	2.70 (2.7,2.8)
Nonspecific chest pain	31341	37.74	20177	24.30	2.10 (2.0,2.1)
Acute upper respiratory infections of multiple or unspecified sites	30716	36.99	24805	29.87	1.40 (1.4,1.5)
Other headache	30126	36.28	13070	15.74	3.20 (3.1,3.3)
Allergic reactions	28909	34.81	22971	27.66	1.40 (1.4,1.5)
Other eye disorders	28567	34.40	21219	25.55	1.60 (1.6,1.6)
Other and unspecified gastrointestinal disorders	27635	33.28	17061	20.54	2.00 (2.0,2.1)
Superficial injury; contusion	26869	32.35	15552	18.73	2.10 (2.1,2.2)
Other ear and sense organ disorders	26352	31.73	18559	22.35	1.70 (1.6,1.7)
Other and unspecified circulatory disease	25911	31.20	15087	18.17	2.30 (2.2,2.4)
Other central nervous system disorders	25633	30.87	4591	5.53	7.80 (7.5,8.1)
Sprains and strains	25339	30.51	20144	24.26	1.40 (1.4,1.4)

CI= Confidence interval; IHCIS= Integrated Healthcare Information Services

Table 8. Prevalence and odds ratios for the top 25 most common comorbidities comparing cases and controls during or before the analysis period in the IHCIS

Comorbidity	Number Cases	Percent Cases	Number Controls	Percent Controls	Odds Ratio (95% CI)
Convulsions	41078	49.46	9	0.01	13688.40 (4415.0,42439.7)
Intellectual disabilities	2010	2.42	17	0.02	143.10 (84.6,241.9)
Cancer of brain and nervous system	1705	2.05	43	0.05	39.60 (29.3,53.6)
Developmental disabilities	1312	1.58	45	0.05	36.20 (26.0,50.4)
Other paralysis	3942	4.75	116	0.14	34.90 (28.9,42.0)
Congenital hip dislocation	217	0.26	9	0.01	26.80 (13.3,54.1)
Other nervous system congenital anomalies	864	1.04	34	0.04	25.40 (18.0,35.8)
Learning disorders	1792	2.16	88	0.11	22.30 (17.8,27.9)
Cerebrovascular anomalies	431	0.52	20	0.02	21.50 (13.7,33.6)
Hemiplegia	1724	2.08	92	0.11	19.30 (15.6,23.9)
Motor skill disorders	304	0.37	17	0.02	18.90 (11.4,31.3)
Encephalitis (except that caused by TB or STD)	340	0.41	19	0.02	17.90 (11.3,28.4)
Benign neoplasm of cerebral meninges	712	0.86	43	0.05	16.90 (12.4,23.1)
Pervasive developmental disorders	1979	2.38	140	0.17	15.40 (12.9,18.4)
Intrauterine hypoxia and birth asphyxia	72	0.09	5	0.01	14.40 (5.8,35.6)
Intracranial hemorrhage	1237	1.49	92	0.11	13.90 (11.2,17.2)
Respiratory distress syndrome	65	0.08	5	0.01	13.00(5.2,32.3)
Congenital anomalies of skull and facial bones	150	0.18	13	0.02	11.50 (6.6,20.3)
Aspiration pneumonitis; food/vomitus	952	1.15	85	0.10	11.30 (9.1,14.2)
Spina bifida	215	0.26	20	0.02	10.80 (6.8,17.0)
Congenital hip deformity	211	0.25	20	0.02	10.60 (6.7,16.7)
Occlusion of cerebral arteries	4102	4.94	456	0.55	9.90 (9.0,11.0)
Late effects of cerebrovascular disease	3354	4.04	375	0.45	9.80 (8.8,11.0)
Other dependence on machines	59	0.07	6	0.01	9.80 (4.2,22.6)
Acute but ill-defined cerebrovascular accident	3526	4.25	437	0.53	9.20 (8.3,10.3)

CI= Confidence interval; IHCIS= Integrated Healthcare Information Services

Table 9. Prevalence and odds ratios for the 25 comorbidities with the highest odds ratios comparing cases and controls during the analysis period in the IHCIS

Comorbidity	Number Cases	Percent Cases	Number Controls	Percent Controls	Odds Ratio (95% CI)
Convulsions	76929	92.64	58	0.07	76870.30 (10828.3,545702.2)
Intellectual disabilities	3836	4.62	52	0.06	79.80 (60.1,106.1)
Microcephalus	818	0.99	12	0.01	67.80 (38.4,119.6)
Congenital hydrocephalus	780	0.94	17	0.02	45.80 (28.4,74.1)
Cancer of brain and nervous system	3219	3.88	121	0.15	27.70 (23.0,33.3)
Developmental disabilities	3129	3.77	153	0.18	24.80 (20.8,29.7)
Other nervous system congenital anomalies	2545	3.06	119	0.14	22.50 (18.6,27.1)
Other paralysis	6590	7.94	315	0.38	22.30 (19.8,25.0)
Hemiplegia	4776	5.75	285	0.34	18.30 (16.2,20.8)
Cerebrovascular anomalies	1506	1.81	87	0.10	17.50 (14.1,21.7)
Intracranial hemorrhage	4660	5.61	307	0.37	17.30 (15.3,19.6)
Learning disorders	4539	5.47	324	0.39	17.10 (15.1,19.4)
Benign neoplasm of cerebral meninges	1530	1.84	98	0.12	16.10 (13.1,19.8)
Coma; stupor; and brain damage	20114	24.22	1715	2.07	16.10 (15.2,17.0)
Encephalitis (except that caused by TB or STD)	1264	1.52	80	0.10	16.00 (12.7,20.1)
Motor skill disorders	1047	1.26	79	0.10	14.60 (11.5,18.6)
Pervasive developmental disorders	2978	3.59	251	0.30	13.70 (12.0,15.8)
Aspiration pneumonitis; food/vomitus	2675	3.22	218	0.26	12.90 (11.2,14.9)
Occlusion of cerebral arteries	11582	13.95	1286	1.55	12.40 (11.6,13.3)
Secondary malignancy of brain/spine	619	0.75	52	0.06	12.30 (9.3,16.5)
Congenital hip dislocation	569	0.69	49	0.06	12.10(9.0,16.2)
Mental disorders due to general medical conditions not elsewhere classified	2139	2.58	192	0.23	11.60 (10.0,13.5)
Dissociative disorders	185	0.22	16	0.02	11.60 (6.9,19.3)
Acute but ill-defined cerebrovascular accident	9617	11.58	1233	1.48	11.00 (10.3,11.9)
Late effects of cerebrovascular disease	7766	9.35	967	1.16	9.80 (9.1,10.6)

CI= Confidence interval; IHCIS= Integrated Healthcare Information Services

Table 10. Prevalence and odds ratios for the 25 comorbidities with the highest odds ratios comparing cases and controls during or before the analysis period in the IHCIS

Drug	N (%)
Anti-Epileptic Drugs	26584 (97.3)
Anti-depressants	4806 (17.6)
Valproic acid	9293 (34.0)
Carbamazepine	8776 (32.1)
Lamotrigine	5020 (18.4)
Phenytoin	4757 (17.4)
Levetiracetam	2977 (10.9)
Phenobarbital	1645 (6.02)
Clobazam	1161 (4.3)
Topiramate	1133 (4.2)
Gabapentin	784 (2.9)
Clonazepam	733 (2.7)
Primidone	570 (2.1)
Pregabalin	507 (1.9)

GPRD= General Practice Research Database. Note: the following anti-epileptic drugs were prescribed to <1% of the patients with epilepsy: zonisamide, oxcarbazepine, ethosuximide, lacosamide, vigabitrin, acetazolamide, rufinamide, tiagabine hydrochloride, paraldehyde, stiripentol, sultiame or mesuximide. No patients were prescribed beclamide, dipotassium clorazepate, eslicarbazepine acetate, or fosphenytoin sodium.

Table 11. Prevalence of use of anti-convulsants and anti-depressants in epilepsy patients during the one-year period of observation from 01 Jan 2009 to 31 Dec 2009 in GPRD

Drug Category	N (%)
Control of epilepsy	26595 (97.3)
Neuropathic pain	14297 (52.3)
Non-opioid analgesics	10861 (39.7)
Antimanic drugs	8859 (32.4)
Non-steroidal anti-inflammatory drugs	8249 (30.2)
Opioid analgesics	6516 (23.8)
Broad-spectrum penicillins	5763 (21.1)
Statins	5530 (20.2)
Urinary-tract infections	5308 (19.4)
Proton pump inhibitors	5244 (19.2)
Topical corticosteroids	4856 (17.8)
Antiplatelet drugs	4587 (16.8)
Selective beta-2-agonists	3983 (14.6)
Anxiolytics	3684 (13.5)
Emollient skin preparations	3535 (12.9)
Osmotic laxatives	3362 (12.3)
Hypnotics	3345 (12.2)
Angiotensin-converting enzyme inhibitors	3274 (12.0)
Skeletal muscle relaxants	3064 (11.2)
Anxiolytics and neuroleptics (in anaesthesia)	3041 (11.1)
Selective serotonin re-uptake inhibitors	2886 (10.6)
Prophylaxis of migraine	2863 (10.5)
Corticosteroids (inhaled for respiratory conditions)	2859 (10.5)
Beta-adrenoceptor blocking drugs	2819 (10.3)
Drugs used in nausea and vertigo	2747 (10.1)

BNF= British National Formulary; GPRD= General Practice Research Database

Table 12. Prevalence of use of the top 25 most frequent medications in epilepsy patients during the one-year period of observation from 01 Jan 2009 to 31 Dec 2009, by BNF Category in GPRD

Drug	N (%)
Anti-depressants	10378 (22.1)
Anticonvulsants- antiepileptics	35543 (75.8)
Lamotrigine	7157 (15.3)
Phenytoin	6877 (14.7)
Carbamazepine	5549 (11.8)
Topiramate	3976 (8.5)
Clonazepam	2973 (6.3)
Gabapentin	2279 (4.9)
Phenobarbital	2070 (4.4)
Valproate	503 (1.1)
Ethosuximide	428 (0.9)
Methsuximide	16 (0.03)

IHCIS= Integrated Healthcare Information Services

Table 13. Prevalence of use of anti-convulsants and anti-depressants in epilepsy patients during the one-year period of observation from 01 Jan 2009 to 31 Dec 2009 in IHCIS

Drug Category	N (%)
Seizure disorders	34723 (74.0)
Codeine & Comb, Non-Inj	10742 (22.9)
Extended spectrum macroli	8784 (18.7)
Benzodiazepines	7715 (16.5)
SSRI	7037 (15.0)
HMG-COA reductase inhibitors	6693 (14.3)
Aminopenicillins	6304 (13.4)
Hormones, Cort plain, oral	5941 (12.7)
Cephalosporins & related	5829 (12.4)
Proton pump inhibitors	5642 (12.0)
Anti-arthritis, plain	5627 (12.0)
Quinolones, systemic	5525 (11.8)
Beta blockers	4332 (9.2)
Steroid, inhaled nasal	4244 (9.1)
B-lactam, increased activity	4212 (9.0)
Mus relx, non-surg,W/O ANA	4150 (8.9)
Hormones,Cort plain, derm	3732 (8.0)
Thyroid hormone, synth	3616 (7.7)
ACE Inhib, alone	3579 (7.6)
Beta agonists, aerosol	3522 (7.5)
Antivirals, other	3482 (7.4)
Sulfa & Trimeth comb	3020 (6.4)
Calcium blockers	2690 (5.7)
Antipsychotics, other	2638 (5.6)
Analeptics	2493 (5.3)

Table 14. Prevalence of use of the top 25 most frequent medications in epilepsy patients during the one-year period of observation from 01 Jan 2009 to 31 Dec 2009, by Universal System Classification Fourth Level in IHCIS

4. Discussion

Electronic medical record systems provide an opportunity to identify treatment patterns and comorbidities in a large diagnosed disease population. They also allow for comparisons between the relative prevalence estimates of various comorbidities within the same data source. The comorbidities were ranked by how prevalent they were in epilepsy cases, and then by the ORs comparing cases to controls. The conditions with the highest ORs have the strongest associations with epilepsy compared to matched controls, therefore these findings may be hypothesis-generating for conditions related to epilepsy, though temporality cannot be established in this cross-sectional study. For instance, these can be tested as risk factors for epilepsy; conversely, epilepsy can be examined as a risk factor for these associated conditions.

The definition of both cases and controls requires that patients are registered throughout the full lead-in and analysis periods. The lead-in period is used to identify existing epilepsy patients to ensure that all cases have epilepsy prior to the start of the observation period. This ensures that patients are "at risk" of receiving management for epilepsy throughout the observation period when the patient's status is being assessed. This cross sectional approach, based on a set calendar index date, means there is no restriction of the duration of epilepsy prior to the start of observation, and the population is likely to contain both prevalent and newly-diagnosed epilepsy cases. The use of an index date tied to an individual patient (such as their first diagnosis on a database) is another possible approach, which is more tailored incident cases (or patients at an earlier stage of the disease) and historical rather than recent management patterns.

Diagnosed prevalence rates were similar in a US insurance claims database (0.5%) and a UK general practice-based electronic medical record system (0.8%), although peak age prevalence differed, likely based on the patient populations covered by these systems. The IHCIS system under-represents the elderly population, because it mainly consists of the employed, insured population. These prevalence estimates are similar to those reported in the literature for studies with records-based methodology, ranging from 3 to 8 per 1000 persons (Banerjee et al., 2009).

Many diagnosed comorbidities, including psychiatric and neurological comorbidities, were more prevalent in the patients with epilepsy compared to matched controls. A previous study in the GPRD also reported that many conditions were associated with epilepsy (Gaitatzis, 2004). The current study supports the evidence that the burden of epilepsy along with its comorbidities is high compared to the general population.

Major depression is a common co-morbidity of epilepsy with at least 20% of epilepsy patients experiencing mild to severe depressive symptoms (O'Donoghue et al., 1999; Mendez et al., 1986; Hermann et al., 1986; Baker et al., 1996; Cramer et al., 2004; Jacoby et al., 1996; Boylan et al., 2004; Beghi et al., 2002). In the current study, 29% of patients with epilepsy in the GPRD (OR= 1.5, 95%CI: 1.4-1.5), and 24% of patients with epilepsy in the IHCIS (OR=2.6, 95%CI: 2.5-2.7) had a diagnosis of depression in the analysis period or before. Studies using structured psychiatric interviews in epilepsy clinics, likely to represent more severe epilepsy patients, have reported a prevalence of major depression of up to 55% (Mendez et al., 1996). However, the cross-sectional nature of most studies prevents inferences concerning the temporal order of disease development. When longitudinal analyses have been completed a history of major depression has been associated with an increased risk for incident epilepsy and first unprovoked seizure (Nilsson et al., 2003; Forsgren & Nystrom 1990; Hesdorffer et al., 2006; Hesdorffer et al., 2000).

Certain epilepsy types may be at increased risk of depression: the mean estimated lifetime prevalence of depression is 30% for patients with temporal lobe epilepsy and refractory epilepsy with corresponding risks in the general population of between 6% and 17% (Glosser et al., 2000). Studies have consistently identified co-morbid depression as a powerful predictor of poor health related quality of life in epilepsy patients even after adjustment for seizure frequency and severity (Kanner, 2009). Depression is also a strong predictor for increased suicidality among epilepsy patients (Kanner, 2009).

The prevalence of anxiety disorders is consistently higher (approximately twofold increased risk) among epilepsy patients than the general population. In the current study, 21% of patients with epilepsy in the GPRD (OR= 1.4, 95%CI: 1.3-1.5), and 26% of patients with epilepsy in the IHCIS (OR=2.1, 95%CI: 2.1-2.2) had a diagnosis of anxiety in the analysis period or before. Studies using a range of disease measurement scales, and capturing patients mainly through cross sectional health surveys, have reported point prevalence estimates in epilepsy patients of 11% to 39% (Gaitatzis et al., 2004; Tellez-Zenteno et al., 2007; Edeh & Toone, 1987; Stirne et al., 2005; Kobau et al., 2006). The variation is likely to reflect the selection of different subsets of the epilepsy population with higher prevalence estimates observed among patients with temporal lobe epilepsy.

The prevalence of psychoses in epilepsy, as reported from population-based studies, ranges from 2% to 7% (Gaitatzis et al., 2004). The prevalence varies by epilepsy type with estimates of 10% to 19% reported among individuals with temporal lobe epilepsy, nearly double the risk associated with generalised epilepsy, though larger differences have been reported in older studies (Gaitatzis et al., 2004; Shukla et al., 1979). Gender differences have also been reported with females at an increased risk of psychoses. An Icelandic study reported 6% prevalence in males with epilepsy versus 9% in females (Gudmundsson, 1966). In the current study, 9% of patients with epilepsy in the IHCIS (OR=9.7, 95%CI: 9.0-10.4) had a diagnosis of psychosis in the analysis period or before.

The incidence of psychoses is reported to be 3 to 12 times higher in epilepsy patients than the general population. The range again depends on the epilepsy population sampled (seizure type and severity) as well as the instrument used to diagnose psychosis (Bredkjaer et al., 1998; Torta & Keller, 1999). Patients undergoing epilepsy surgery are at particular risk of developing psychoses for the first time. Interictal psychoses can develop in 3% to 12% of patients following anterior temporal lobectomy and seizure-related psychoses can affect 1% to 13% of patients (Gaitatzis et al., 2004; Gaitatzis et al., 2004 (2)).

Studies concentrating solely on schizophrenia have reported prevalence estimates of 4% to 18% among patients with epilepsy (the majority suffering from temporal lobe epilepsy) (Gaitatzis et al., 2004; Gaitatzis et al., 2004 (2)). The expected prevalence of schizophrenia in the general population is 1% (Toone, 2000). Patients with schizophrenia are also at an increased risk of seizures related to the condition itself and to exposure to psychotropic medications that lower seizure threshold (e.g. clozapine) (Torta & Keller, 1999). In the current study, 1% of patients with epilepsy in the GPRD (OR=2.8, 95%CI: 2.5-3.1) had a diagnosis of schizophrenia in the analysis period or before.

Suicide is a much discussed cause of death in epilepsy patients, especially with the recent analysis by the US Food and Drug Administration in 2008 that showed an association between AEDs and suicidality in pooled clinical trials. Population-based studies report that between 0% and 9% (Sweden and Iceland, respectively) of deaths among patients with epilepsy result from suicide (Tomson et al., 2004). However it is not clear whether epilepsy or its treatment increases the risk of suicide: suicide attempt has been associated with an increased risk for developing epilepsy indicating the association could represent the recurrence, post epilepsy diagnosis, of an underlying suicidality risk 74. The GPRD and IHCIS results indicate an association between epilepsy diagnosis and suicidality, with an OR of 2.8 (95% CI: 2.5-3.1) in GPRD and 5.5 (95% CI: 5.2-6.0) in IHCIS for during or ever before the analysis period.

The reported prevalence of migraine among epilepsy patients ranges from 8% to 23% (Marks & Ehrenberg, 1993) compared with 12% in the general population (Lipton et al., 2007). While the majority of studies report the risk of migraine to be two-fold greater among epilepsy patients (Lipton et al., 1994), two studies failed to confirm this association (Karaali-Savrun et al., 2002; Nuyen et al., 2006). This discordance is most likely due to differences in migraine definition and the absence of well defined control groups in some studies. Recent studies indicate that the association is primarily with migraine with aura, though the absolute prevalence of migraine with aura among epilepsy patients has yet to be reported (Piccinelli et al., 2006).

The IHCIS and GPRD database studies supported a positive association between epilepsy and migraine. A history of diagnosed migraine was present in 16% of epilepsy cases and 5% of controls in the IHCIS database study (OR = 3.7, 95% CI: 3.6-3.8). In the GPRD database, 9% of cases and 7% of controls had a history of diagnosed migraine (OR= 1.3, 95% CI: 1.3-1.4). The differential prevalences between the databases likely reflect between-country differences in diagnostics, awareness and treatment of migraine.

The current medication data was only reported for the patients with epilepsy to determine the most commonly used medications among patients with epilepsy. The most common AEDs varied between the US and UK databases. This is likely due to different treatment patterns and guidelines in the two countries. It has previously been shown that there is an association between the first AED prescribed after diagnosis of and history of psychiatric disorders, including depression and bipolar disorder, and the differential prescribing varied between the US and UK (Ishihara et al., 2010). One potential use of these data is to characterise polypharmacy patterns to inform potential drug interaction studies. Since the majority of patients are prescribed AEDs, the list identifies other medication types that are commonly used among the epilepsy patients.

The study should be interpreted in the context of its strengths and potential limitations. The strengths of the study include the large sizes of the databases, and the availability of detailed diagnosis and medication records. The GPRD is representative of the general population of the UK, and the IHCIS is representative of the US insured population. The IHCIS database is a large sample of people in the US covered by private insurance plans. Therefore results of this study may not be representative of US patients who receive healthcare through government organizations (e.g., Medicare, Medicaid) or who lack health insurance; for instance, these patients may be more likely to receive generic or older AEDs. In both databases, only diagnosed diseases are recorded, and therefore patients had to present to healthcare to be diagnosed with conditions or prescribed medications. There is a possibility of confounding by consultation frequency because patients with epilepsy or other chronic medical conditions will be more likely to be seen by healthcare providers compared to the general population.

The results of this study can be used to generate hypotheses about which medical conditions may be associated with epilepsy (either as risk factors for epilepsy, or resulting from epilepsy). Understanding the comorbidities and medication patterns in epilepsy also informs the effects of eligibility criteria on clinical trial recruitment, and facilitates assessments of potential safety signals that may arise in clinical trials (e.g. if a conditions is more common within the disease population at baseline, then this should be taken into account in evaluating whether exposure to a medication is associated with that condition).

5. Conclusion

In conclusion, psychiatric, neurological and other comorbidities are more common in patients with epilepsy, compared to age-, sex-matched controls. The results of this study provide hypotheses about conditions which may be associated with epilepsy, and these may be the subject for further investigation.

Among patients with epilepsy, the most commonly prescribed medications varied between the UK and US. Two of the older AEDs, valproate and carbamazepine, were the most commonly prescribed AEDs in 2009 amongst epilepsy patients in GPRD. Lamotrigine and phenytoin were the most commonly prescribed AEDs to patients with epilepsy in 2009 within IHCIS.

The most commonly prescribed medications among the epilepsy patient population, aside from AEDs, included analgesics, non-steroidal anti-inflammatory drugs, extended spectrum macroli (anti-biotics), selective serotonin reuptake inhibitors, and statins. The list of commonly prescribed medications in the epilepsy patient population can give an indication as to which drugs to consider for possible drug-drug interactions.

6. References

Baker, G.A., Jacoby, A., Chadwick, D.W. (1996). The associations of psychopathology in epilepsy: a community study. *Epilepsy Res*. Vol. 25, No. 1, pp. 29-39

Banerjee PN, Filippi D, Hauser WA. The descriptive epidemiology of epilepsy – a review. *Epilepsy Res*. 2009; 85: 31-45.

Beghi, E., Spagnoli, P., Airoldi, L., Fiordelli, E., Appollonio, I., Bogliun, G., et al. (2002). Emotional and affective disturbances in patients with epilepsy. *Epilepsy Behav*. Vol. 3, No. 3, pp. 255-261

Boylan, L.S., Flint, L.A., Labovitz, D.L., Jackson, S.C., Starner, K., Devinsky, O. (2004). Depression but not seizure frequency predicts quality of life in treatment-resistant epilepsy. *Neurology*. Vol. 62, No. 2, pp.258-261

Bredkjaer, S.R., Mortensen, P.B., Parnas, J. (1998). Epilepsy and non-organic non-affective psychosis. National epidemiologic study. *Br J Psychiatry*. Vol. 172, No. 3, pp. 235-238

Cramer, J.A., Blum, D., Fanning, K., Reed, M. (2004) The impact of comorbid depression on health resource utilization in a community sample of people with epilepsy. *Epilepsy Behav*. Vol. 5, No. 3, pp. 337-342

de Boer, H.M., Mula, M., & Sander, J.W. (2008). The global burden and stigma of epilepsy. *Epilepsy Behav*. Vol. 12, No.4, pp.540-546

Edeh, J., Toone, B. (1987). Relationship between interictal psychopathology and the type of epilepsy. Results of a survey in general practice. *Br J Psychiatry*. Vol. 151, No.1, pp. 95-101.

Forsgren, L., Nystrom, L. (1990). An incident case-referent study of epileptic seizures in adults. *Epilepsy Res*. Vol. 6, No. 1, pp. 66-81.

Gaitatzis, A., Carroll, K., Majeed, A., Sander, J.W. (2004)(2). The epidemiology of the comorbidity of epilepsy in the general population. *Epilepsia*. Vol. 45, No. 12, pp. 1613-1622

Gaitatzis, A., Trimble, M.R., Sander, J.W. (2004). The psychiatric comorbidity of epilepsy. *Acta Neurol Scand*. Vol. 110, No. 4, pp. 207-220.

Glosser, G., Zwil, A.S., Glosser, D.S., O'Connor, M.J., Sperling, M.R. (2000). Psychiatric aspects of temporal lobe epilepsy before and after anterior temporal lobectomy. *J Neurol Neurosurg Psychiatry*. Vol. 68, No. 1, pp. 53-58.

Gudmundsson, G. (1966). Epilepsy in Iceland. A clinical and epidemiological investigation. *Acta Neurol Scand* Vol. 43, Supp. L, p. 124.

Healthcare Cost and Utilization Project (HCUP, 2011). HCUP Clinical Classifications Software (CCS). Agency for Healthcare Research and Quality, Rockville, MD. Internet Citation: www.hcup-us.ahrq.gov/toolssoftware/ccs/ccs.jsp

Hermann, B.P., Seidenberg, M., Haltiner, A., Wyler, A.R. (1991). Mood state in unilateral temporal lobe epilepsy. *Biol Psychiatry*. Vol. 30, No. 12, pp. 1205 - 1218.

Hesdorffer, D.C., Hauser, W.A., Annegers, J.F., Cascino, G. (2000). Major depression is a risk factor for seizures in older adults. *Ann Neurol*. Vol. 47, No. 2, pp. 246 - 249.

Hesdorffer, D.C., Hauser, W.A., Olafsson, E., Ludvigsson, P., & Kjartansson, O. (2006). Depression and suicide attempt as risk factors for incident unprovoked seizures. *Ann Neurol*. Vol. 59, No. 1, pp. 35-41

Ishihara L, Webb DJ, Irizarry M, Weil J. (2010) Exploring differential prescribing between anti-epileptic drugs in epilepsy patients with a history of mood disorders. *Pharmacoepidemiol Drug Saf* Vol. 19, No. 2, pp.289-295.

Jacoby, A., Baker, G.A., Steen, N., Potts, P., Chadwick, D.W. (1996). The clinical course of epilepsy and its psychosocial correlates: findings from a U.K. Community study. *Epilepsia* Vol. 37, No. 2, pp.148-161.

Jick, S.S., Kaye, J.A., Vasilakis-Scaramozza, C, Garcia Rodriguez, L.A., Ruigomez, A., Meier, C.R., Schlienger, R.G., Jick, J.(2003). Validity of the general practice research database. *Pharmacotherapy*; Vol. 23, No. , pp. 686-689.

Kanner, A.M. (2009). Suicidality and epilepsy: a complex relationship that remains misunderstood and underestimated. *Epilepsy Curr*. Vol. 9, No. 3, pp. 63 - 66.

Karaali-Savrun, F., Goksan, B., Yeni, S.N., Ertan, S., Uzun, N. (2002). Seizure-related headache in patients with epilepsy. *Seizure*. Vol. 11, No. 1, pp. 67-69.

Kobau, R., Gilliam, F., Thurman, D.J. (2006). Prevalence of self-reported epilepsy or seizure disorder and its associations with self-reported depression and anxiety: results from the 2004 HealthStyles Survey. *Epilepsia*. Vol. 47, No. 11, pp. 1915-1921.

Lipton, R.B., Bigal, M.E., Diamond, M., Freitag, F., Reed, M.L., Stewart, W.F. (2007). Migraine prevalence, disease burden, and the need for preventive therapy. *Neurology*. Vol. 68, No. 5, pp. 343-349.

Lipton, R.B., Ottman, R., Ehrenberg, B.L., Hauser, W.A. (1994). Comorbidity of migraine: the connection between migraine and epilepsy. *Neurology*. Vol. 44, No. 10 Suppl 7, pp. S28-S32.

Marks, D.A., Ehrenberg, B.L. (1993). Migraine-related seizures in adults with epilepsy, with EEG correlation. *Neurology*. Vol. 43, No. 12, pp. 2476-2483.

Mendez, M.F., Cummings, J.L., Benson, D.F. (1986). Depression in epilepsy. Significance and phenomenology. *Arch Neurol*. Vol. 43, No. 8, pp. 766-770.

Nilsson, F.M., Kessing, L.V., Bolwig, T.G. (2003). On the increased risk of developing late-onset epilepsy for patients with major affective disorder. *J Affect Disord*. Vol. 76, No. 1-3, pp. 39-48.

Nuyen, J., Schellevis, F.G., Satariano, W.A., Spreeuwenberg, P.M., Birkner, M.D., van den Bos, G.A., et al. (2006) Comorbidity was associated with neurologic and psychiatric diseases: a general practice-based controlled study. J Clin Epidemiol. Vol. 59, No. 12, pp. 1274-1284.

O'Donoghue, M.F., Goodridge, D.M., Redhead, K., Sander, J.W., Duncan, J.S. (1999) Assessing the psychosocial consequences of epilepsy: a community-based study. *Br J Gen Pract*. Vol. 49, No. 440, pp. 211-214.

Ottman, R., Lipton, R.B. (1994). Comorbidity of migraine and epilepsy. *Neurology*. Vol. 44, No. 11, pp. 2105-2110

Piccinelli, P., Borgatti, R., Nicoli, F., Calcagno, P., Bassi, M.T., Quadrelli, M., et al. (2006). Relationship between migraine and epilepsy in pediatric age. *Headache*. Vol. 46, No. 3, pp. 413-421.

Shukla, G.D., Srivastava, O.N., Katiyar, B.C., Joshi, V., Mohan, P.K. (1979). Psychiatric manifestations in temporal lobe epilepsy: a controlled study. *Br J Psychiatry*. Vol. 135, No. 5, pp. 411-417.

Strine, T.W., Kobau, R., Chapman, D.P., Thurman, D.J., Price, P., Balluz, L.S. (2005). Psychological distress, comorbidities, and health behaviors among U.S. adults with seizures: results from the 2002 National Health Interview Survey. *Epilepsia*. Vol. 46, No. 7, pp. 1133-1139.

Tellez-Zenteno, J.F., Patten, S.B., Jette, N., Williams, J., Wiebe, S. (2007). Psychiatric comorbidity in epilepsy: a population-based analysis. *Epilepsia*. Vol. 48, No. 12, pp. 2336-2344.

Tomson, T., Beghi, E., Sundqvist, A., Johannessen, S.I. (2004). Medical risks in epilepsy: a review with focus on physical injuries, mortality, traffic accidents and their prevention. *Epilepsy Res*; Vol. 60 No. 1; pp. 1-16.

Toone, B. (2000). The psychoses of epilepsy. *J Neurol Neurosurg*. Vol. 69, No. 1, pp. 1-4

Torta, R., Keller, R. (1990). Behavioral, psychotic, and anxiety disorders in epilepsy: etiology, clinical features, and therapeutic implications. *Epilepsia* Vol. 40, Suppl. l0, pp. S2-20.

10

Epilepsy and Anticonvulsant Therapy During Pregnancy

Eva Maňáková and Lucie Hubičková
3rd Faculty of Medicine, Charles University in Prague, Czech Republic

1. Introduction

Epilepsy is one of the most common chronic diseases accompanying mankind for centuries. Approximately 1% children in Europe have been born to the women suffering from epilepsy. For epileptic women is important to obtain appropriate information about possibility to have children and about risks connected with their pregnancy. A population-based cohort study in Finland (Artama et al., 2006) suggested decreased birth rate among patients with epilepsy. As both, disease and treatment, may induce inborn defect, it is essential to diminish their negative effects. Every chronic treatment during pregnancy increases estimation of the risk to offspring. Risk perception during pregnancy is individual, however almost 35% of women according to the study (Helbig et al., 2010) investigating factors important in the family planning decided to have fewer children. They were afraid about transfer epilepsy onto the offspring or disability to care for a child. Another factor having effect on their decision is teratogenicity of drugs used for treatment. Women with epilepsy may benefit from discussion with their healthcare provider about the impact their epilepsy may have on children. As almost 50% pregnancies in women with epilepsy in USA (Davis et al., 2008) are not intended, relevant information in right time may decrease the number of elective abortion.

Every physician should be informed about risk to the fetus that is associated with seizures and drugs used for treatment during pregnancy. Drug used in girls and young women should be chosen with the respect to the future reproduction, because the use of anti-epileptic drugs (AED) in women with epilepsy is in fact a balance between seizure control and adverse effects of drugs.

2. History

Modern treatment of epilepsy started during the19th century. The first drug introduced for treatment of epilepsy was potassium bromide that was widely used in USA and Europe during the second half of the 19th century. Another drug that was introduced at the beginning of 20th century was phenobarbital. Hydantoins has been used since 1938. Many new drugs were discovered subsequently. Apart from the fact, that anticonvulsant drugs have been used for many years, their embryotoxicity was not be described before 60th, when first case reports were published (Meadow, 1968; Müller-Küppers, 1963; Centa & Rasore-Quartino, 1965; Massey, 1966). Fetal hydantoin syndrome was described in 1975 by

Hanson and Smith. Similar inborn defects were described for all older anticonvulsant drugs (primidone, valproate, phenobarbital, phenytoin, carbamazepine, trimethadion). The frequency and severity of defects associated with use trimethadion were so high to warrant consideration of early elective termination of pregnancy. The teratogenic mechanism of AEDs is only partially understood.

2.1 Fetal anticonvulsant syndrome

Fetal anticonvulsant syndrome is associated with exposure to dilantin, diphenylhydantoin, phenytoin, hydantoin, and valproic acid during 1st trimester of pregnancy, in lower degree also with other (carbamazepine). The abnormalities include (Jones, 1997; Žižka, 1997; Ornoy, 2009):

a. An increase of major congenital anomalies: congenital heart defects (septal defects, tetratology of Fallot, aortic coarctation etc.), cleft lip and palate, limb defects with hypoplasia of nails and distal phalanges, finger-like thumbs, abnormal palmar creases, dislocation of hip, malformation of brain, especially neural tube defects.
b. Specific syndrome including facial dysmorphy with wide anterior fontanel, ocular hypertelorism, broad, depressed nasal bridge, short nose with bowed upper lip, midface hypoplasia, epicantus, often also malformation of external genitalia and neural tube.
c. Intrauterine growth retardation.
d. Developmental disorders mainly affecting cognitive functions and behaviour.

Small variations were noted according to the drug used. A significant association was seen between maternal use of valproic acid and spina bifida, and a weaker, non-significant one between carbamazepine and spina bifida. Facial clefts were associated with both diphenylhydantoin and phenobarbitone use and also with polytherapy (Källén et al., 1989). As AEDs have effect also on cognitive development, children exposed to valproate have increased risk of delayed early development in comparison to the control group (Bromley et al., 2010). It seems, that a distinctive pattern of abnormalities in infants is associated with the use of anticonvulsant drugs during pregnancy rather than with epilepsy itself (Holmes et al., 2001).

3. Embryotoxicity and its evaluation

3.1 Animal studies

How embryotoxic potential of drug may be detected? The first opportunity is an animal study. Every drug has to be tested in animal studies with a respect to protect the unborn child from adverse effects. Animal studies can, but do not always, predict whether a drug will be teratogenic in humans. Unfortunately, animal studies have shown as poor predictors in the case of thalidomide that did not produce malformations in rats and mice. On the other hand, some drugs have been found teratogenic in animals and not in humans. Therefore, minimally two different animal models are required for routine testing. Animals are often given far higher doses of drugs than humans would ever receive. Interspecies differences regarding the teratogenicity of drugs, that can increase doubts about results, result from differing pharmacokinetic processes, different metabolites, concentration-time relationships in an embryo, placental transfer and elimination rate. The only way to ascertain the ultimate risk or safety of drugs during pregnancy is to verify them in human studies (Einarson & Koren, 1999).

3.2 Epidemiological studies

As pregnant women cannot be enrolled in randomized, controlled studies from obvious ethical reasons, the teratogenicity have to be established in prospective or retrospective epidemiological studies. Data have been collected in a registry of birth defects (CDC- The International Clearinghouse for Birth Defects Monitoring Systems, EUROCAT - A European Network of Population-based Registries for the Epidemiological Surveillance of Congenital Anomalies), by specific registry collecting data about AEDs exposure (EURAP- European and International Registry of Antiepileptic Drugs in Pregnancy, NAAPR - North American AED Pregnancy Registry) or by services offering consultation about drug safety (OTIS - Organisation of Teratology Information Specialists, and ENTIS - European Network of Teratology Information Services). Criterion for inclusion enrolment in prospective studies is AED use at time of conception or during first trimester, however before ultra-sonographic examination of normal development of child. Registry data can be used for monitoring that can identify specific risk.

Retrospective studies using data from registry are utilized for case-control studies, where drug use among mothers whose babies express a specific malformation is compared with that of mothers whose babies do not. This method has a high sensitivity, but is more prone to bias. It is difficult to identify all concomitant factors those may affect development of birth defect. There is the evidence of partial memory and bias in the way women recall the drugs they took during pregnancy. Women suffering from chronic disease tend to recall their treatment better than women who took an over-the-counter drug.

Prospective, controlled, epidemiological studies of the pregnancy outcomes of women who were treated by a particular drug during pregnancy are another possibility how is possible to evaluate risk. Even this type of research is not ideal, because the limited size of the studies means they do not have the statistical power to detect increased risk of rare malformations. Moreover indications for treatment and concurrent exposures are not standardized.

The information received by drug manufactures is often a mix of prospective and retrospective case reports. The quality of the information about exposure is usually poor, reports of adverse fetal outcomes are more frequent as uneventful ones.

The group of exposed pregnancies is usually compared to the control group performed by the pregnancies with normal outcome. The second possibility is the use of baseline risk of major malformation in population, that is 2.75% in USA (according to CDC) and 2-3% in Europe (according to EUROCAT). Finally, the group of pregnant women exposed to drugs with minimal or no risk, represents the third type of control group.

To monitor malformations, the statistical approach is used, that compares number of observed infants with specific type the inborn defect born during a specific time period with the number of infants expected to be born during that period. However, difference between the observed and the expected number can have many explanations: real change caused by introduction of a teratogenic agents, changes in detection and registration, fluctuation of specific malformation in time, wrong estimation of expected number of malformation etc. Therefore only limited number of conditions and set of standard malformations may be monitored.

Teratological approach is focused on occurrence of specific malformations or their combinations (syndromes) those are present in exposed population or in all pregnant women. If malformation is very specific as phocomelia in thalidomide exposure, no baseline level of birth defects is needed (Källén & Hay, 1991).

Published case-reports have only limited significance, because causality between malformation and exposure can be only accidental. We need large exposed group for risk evaluation. The international cooperation is useful, because it allows collect many cases in relatively short time. For example, if the risk of major malformations in a given population is 3 percent, then at least 220 pregnancies with specific exposure and similar number of control pregnancies will be required to show that is increased risk by factor of 2.5, with a power of 80 percent (Koren, 2001). More than one thousand of cases are needed for risk assessment lower than 1%.

It is generally accepted that assessing the risk of a substance to humans we need today:

Case reports describing repeatedly a typical malformation pattern (syndrome).

At least two large and well controlled epidemiological studies.

Results of testing in laboratory mammals following the Good Laboratory Practice and WHO criteria, that serves only for confirming biological plausibility (Jelinek, 2005).

FDA classification dividing drugs in 5 groups according to its impact to fetus is greatly simplifying. Merlob and Stahl (2002) concluded that this classification of drugs for teratogenic risk must be considered as anachronistic and misleading way of approach and counselling, because the causation of inborn defects is multi-factorial and could not be limited to the qualification (if known) of a single factor, only. It is necessary perform the separate analysis of any individual case collecting as much relevant data as possible.

3.3 Genetic background as a factor for inborn defect

Drug metabolising enzymes and the genetic variants they carry are one of the factors that might be responsible for the efficacy and side effect of AED treatment in individual patients. They also modulate development and induce embryotoxicity. The speed and differences in metabolic inactivation may increase plasma level of AEDs up to embryotoxic threshold. Polymorphy in genes for enzymes involved in metabolic pathways for detoxification is suspected cause for development of birth defect in certain cases. For example, phenytoin toxicity is dependent on epoxide hydrolase activity, i.e. arena oxidase (Strickler et al., 1985) or on CYP2C19 specific cytochrome P-450 isoenzyme deficiency (Maier & Mayer, 1987). Valproate toxicity is increased in ornithine trans-carbamylase deficiency. Drug competition or the induction of microsomal enzymes may change AED plasma level and increase the risk. Higher risk for neural-tube defects such spina bifida and anencephaly after valproate or carbamazepine exposure has been assigned to the deficiency in folate dependent homocystein metabolism. Polymorphism of MTHFR (methylenetetrahydrofolate reductase) is associated with higher risk for anticonvulsant syndrome. Mothers who are homozygous for MTHRF genotype 677T were found to have three to four higher risk compared with those, that were homozygous for allele 677C. Other genes, for example MTR 2756, are involved in susceptibility to embryotoxic impairment (Steinlein, 2010). In present, we may conclude those woman having a child with vaproate fetal syndrome is in higher risk of malformed child for the next pregnancy (Tripp, 1981; Malm et al., 2002). In future, the genetic profile will be a goal for the optimal treatment of epileptic patients.

3.4 Ischemia and re-perfusion injury

The role of ischemia and re-perfusion producing tissue damage linked for example to neural tube defect has to become more evident in the past years. During an ischemic event, intracellular xantin dehydrogenase is converted to xantin oxidase. When the ischemia resolves, xantin oxidase metabolised purines in uric acid. By-products of this reaction are super-oxide radicals. They produce tissue damage directly or indirectly. As convulsions results in anoxia, higher rate of malformation was demonstrated in epileptic women without treatment and without seizure control in comparison with healthy population. Combination anoxia with teratogenic potential of drug even increases risk (Verrotti et al., 2006).

4. Embryotoxicity of antiepileptic drugs (AEDs)

4.1 First generation of antiepileptic drugs

4.1.1 Phenytoin

Phenytoin is the most widely used hydatoin derivate with antiepileptic effect. The teratogenic potential of hydantoin and its derivatives is known since 1968 (Meadow). The anomalies observed were described as "fetal hydantoin syndrome" (see above). In the case of phenytoin, it appears that fetal susceptibility correlates with the fetal level of the microsomal detoxifying enzyme epoxide hydrolase (Buehler et al., 1994). Developmental toxicity is probably caused by concentration-dependent bradycardia and hypoxia related damage of embryonic tissue (Azarbayjani & Danielson, 1998; Danielsson et al., 2000) resulting in alteration of gene expression minimally, if not everywhere, in craniofacial region (Gelineau-van Waes et al., 1999). In comparison with other AEDs, phenytoin produced higher incidence of fetal defects (20,9%) in animal study (Sullivan & McElhatton, 1977), however risk occurring in epidemiological studies was lower.

The risk of phenytoin exposure during pregnancy has been well documented. It has been estimated to be two to three folds higher that than of mothers without treatment as has been confirmed in several studies (Kluger & Meador, 2008; Schaefer et al., 2001). The prospective observation study made by 25 epilepsy centres in USA and UK from 1999 to 2004 determine risk of adverse outcomes for phenyltoin on 10.7% (including fetal death), and major malformation on 7.1% (Meador et al., 2006). Phenytoin mono-therapy increases the risk for cleft palate, but it has not been associated with microcephaly (Almgren et al., 2009).

4.1.2 Barbiturates

Barbiturates used for epilepsy treatment are phenobarbital, methylphenobarbital, and primidone, the pro-drug of phenobarbital to which is largely metabolized. In higher doses (50 mg/kg/day and more) primidone was teratogenic in mice increasing the incidence of cleft palate, other defects as exencephaly, fused ribs, and undescended testes were observed less frequently. The incidence of major malformation was dose dependent in primidone as well as phenobarbital (McElhatton & Sullivan, 1975; McElhaton et al., 1976; Fritz et al., 1976). After exposure to primidone, the malformation typical for AEDs have been described in many case reports and studies (Rating et al., 1982; Battino et al., 1998; Akšamija et al., 2009). Increased risk for major malformations associated with primidone exposure was demonstrated in large prospective study (Jones et al., 1992). North American Registry demonstrated a 6.5% risk after phenobarbital mono-therapy in comparison with 1.6% for control population (Kluger & Meador, 2008).

4.1.3 Ethosuximide

Ethosuximide is recommended drug for petit mal treatment, only. In animal studies the risk of major malformation was approximately as high as in primidone (Sullivan & McElhatton, 1977). There are only a few report of the ethosuximide therapy during pregnancy. Study reporting on pregnancy outcome in ten women described two major malformation cleft lip in mothers treated ethosuximide in combination with primidone or phenobarbital (Kuhnz et al., 1984).

4.2 Second generation of antiepileptic drugs

4.2.1 Valproic acid (VPA)

Valproic acid is widely used for treatment of a broad spectrum of epilepsy types, migraine as well as bipolar disorder. In utero exposure results in higher incidence of major and minor malformations. Proposed mechanism of action is related to the changes in methylation of histones (Tung & Winn, 2010). Epigenetic modification of them with hyperacetylation is accompanied with induction of apoptosis (Menegola et al., 2005; Di Renzo at al., 2010). Malformations occurred not only after valproic acid but also after valproate conjugates with anticonvulsant activity in animal model with different intensity (Spiegelstein et al., 2003; Okada et al., 2009).

Fetal valproate syndrome was described in 1968 (Meadow, 1968). Drug teratogenicity was documented in many studies (Arpino at al., 2000; Bromfield et al., 2008). Dansky and Finnel (1991) summarized the knowledge on the reproductive outcome of patients treated with antiepileptic drugs during pregnancy that covered over 30 years in their meta-analysis. They demonstrated twofold to threefold increased risk of congenital malformation in epileptic women as compared with the general population. Similar finding, i.e. 2.5 times higher risk of having baby with malformation after valproic acid mono-therapy, was published in another large meta-analysis (Koren at al., 2006). Prospective observation study (Meador et al., 2006) that enrolled mother-child pairs from USA and UK demonstrated 17.4% malformations and 20.3% of serious adverse outcomes, that included fetal death in addition to malformations. Chong and Bazil (2010) published meta-analysis including 59 studies and more than 65 000 pregnancies. They demonstrated high rate (10.73%) of malformations after VPA mono-therapy and after poly-therapy even 16.78%. Meador et al. (2009) published similar findings, i.e. 10.73% (95% CI: 8.16-13.29). The most frequent malformations were hernia, ear/neck/face malformations, cleft lip, and spina bifida. Nowadays, the studies have been focused on the correlation between dose and teratogenic effect. Higher doses than 1400 mg/day have been proved to be more teratogenic (Vajda & Eadie, 2005). The evidence for higher risk is lacking for doses that are lower than 600mg per day, and risk gradually increases (Tomson & Battino, 2009; Diav-Citrin et al., 2008) and becomes more prominent at doses above 1000mg (Koren et al., 2006). EUROCAT study published in 2010 reveals significantly higher risk for those malformations after valproic acid mono-therapy. The adjusted odds ratios were as follows: spina bifida 12.7, atrial septal defect 2.5, cleft palate 5.2, hypospadia 4.8, polydactyly 2.2., craniosynostosis 6.8 (Jentink et al., 2010).

4.2.2 Carbamazepine (CBZ)

Carbamazepine is efficacious in treatment of a variety of CNS disorders, as well as epileptic seizures. CBZ is usually well tolerated and therefore is also used in pregnant women. Carbamazepine in dose that is corresponding to the therapeutic range in humans was not associated with negative pregnancy outcome in mice. It had no effect on fertility. Higher number of resorptions or higher risk of malformation was not detected (Christensen et al., 2004). Similar findings were found in study after the exposure to higher doses (1.000, 1.500 and 2.000 mg/kg). In those doses no specific pattern of malformation and no correlation between detected anomalies and dose were found (Finnel et al., 1986). The finding was supported also by following studies (Wray et al., 1982; Fritz et al., 1976). On the other hand, Sullivan and McElhatton (1977) demonstrated higher frequency of malformation in exposed mice (4.7% compared with 1.3% in controls). Afshar end co-workers (2010) described specific eye malformations in mice after carbamazepine exposure at clinically comparable doses.

Exposure to the carbamazepine was found to increase malformation rate in several studies (Diav-Citrin et al., 2001). Ornoy and Cohen (1996) described typical carbamazepine syndrome characterized by facial dysmorphic features and mild mental retardation, that did not seem to be related to presence of maternal convulsions but more to the hereditary factors. Rosa (1991) found higher (1%) risk for spina bifida in women used carbamazepine, that is ten times higher than in unexposed population. Many case reports describing occurrence of spina bifida or eye malformation may support the opinion (Akšamija et al., 2007; Källén, 1994; Sutcliffe et al., 1998). Meta-analysis using 16 prospective studies compared the risk of major malformation for CBZ mono-therapy and CBZ with other antiepileptic drugs, both in comparison to matched control pregnancies and to untreated epileptic pregnancies. It included 1255 CBZ exposed pregnancies. Study proved 2.89 fold-increased risks of major congenital anomalies in children treated with CBZ as compared with children of healthy control. Rate of malformations was 2.34% in control population. The rate of major malformations was further increased in cases of women treated with combination of CBZ and other antiepileptic drugs, that was about 2-fold higher. Anomalies that risk was increased were neural tube defects, however cleft lip and cardiac defects were found, too. Decrease in gestational age at delivery was also revealed (Matalon et al., 2002). Case-control study published by Jentink et al. (2010) using literature review and EUROCAT database demonstrated higher risk for spina bifida, only (odds ratio 2.6; 95% confidence interval 1.2 to 5.3). Difference was in classification of major malformations and exclusion of cases as compared with meta-analysis mentioned above.

4.2.3 Oxcarbazepine (OCZ)

Oxcarbazepine is similar to carbamazepine in chemical structure, but it is metabolized in different metabolic pathway. A monohydroxy-derivative (MHD) is responsible for its clinical efficacy. Premarketing studies showed an increase in congenital malformations in the offspring of rats treated with oxcarbazepine at doses similar to those used in humans on a surface area basis. The abnormalities in the offspring included craniofacial, cardiovascular, and skeletal abnormalities. In rabbits, an increase in fetal mortality was noted at similar doses (Micromedex® 2.0, 2011). Higher frequency of malformation was found also in mice (Bennet at al., 1996).

In one report, mother using oxcarbazepine during all pregnancy gave birth to normal healthy girl and second pregnancy on the same therapy resulted also in healthy infant (Eisenschenk, 2006). Data from Argentina register revealed 35 pregnancies exposed to oxcarbazepine in mono-therapy resulted in the delivery of healthy infants. Of the 20 pregnancies exposed to oxcarbamazepine in combination with other AEDs only one malformed child was reported: a cardiac malformation in a newborn exposed to phenobarbital and oxcarbamazepine (Meischenguiser et al., 2004). An analysis of 248 published pregnancies involving maternal exposure of oxcarbamazepine in mono-therapy and 61 in poly-therapy did not find an increased incidence of malformations in exposed infants. Malformation rate was 2.4%, the same as malformation rate reported in the general population. In poly-therapy the risk was 6.6% (Montouris, 2005). The author notes that the available data are not sufficiently large to draw definitive conclusions.

4.2.4 Benzodiazepines

Benzodiazepines are widely used as tranquilisers, hypnotics as well as AEDs. For epilepsy treatment are used currently diazepam, clonazepam, clobazam, and sultiam. Diazepam cross easily placenta and it is present in blood in three time higher level than in mother. Case control studies indicate higher risk of major malformation, especially oral cleft, however meta-analysis demonstrated no association between benzodiazepine exposure and major malformations. Short exposure is possible, however long term treatment is associated with withdrawal symptoms (Robert-Gnansia & Schaefer, 2007). Shepard and Lamire (2004) refer that clonazepam in animal studies demonstrated no fetal effect. There are only few epidemiological studies. Ornoy et al. (1998) found no increase of malformation in 69 women. No relevant information was published about clobazam and sultiam.

4.3 Third generation of antiepileptic drugs

4.3.1 Lamotrigine (LTG)

The manufacturer (GlaxoSmithKline, Research Triangle Park, NC, USA) reported teratology testing in mice, rats, and rabbits at oral doses. There was no increase in congenital malformations in any of these species. Top doses were 1.3 (mice), 0.5 (rats), and 1.1 (rabbits) times the maintenance dose recommended for humans on a mg/m^2 basis. Maternal and fetal toxicity (delayed ossification and decreased weight) were seen at the high doses in the rodent studies (Micromedex® 2.0, 2011). Lamotrigine in reproductive toxicity study given intravenously in the mouse did not produce malformation except for highest doses that were toxic for mother (50 - 300 mg/kg/day). Resorption and reduction of fetal weight were seen both being dose dependent. Skeletal malformation found in these studies were assigned to the maternal toxicity, however neural tube defects (anencephaly), malformation related to the cranial crest cells, and caudal dysgenesis were probably induced by lamotrigine (Padmanabhan et al., 2003). Prenatal exposure to LTG induced altered brain structure in a dose-dependent manner at maternal plasma concentrations within the clinically occurring range (Manent et al., 2008).

The manufacturer set up a registry to collect information on pregnant women exposed to lamotrigine. A report from this registry extending till 31 March 2009 included 1439 pregnancy outcomes after first trimester exposure to lamotrigine mono-therapy. There were 35 pregnancies with congenital malformations, for a rate of 2.4% (95% CI 1.7- 3.4%). Among the defects reported were cleft lip and palate, clubfoot, hydronephrosis with megaureter, anencephaly, anal atresia, cardiac defects, limb defects, and an esophageal malformation. No relationship of malformation rate to lamotrigine dose was evident, and an evaluation of exposure level and malformation did not suggest a dose-response relationship. The Advisory Committee noted that the registry did not replicate a signal for orofacial clefts such as that reported from the AED Pregnancy Registry (discussed below) and that with more than 1000 pregnancies enrolled, the confidence was sufficiently narrow to exclude an appreciable increase in malformation risk (Cunnington & Messenheimer, 2007). Australian Pregnancy Register of Antiepileptic Drugs included 243 pregnancies exposed to lamotrigine. The analysis did not show statistically significant difference between the risk of fetal malformation and exposure to lamotrigine mono-therapy (Vajda et al., 2010). UK Epilepsy and Pregnancy Register enrolled 647 pregnancies exposed to lamotrigine. Malformation rate was 3.2%. When adjusted for age, parity, family history of malformations, periconceptional folic acid exposure and sex of infant odds ratio was 1.71 (95%CI 0.88 - 3.32). This study revealed positive dose response with malformation rate of 5,4 (95% CI 3.3-8.7%) for total daily doses more than 200mg. Results of five registries and one large prospective study were published up to 2007. The prevalence of major malformations in North American AED Pregnancy Registry (NAAPR) was 2.7%, however higher prevalence of cleft lip and palate than that observed in control group (Holmes et al., 2006). In contrast the EUROCAT did not find an increased risk of orofacial clefts for mono-therapy, but for poly-therapy it was increased (OR: 1.43; 95%CI: 1.03-1.93). However, observed rate was low and absolute risk is minimal (Shor et al., 2007; Meador & Penovich, 2008). Later, Miskov et al. (2009) did not find an increase of birth defect in their small prospective study (23 pregnancies).

4.3.2 Levetiracetam

In preclinical studies presented by the sponsor, levetiracetam did not produce fertility impairment in male and female rats given up to 1800 mg/kg/d, which is six times the recommended human dose on a surface area basis. Pregnant rats given levetiracetam at doses similar to the human dose were born fetuses with an increased incidence of intrauterine growth retardation and minor skeletal abnormalities. No maternal toxicity was noted at this dose (Micromedex® 2.0, 2011). Saillenfait et al. (2007) described higher incidence of resorptions in rats at dose 500mg/kg/day and dose related decrease in fetal weight. They demonstrated malformations as super-numerable ribs, absent tail, anal atresia, cardiovascular defects, and impairment of ossification at dose 250mg/kg /day and higher, that was six fold higher than therapeutic dose for human and that was toxic for mother. Study in a mouse model did not reveal higher incidence of major malformations after levetiracetam treatment up to dose 2000mg/kg/day. There was higher frequency of resorptions at high doses (Isoherranen et al., 2003).

Case reports on 3 pregnancies exposed to levetiracetam (Long, 2003) showed no adverse outcome. French et al. (2001) reported 23 women became pregnant during clinical trials. Eight pregnancies results in nine healthy offspring. Two babies had malformations, but both mothers were exposed also to other AEDs. Seven pregnancies resulted in spontaneous abortion and three women had voluntary termination. Prospective study (Johannessen et al., 2005) described 7 children (2 pregnancies with mono-therapy, 5 pregnancies with poly-therapy) without any malformation. EURAP in Netherlands (ten Berg et al., 2005) reported 11 pregnancies exposed to levetiracetam: one woman had the spontaneous abortion, and one pregnancy was elective terminated from social reasons. Nine live born children were without any malformations. The UK Epilepsy and Pregnancy Register (Hunt et al., 2006) identified 39 pregnancies exposed to levetiracetam mono-therapy and 78 in combination with at least one other AED. There were no congenital malformations in group with mono-therapy. Longo et al. (2009) summarized accessible data revealing 147 patients. Of these patients 2% experienced a major malformation, 4.8% a minor anomaly. All of them were receiving poly-therapy.

4.3.3 Topiramate

As reported by the manufacturer (Janssen-Cilag), topiramate is teratogenic in mice, rats and rabbits. Similar findings revealed a study describing an adverse effect of topiramate (100mg/kg/day) on developing embryos in rats increasing number of resorptions (Khouri, 2005).

Gentile (2009) reported on one pregnancy with normal outcome. Ornoy et al. (2008) reported on the outcome of 52 pregnancies where the mothers used topiramate at least during the first trimester of pregnancy. The rate of spontaneous abortions (11.3%) was significantly higher in comparison to controls (2,8%). Although rate of major malformation was higher (9.8%), two cases were genetic in origin. One case from non-genetic was a baby whose mother used also valproic acid and clonazepam. Another case report (Vila Cerén et al., 2005) described the case of a neonate whose mother treated with topiramate during pregnancy at doses of 300 mg per day was born malformed child with oligodactyly and syndactyly. Prospective study (Hunt et al., 2008) following 203 pregnancies exposed to topiramate resulted in 178 live birth babies, 16 had major malformations. Three occurred in 70 pregnancies in which the drug was in mono-therapy. Two other newborns were exposed to the drug as poly-therapy. Overall, the rate for oral clefts was 11 times the background rate. Hernandez-Diaz and co-workers (2010) reported 3.8% major malformations among 289 women taking the drug in the first trimester that were enrolled by the North American AED Pregnancy Register. Risk ratio for major malformation was 2.8. They found also higher risk for cleft lip and lower birth weight. FDA now alerts on higher risk of cleft lip and palate.

4.3.4 Other new antiepileptic drugs

Risk assessment for following new antiepileptic drugs is not possible due to lack of experience. Information on few case reports was hardly even published. Only preclinical studies on animals performed by producer have been accessible for some of them.

Gabapentin: Small ENTIS study identified five normal infants after exposure to gabapentin (De Santis et al., 2004).

Vigabatrin (VGB): The animal experiments demonstrated significant teratogenic effect when drug was administered to mice during organogenesis (Padmanabhan et al., 2010). Lower doses were associated with disturbance of motor-cognitive behaviour and lower weight of pups, however higher caused abortions (Lombardo et al., 2005). Since vigabatrin exposure has been associated with retina damage, two small studies examined children exposed in utero to drug demonstrated no clear ophthalmic abnormalities, However, sample was to small to be able to confirm safety for fetus (Sorri et al., 2005; Lawthom et al., 2009). According to the FDA recommendation, the treatment may be only short-term (Chong & Bazil, 2010).

Zonisamid teratogenicity was evaluated in six pregnant women. Five patients, two on mono-therapy and three on poly-therapy delivered healthy children. Malformed child with anencephaly was reported after zonisamid in combination with phenytoin. Together with above mentioned, there were 26 pregnancies reported, only. Two of them had malformations (7.7%) The other child was born with an atrial septal defect to the woman treated poly-therapy that included phenytoin and valproate (Ohtahara & Yamatogi, 2007).

Pregabalin is a GABA analogue that inhibits with high affinity and selectivity the voltage dependent calcium channels. Animal study revealed increasing incidence of a specific tumour type (Selak, 2001)

No information about **rufinamide, lacosamide, stripentol** and **tiagabin** embryotoxicity has been published, yet.

5. Trends in epilepsy treatment and our experience

Study characterizing trends in prescribing antiepileptic drugs in Czech Republic in comparison with European countries and Australia compared used drug spectra from 1987 to 2000. Utilization of barbiturates and succimide derivatives was decreasing. Hydantoins, that utilization in Australia was steady, were in Europe decreasing, too. The valproic acid consumption was increasing as well as utilisation of third generation AEDs (Kořístková & Grundmann, 2005). The trends in usage corresponds to recommendation for general population, however valproic acid is the most teratogenic AEDs. Studies focused on girls or women in childbearing age demonstrated also changes in prescribed drugs and increase of lamotrigine prescribing in female (Ackers et al., 2009; Vajda et al., 2007). Proportion of women that were exposed to topiramate and levetiracetam was increasing, too (Vajda et al., 2010). We recorded the same trends in treatment of epilepsy during pregnancy in our ten years experience of Czech Teratology Information Service (CZTIS) with inquiries about epilepsy treatment during pregnancy (Maňáková et al., 2006).. Lamotrigine was used in almost 30% of pregnant women, carbamazepine in 23.4%, and valproic acid in 21.3%, that correspond with above mentioned studies. New drugs as levetiracetam and topiramate were used for treatment of pregnant women in last years, too.

6. Conclusions

The management of the pregnant women suffering from epilepsy requires close cooperation between the neurologist and obstetrician. Women with epilepsy have a low complication rate except of that related to AEDs exposure (Borthen et al., 2009). All of them in childbearing age should be informed about the rates of teratogenicity of AEDs, possibility of increased seizure frequency during pregnancy, and the risks of the pregnancy and labour. If almost half of pregnancies are not planned, the optimalization of treatment and consultation should be discussed with girls on beginning of their childbearing age. Since unplanned pregnancy is very often diagnosed after the most sensitive period of embryo development, when malformations are already developed, it makes no sense to change treatment. Exposure to antiepileptic drugs is not an indication for therapeutic abortion, even if they are teratogenic. Counselling is very important, because it helps to gain a realistic perspective of risk.

The frequency of seizures is essentially the same as before pregnancy, however tonic-clonic convulsions should be avoided, because they are risky for mother and fetus. Seizures can cause trauma leading to ruptured fetal membranes or abruptio placentae (Pennell, 2003). Fortunately, with close monitoring and proper management, more than 90 percent of pregnancies in women with epilepsy will be uncomplicated.

6.1 Optimization of treatment

Optimization of treatment should be made before pregnancy. Diagnosis of epilepsy should be confirmed and indication for treatment with AEDs re-assessed. The possibility of AED gradual withdrawal should be considered in appropriate clinical setting prior to conception. The AED treatment should be optimized also prior to conception. Selection should be made the most appropriate for patient. Changing during pregnancy is rarely justified, risk probably overweight potential gain (Tomson & Hiilesmaa, 2007). To ascertain whether epilepsy remains in remission enough time before conception is required.

Drugs of choice during pregnancy are considered lamotrigine and carbamazepine. Drugs should be given in mono-therapy with the lowest effective dose. Poly-therapy should be avoided because of proved increase of risk. Effective dose and optimal concentration of the drug before pregnancy should be documented. Monitoring of drug plasma concentration have to be more frequent, minimally once during trimester. Good compliance with

treatment is essential. Lamotrigine, levetiracetam, and topiramate plasma levels are changing (decreasing) during pregnancy, so adjustment of therapeutic dose during pregnancy is needed. Valproic acid should be avoided, if it is possible. However, adequate seizure control is the primary goal. If it is only drug giving satisfactory control of seizures, valproic acid should be used of the lowest possible day dose (optimum under 600mg/day) divided into three doses to minimize negative influence to fetus. Pregnancy should be considered of high risk and must have appropriate follow up (Ornoy, 2009).
The second level (expert) ultra-sonography may justified normal development or detect most neural tube defects and about two third of other major malformations.

6.2 Folic acid supplementation and its profit

Low serum folic acid level in epileptic mothers is associated with an increased risk of congenital malformations in their offspring (Ogava et al., 1991). Population studies demonstrate benefit from fortification of cereal products by folic acid (De Walls et al., 2007) or supplementation before planed pregnancy. Daily consumption of supplements containing 400 micrograms of folic acid in the periconception period may reduce the risk of neural tube defects in general population by as much as 70% (Morin et al., 2002). If risk of malformation is higher in women with low plasma level of folic acid, periconceptional supplementation with minimally 0.4 mg folic acid per day in AEDs exposed population is considered prophylactic. The measurement that determines intra-erythrocythal level of folic acid may help with definition of optimal dose. Results suggest, that 5 mg/day folic acid as preconception supplementation in women with epilepsy is effective to balance the impact of AEDs on folate metabolism (Bauer et al., 2010). Folate profylaxis is recommended to all women taking antiepileptic drugs. Treatment with dose up to 5mg/day should start before planned pregnancy and continued minimally to the end of first trimester.

6.3 Vitamin K supplementation

Management strategies include also the prenatal use vitamin K. Vitamin K 10 mg per day orally should be administered in the last 4 weeks of pregnancy for women taking hepatic enzyme-inducing AEDs (phenytoin, phenobarbital, primidone, carbamazepine, topiramate, and oxcarbazepine). The newborn should receive vitamin K 1 mg intravenously or intramuscularly regardless of maternal AED exposure.

7. Acknowledgement

Work was supported by Ministry of Education of Czech Republic, grant INGO LA 08034.

8. References

Ackers, R., Besaq, F.M.C., Wade, A., Murray, M.L., Wong, I.C.K. (2009).Changing trends in antiepileptic drug prescribing in girls of child-bearing potential. *Archived of Disease in Childhood.* Vol.94, No.6, (June 2009), pp.443-447, ISSN: 0003-9888

Akšamija, A., Habek, D., Stanojevic, M., Ujevic, B. (2009). Fetal malformation associated with the use of methylphenobarbital and carbamazepine during pregnancy. *Fetal Diag Ther.* Vol.25, No.1, (Feb 2009), pp.79-82, ISSN: 1015-3837

Almgren, M., Källén, B., Levebratt, C. (2009). Population-based study of antiepileptic drug exposure in utero- Influence on head circumference in newborns. *Seizures.* Vol.18, No.10, (December 2009), pp. 672-675, ISSN: 1059-1311

Arpino, C., Brescianini, S., Robert, E., Castilla, E.E., Cocchi, G., Cornel, M.C., de Vigan, C., Lancaster, P.A., Merlob, P., Sumiyoshi, Y., Zampino, G., Renzi, C., Rosano, A., Mastroiacovo, P. (2000). Teratogenic effect of antiepileptic drugs: use of an International Database on Malformations and Drug Exposure (MADRE). *Epilepsia.* Vol.41, No.11, (November 2000), pp. 1436-1443, ISSN: 0013-9580

Artama, M., Isojärvi, J.I.T., Auvinen, A. (2006). Antiepileptic drugs use and birth rate in patients with epilepsy - a population- based cohort study in Finland. *Human Reproduction.* Vol.21, No.9, (September 2006), pp.2290-2295. ISSN: 0268-1161

Azarbayjani, F., Danielsson, B.R. (1998). Pharmacologically induced embryonic dysrythmia and episodes of hypoxia followed by reoxygenation: A common teratogenic mechanism for antiepileptic drugs? *Teratology.* Vol. 57, No.3, (March 1998), pp.117-126, ISSN: 0040-3709

Battino, D., Kaneko, S., Andermann, E., Avanzini, G., Canevini, M.P., Canger, R., Croci, D., Fumarola, C., Guidolin, L., et al. (1999) Intrauterine growth in the offspring of epileptic wome: a prospective multicenter study. Epilepsy Research. Vol 36, No.1 (August 1999), pp.53-60, ISSN:0920-1211

Bauer, J., Bös, M., Rück, J., Stoffel-Wagner, B. (2010). Folsäuresubstitution bei Frauen mit Epilepsie. Evaluation des Substitutionseffektes durch intraerythrozytäre Folsäurebestimmung. Nervenartzt (July 2010). DOI: 10.1007/s00115-010-3077-6, ISSN: 0028-2804, 15.3.2011. Available on www.springerlink.com/content/u381561731q24027/fulltext.pdf

Bennett, G.D., Amore, B.M., Finnell, R.H., Wlodarczyk, B., Kalhorn, T.F., Skiles, G.L., Nelson, S.D., Slattery, J.T. (1996). Teratogenicity of carbamazepine-10, 11-epoxide and oxcarbazepine in the SWV mouse. *J Pharmacol Exp Ther.* Vol.279, No.3, (Dec 1996), pp.1237-1242, ISSN: 0022-3565

Borthen, I., Eide, M.G., Veiby, G., Daltveit, A.K., Gilhus, N.E. (2009). Complications during pregnancy in women with epilepsy: population-based cohort study. *BJOG* Vol.116, No.13, (December 2009), pp. 1736-1742, ISSN: 1470-0328

Bromfield, E.B., Dworetzky, B.A., Wyszynski, D.F., Smith, C.R., Baldwin, E.J., Holmes, L.B. (2008). Valproate teratogenicity and epilepsy syndrome. *Epilepsia.* Vol.49, No.12, (December 2008), pp. 2122-2124, ISSN: 0013-9580

Bruno, M.K., Harden, C.L.(2004). Epilepsy in pregnant women. *Expert Opin Drug Saf.* Vol.3, No.5, (September 2004), pp.415-24, ISSN: 1474-0338

Buehler, B.A., Delimont, D., van Waes, M., Finnel, R.H.(1990). Prenatal prediction of risk of the fetal hydantoin syndrome. *New Eng J Med.* Vol.322, No.22, (May 1990), pp. 15671572, ISSN: 0028-4793

Buehler, B.A., Rao, V., Finnell, R.H. (1994). Biochemical and molecular teratology of fetal hydantoin syndrome. *Neurol Clin.* Vol.12, No.4, (November 1994), pp.741-748, ISSN: 0733-8619

Centa, A., Rasore-Quartino, A. (1965). The "digito-cardiac" malformative syndrome (Holt-Oram): genetic forms and phenocopy. Probable action of antiepileptic drugs. *Pathologica.* Vol.57, No.853, (Sep-Oct 1965), pp.227-232, ISSN: 0031-2983

Chong, D.J., Bazil, C.W. (2010). Update on Anticonvulsant Drugs. *Curr Neurol Neurosci Rep.* Vol.10, No.4, (July 2010), pp. 308-308. ISSN: 1528-4042

Christensen, H.D., Rayburn, W.F., Parker, K.M., Gonzales, C.L., Gold, K.P. (2004). Chronic prenatal exposure to carbamazepine and perinatal outcome of C3H/HE mice.

American Journal of Obstetricy and Gynecology. Vol.190,No.1, (January 2004), pp.259-263, ISSN: 0002-9378

Cunnington, M.C., Messenheimer J.A. (2007). Fourteen year interim results from an international observation study of pregnancy outcomes following exposure to lamotrigine. *Epilepsia.* Vol. 48, Suppl 6, (n.d.), pp.322-323, ISSN: 0013-9580

Danielsson, B., Sköld, A.C., Azarbayjani, F., Ohman, I., Webster, W. (2000). Pharmacokinetic data support pharmacologically induced embryonic dysrhythmia as explanation to Fetal Hydantoin Syndrome in rats. *Toxicol Appl Pharmacol.* Vol.163, No.2, (March 2000), pp.164-175, ISSN: 0041-008X

Dansky, L.V., Finnel, R.H. (1991). Parental epilepsy, anticonvulsant drugs, and reproductive outcome: Epidemiologic and experimental Findings spanning three decades; 2: Human studies. *Reproductive Toxicology.* Vol.5, No.4, (n.d.), 301- 335, ISSN: 0890-6238

Davis, A.R., Pack, A.M., Kritzer, J., Yoon, A., Camus, A. (2008). Reproductive history, sexual behavior and use of contraception in women with epilepsy. *Contraception.* Vol.77, No.6, (June 2008), pp.405-409, ISSN: 0010-7824

De Santis, M., Straface G, Cavaliere, G.A.F., Nobili, E., Carducci, B., Caruso, A.(2004). New Antiepileptic drugs: Case series of pregnancy exposure. *Reproductive Toxicology.* Vol.19, No.2, (n.d.), pp. 256-257, ISSN: 0890-6238

De Wals, P., Tairou, F., Van Allen, M.I., Uh, S.H., Lowry, R.B., Sibbald, B., Evans, J.A., Van den Hof, M.C., Zimmer, P., Crowley, M., Fernandez, B., Lee, N.S., Niyonsenga, T. (2007). Reduction in neural-tube defects after folic acid fortification in Canada. *N Engl J Med.* Vol.357, No.2, (July 2007), pp.135-142. ISSN: 0028-4793

Di Renzo, F., Broccia, M.L., Giavini, E., Menegola, E. (2010). VPA-related axis skeletal defects and apoptosis: A proposed event cascade. *Reproductive Toxicology* Vol.29, No.1, (January 2010), pp.106-112, ISSN: 0890-6238

Diav-Citrin, O., Shechtman, S., Bar-Oz, B., Cantrell, D., Arnon, J., Ornoy, A. (2008). Pregnancy outcome after in utero exposure to valproate: evidence of dose relationship in teratogenic effect. *CNS drugs.* Vol.22, No.4, (n.d.), pp.325-334, ISSN: 1172-7047

Diav-Citrin, O., Shetchman, S., Arnon, J., Ornoy, A.(2001). Is carbamazepine teratogenic? A prospective controlled study of 210 pregnancies. *Neurology.* Vol.57, No.2, (July 2001), pp.321-324, ISSN: 0028-3878

Einarson, A.R.N., Koren, G. (1999). Dextromethorphan: Extrapolation of findings from reproductive studies in animals to humans. *Canadian Family Physician.* Vol. 45, (October 1999), pp. 2053-7, ISSN: 0008-350X

Eisenschenk, S. (2006). Treatment with oxcarbazepine during pregnancy. *Neurologist.* Vol..12, No.5, (September 2006), pp.249-254, ISSN: 1074-7931.

Finnel, R.H., Mohl, V.K., Bennet, G.D., Taylor, S.M. (1986). Failure of epoxide formation to influence carbamazepine- induced teratogenesis in a mouse model. *Teratol Carcinog Mutagen.* Vol.6, No.5, (n.d.), pp.393-401, ISSN: 0270-3211

French, J., Edrich, P., Cramer, J.A.(2001). A systematic review of the safety profile of levetiracetam: a new antiepileptic drug. *Epilepsy Research.* Vol. 47, No. 1-2, (November 2001), pp.77-90, ISSN: 0920-1211

Fritz, H., Müller, D., Hess, R. (1976). Comparative study of the teratogenicity of phenobarbitone, diphenylhydantoin and carbamazepine in mice. *Toxicology.* Vol.6, No.3, (November-December 1976), pp.323-330, ISSN: 0300-483X

Gelineau-van Waes, J., Bennett, G.D., Finnell, R.H. (1999). Phenytoin-induced alterations in craniofacial gene expression. *Teratology.* Vol.59, No. 1, (January 1999), pp.23-34, ISSN 0040-3709

Gentile, S.(2009). Topiramate in pregnancy and breastfeeding. *Clin Drug Investig*. Vol. 29. No.2, (n.d.), pp. 139-141. ISSN: 1173-2563

Hanson, J.W., Smith, D.W. (1975). The fetal hydantoin syndrome. *J Pediatr*. Vol.87, No.2, (August 1975), pp.85-90. ISSN: 0022-3476

Helbig, K.L., Bernhardt, B.A., Conway, L.J., Valverde, K.D., Helbig, I., Sperling, M.R. (2010). Genetic risk perception and reproductive decision making among people with epilepsy. *Epilepsia*. Vol. 51, No.9, (September 2010), pp.1874-1877, ISSN: 0013-9580

Hernandez-Diaz, S. Mittendorf, R., Holmes, L.B. (2010). W9. Comparative safety of topamirate during pregnancy. Teratology society program. (abs). *Birth Defects Research (Part A)*. Vol.88, No.5, (May 2010), pp.408, ISSN: 1542-0752

Holmes, L.B., Harvey, E.A., Coull, B.A., Huntington, K.B., Khoshbin, S., Hayes, A.M., Ryan, L.M. (2001). The teratogenicity of anticonvulsant drugs. N Engl J Med. Vol.344, No.15, (April 2001), pp. 1132-1138, ISSN: 0028-4793

Holmes, L.B., Wyszynski, D.F., Baldwin, E.J., Habecker, E., Glassman, L.H., Smith, C.R. (2006). Increased risk for non-syndromic cleft palate among infants exposed to lamotrigine during pregnancy. *Birth Defects Res A Clin Mol Teratol*. Vol.76, No.5 (May 2006), p.318, ISSN: 1542-0752

www.eurocat-network.eu/content/Special-Report-Env-Risk-I-and-II.pdf, access 18.3.2011.

Hunt, S., Craigh, J., Russell, A., Guthrie, E., Parsons, L., Robertson, I., Waddel, R., Irwin, B., Morrison, P.J., Morrow, J. (2006). Levetiracetam in pregnancy: Preliminary experience from the UK Epilepsy and Pregnancy Register. *Neurology*. Vol. 67, No.10 (November 2006), pp.1876-1879, ISSN: 0028-3878

Hunt, S., Russell, A., Smithson, W.H., Parsons, L., Robertson, I., Waddell, R., Irwin, B., Morrison, P.J., Morrow, J., Craig, J. (2008). Topiramate in pregnancy. Preliminary experience from The UK Epilepsy and Pregnancy Register. *Neurology*. Vol.71, No.4, (July 2008), pp.272-276, ISSN: 0028-3878

Isoherranen, N., Spiegelstein, O., Bialer, M., Zhang, J., Merriweather, M., Yagen, B., Roeder, M. Triplett, A.A., Schurig, V., Finnell, R.H. (2003). Developmental outcome of levetiracetam, its major metabolite in humans, 2-pyrrolidinone N-butyric acid, and its enantiomer (R)-alp a-ethyl-oxo-pyrrolidine acetamide in a mouse model of teratogenicity. *Epilepsia*. Vol.44, No.10, (October 2003), pp.1280-1288, ISSN: 0013-9580

Jelínek, R. (2005). The contribution of new findings and ideas to the old principles of teratology. *Reproductive Toxicology*. Vol.20, No.3 (September-October 2005), pp. 295–300, ISSN: 0890-6238

Jentink, J., Dolk, H.D., Loane, M.A., Morris, J.K., Wellesley, D., Garne, E., de Jong-van den Berg, L. (2010). Intrauterine exposure to carbamazepine and specific congenital malformations: systematic review and case-control study. *British Medical Journal*. Vol.341-c6581, ISSN: 0959-535X 15.3.2011 Available on www.bmj.com/content/341/bmj.c6581.full.pdf

Jentink, J., Loane, M.A., Dolk, H., Barisic, I., Garne, E., Morris, J.K., de Jong-van den Berg, L.T.W. (for EUROCAT). (2010). Valproic acid monotherapy in pregnancy and major congenital malformations. *N Engl J Med*. Vol.362, No.23 (June2010), pp.2185-2193, ISSN: 0028-4793

Johannessen, S.I., Helde, G., Brodtkorb, E. (2005). Levetiracetam concentrations in serum and in breast milk at birth and during lactation. *Epilepsia*. Vol.46, No.5, (May 2005), pp.775-7, ISSN: 0013-9580

Jones KL (1997) Fetal hydantoin syndrome, Fetal valproate syndrome In: *Smith´s Recognizable Patters of Human Malformation* (5th ed). pp. 559-567. WB Saunders co. ISBN 0-72166115-7. Philadelphia, Pennsylvania, USA

Jones, K.L., Johnson, K.A., Chambers, C.C. (1992). Pregnancy outcome in women treated with phenobarbital monotherapy. *Teratology.* Vol.45, No.5, (May 1995) , pp.452-453, ISSN 0040-3709

Kaaja, E., Kaaja, R., Hiilesmaa, V. (2003). Major malformations in offspring of women with epilepsy. *Neurology.* Vol.60, No.4 (February 2003), pp.575-579. ISSN: 0028-3878

Källén, A.J. (1994). Maternal carbamazine and infant spina bifida. *Reproductive Toxicology.* Vol.8, No.3, (May-June 1994), pp. 203-205. ISSN: 0890-6238

Källén, B., Hay, S. (1991). *Congenital malformation worldwide A Report from The International Clearinghouse for Birth Defects Monitoring systems.* Elsevier. ISBN 0-444-89137-4, Amsterdam, The Netherlands

Källén, B., Robert, E., Mastroiacovo, P., Martinez-Frías, M.L., Castilla, E.E., Cocchi, G.(1989). Anticonvulsant drugs and malformations, is there a drug specificity? *Eur J Epidemiol.* Vol.5, No.1, (March 1989), pp. 31-6, ISSN 0393-2990

Kalter, H. (2003). *Teratology in the twentieth century.* pp.215-222. Elsevier, ISBN 0-444-51364-7, Amsterdam, The Netherlands

Khouri, N.A. (2005). Reproductive toxic effects of Topamax ingestion in female Sprangue Dawley rats. *Neuroendocrinology Letters* Vol.26, No.6, (December 2005), pp.843-7. ISSN 0172-780X

Kluger, B.M,, Meador, K,J. (2008). Teratogenicity of antiepileptic medications. *Semin Neurol.* Vol.28, No.3, (July 2008), pp.328-35, ISSN: 0271-8235

Koren, G., Nava-Ocampo, A.A., Moretti, M.E., Sussman, R., Nulman, I. (2006). Major malformations with valproic acid. *Canadian Family Physician* Vol. 52, No.4, (April 2006), pp. 441-447, ISSN 0008-350X

Kořístková,B., Grundmann, M. (2005). Comparison of the consumption of antiepileptic drugs in the Czech Republic, Scandinavia and Australia. *Česká a Slovenská Farmacie.* Vol.54, No.3, (May 2005), pp. 130-136, ISSN: 1210-7816

Kuhnz, W., Koch, S., Jakob, S., Hartmann, A., Helge, H., Nau, H.(1984). Ethosuximide in epileptic women during pregnancy and lactation period. Placental transfer, serum concentration in nursed infants and clinical status. *British Journal of Clinical Pharmacology* Vol.18, No.5, (November 1984), pp.671-677. ISSN: 0306-5251

Lamotrigine Pregnancy Registry. Interim Report. 1 September 1992 through 31 March, 2009. (July, 2009). Kendle International Inc, Wilmington NC,

Lawthom, C., Smith, P.E.M., Wild, J.M. (2009) In utero exposure to vigabatrin: No indication of visual field loss. *Epilepsia.* Vol.50, No.2, (February 2009), pp. 318-321, ISSN: 0013-9580

Lombardo, S.A., Leanza, G., Meli, C., Lombardo, M.E., Mazzone, L., Vincenti, L., Cioni, M. (2005). Maternal exposure to the antiepileptic drug vigabatrin affects postnatal development in the rat. *Neurol Sci.* Vol.26, No.2, (June 2005), pp.89-94, ISSN1590-1874

Long, L. (2003). Levetiracetam monotherapy during pregnancy: a case series. *Epilepsy Behaviour.* Vol.4, No.4, (August 2003), pp.447-8. ISSN: 1525-5050

Longo, B., Forinash, A.B., Murphy, J.A. (2009). Levetiracetam use in pregnancy. *Ann Pharmacother.* Vol.43, No.10, (October 2009), pp. 1692-1695, ISSN: 1060-0280

Malm, H., Kajantie, E., Kivirikko, S., Kääriäinen, H., Peippo, M., Somer, M. (2002). Valproate embryopathy in three sets of siblings: further proof of hereditary susceptibility. *Neurology.* Vol.59, No.4, (August 2002), pp.630-633, ISSN: 0028-3878

Maňáková, E., Hubičková-Heringová, L., Jelínek, R. (2006). Czech Teratology Information Service: Comparison of treatments by psychotropic and antiepileptic drugs.

Neuroendocrinology Letters. Vol.27, Suppl.2 (December 2006), pp.74-77, ISSN: 0172-780X

Manent, J.B., Jorquera, I., Franco ,V., Ben-Ari, Y., Perucca, E., Represa, A. (2008). Antiepileptic drugs and brain maturation: fetal exposure to lamotrigine generates cortical malformations in rats. *Epilepsy Res.* Vol.78, No.2-3, (February 2008), pp.131-139, ISSN 0920-1211

Massey, K.M. (1966). Teratogenic effects of diphenylhydantoin sodium. *J Oral Ther Pharmacol.* Vol.2, No.5, (March 1966), pp. 380-385.

Matalon, S., Schechtman, S., Goldzweig, G., Ornoy, A. (2002) The teratogenic effect of carbamazepine: a meta-analysis of 1255 exposures. *Reproductive Toxicology.* Vol.16, No.1, (January -February 2002), pp. 9-17, ISSN: 0890-6238

McElhatton, P.R. Sullivan, F.M. (1975). Procceding: Teratogenic effect of primidone in mice. *Br J Pharmacol.* Vol.54, No.2, (June 1975), pp.267P-268P, ISSN 0007-1188

Meador, K.J., Baker, G.A., Finnel, R.H., Kalayjian, L.A., Liporace, J.D., Loring, D.W., Mawer, G., Pennel, P.B., Smith, J.C., Wolff, M.C. (2006). In utero antiepileptic drugs exposure: Fetal death and malformations. *Neurology* Vol.67, No.3, (August 2006), pp.407-412, ISSN: 0028-3878

Meador, K.J., Penovich, P. (2008). What is the risk of orofacial clefts from lamotrigine exposure during pregnancy? Comment on. *Neurology.* Vol.71, No.10, (September 2008), pp.706-707, ISSN: 0028-3878

Meador, K.J., Penovich, P., Baker, G.A., Pennell, P.B., Bromfield, E., Pack, A., Liporace, J.D., Sam, M., Kalayjian, L.A., Thurman, D.J., Moore, E., Loring, D.W. (2009). Antiepileptic drug use in women of childbearing age. *Epilepsy Behav.* Vol.15, No.3, (July 2009), pp.339-343, ISSN:1525-5050

Meadow, S.R. (1968). Anticonvulsant drugs and congenital abnormalities. *Lancet.* Vol.14, No.2 (7581), (December 1968), pp.1296, ISSN: 0140-6736

Meier, U.T., Meyer, U.A. (1987). Genetic polymorphism of human cytochrome P-450 (S)-mephenytoin 4-hydrolase. Studies with human autoantibodies suggest a functionally altered cytochrome P450 isozyme as a cause of the genetic deficiency. *Biochemistry.* Vol.26, No.25, (December 1987), pp.8466-8474, ISSN: 0006-2960

Meischenguiser, R., D´Giano, C.H., Ferraro, S.M. (2004). Oxcarbazepine in pregnancy: clinical experience in Argentina. *Epilepsy and Behaviour.* Vol.5, No.2, (April 2004), pp.163-167, ISSN:1525-5050

Menegola, E., Di Renzo, F., Broccia, M.L., Prudenziati, M., Minucci, S., Massa, V., Gaviani, E. (2005). Inhibition of histone deacetylase activity on specific embryonic tissue as a new mechanism for teratogenicity. *Birth Defect Research (Part B).* Vol.74, No.5, (October 2005), pp.392-398, ISSN: 1542-9741

Merlob, P., Stahl, B. (2002). Classification of drugs for teratogenic risk: an anachronistic way of counselling. *Teratology.* Vol.66, No.2 (August 2002), pp.61–62, ISSN: 0040-3709

Micromedex® 2.0 (electronic version). Thomson Reuters (Healthcare) Inc., Greenwood Village, Colorado,USA. Avaible at: http://www.thomsonhc.com.ezproxy.is.cuni.cz (cited: *March/15/2011*).

Miskov, S., Gjergja-Juraski, R., Cvitanovic-Sojat, L., Bakulic, T.I., Fucic, A., Bosnjak-Pasic, M., Mikula, I., Demarin, V. (2009). Prospective surveillance of Croatian pregnant women on lamotrigine monotherapy- aspects of pre-pregnancy counselling and drug monitoring. *Acta Clin Croat.* Vol.48, No.3, (September 2009), pp.271-281, ISSN: 0353-9466

Montouris, G. (2005). Safety of the newer antiepileptic drug oxcarbazepine during pregnancy. *Curr Med Res Croat.* Vol.48, No.5, (May 2005), pp. 693-701, ISSN: 0300-7995

Morin, P., De Wals, P., St.Cyr-Tribble, D., Niyonsenga, T., Payette, H. (2002). Pregnancy planning: a determinant of folic acid supplements use for the primary prevention of neural tube defects. *Can J Public Health.* Vol.93, No.4, (Jul-Aug 2002), pp.259-263. ISSN: 0008-4263

Morrow, J.I., Russell, A., Gutherie, E., Parsons, L., Robertson, I., Waddell, R., Irwin, B., Morrison, P., McGivern, C.R., Craig, J. (2006). Malformation risks of antiepileptic drugs in pregnancy: A prospective study from UK Epilepsy and Pregnancy Register. *Journal of Neurology, Neurosurgery, and Psychiatry.* Vol.77, No.2,, (February2006), pp.193-198, ISSN: 0022-3050

Müller-Küppers, M. (1963). On problems of fetal damage during pregnancy caused by intake of anticonvulsants. *Acta Paedopsychiatr.* Vol.30, (Nov-Dec 1963), pp.401-405, ISSN: 0001-6586

Nulman, I. (2010). Carbamazepine in pregnancy. *BMJ.* Vol.341:c6582, ISSN: 0959-535X 15.3.2011. Available on www.bmj.com content/341/bmj.c6582.long

Nulman, I., Laslo, D., Koren, G. (2001). Treatment for epilepsy in pregnancy. In: Koren, G. (Ed.) *Maternal-fetal toxicology. A Clinician´s Guide.*(3rd ed). Marcel Dekker Inc. ISBN 0-8247-0378-2, New York, NY, USA

Ogawa, Y., Kaneko, S., Otani, K., Fukushima, Y. (1991). Serum folic acid levels in epileptic mothers and their relationship to congenital malformations. *Epilepsy Res.* Vol.8, No.1, (January 1991), pp.75-78, ISSN: 0920-1211

Ohtahara, S., Yamatogi, Y. (2007) Erratum to "Safety of zonisamide therapy: Prospective follow-up survey." *Seizures.* Vol. 16,No.1,(January 2007), pp. 87-93, ISSN: 1059-1311

Okada, A., Noyori, H., Yagen, B., Shimshoni, J.A., Bialer, M., Fujiwara, M. (2009). Anticonvulsant profile and teratogenic evaluation of potent new analogues of a valproic acid urea derivative in NMRI mice. *Birth defect research (Part B) Dev Reprod Toxicol.* Vol.86 No. 5, (October 2009), pp.394-401, ISSN: 1542-9741

Ornoy, A. (2009). Valproic acid in pregnancy: How much are we endangering the embryo and fetus? *Reprod Toxicol.* Vol.28, No.1, (July 2009), pp.1-10, ISSN 0890-6238

Ornoy, A., Arnon, J., Shechtman, S., Moerman, L., Lukashova, I. (1998). Is benzodiazepine use during pregnancy really teratogenic? *Reprod Toxicol* . Vol.12, No.5, (September - October 1998), pp. 511-515, ISSN 0890-6238.

Ornoy, A., Cohen, E. (1996). Outcome of children born to epileptic mothers treated with carbamazepine during pregnancy. *Archives of Disease in Childhood.* Vol.75, No.6, (December 1996), pp.517-520, ISSN: 0003-9888

Ornoy, A., Zvi, N., Arnon, J., Wajnberg, R., Schechtman, S., Diav-Citrin, O. (2008). The outcome of pregnancy following topiramate treatment:A study on 52 pregnancies. Reproductive Toxicology Vol.25, No.3,(April 2008), pp.388-389, ISSN: 0890-6238

Padmanabhan, R., Abdulrazzaq, Y.M., Bastaki, S.M.A., Nurulain, M., Shafiullah, M.(2010). Vigabatrin (VGB) administered during late gestation lowers maternal folate concentration and causes pregnancy loss, fetal growth restriction and skeletal hypoplasia in the mouse. *Reprod. Toxicol.* Vol.29, No.3, (June 2010), pp. 366-377, ISSN 0890-6238.

Padmanabhan, R., Abdulrazzaq, Y.M., Bastaki, S.M.A., Shafiullah, M.,Chandranath, S.I. (2003). Experimental studies on reproductive toxicologic effects of lamotrigine in mice. *Birth Defect Research (Part B).* Vol.68, No.5, (October 2003), pp.428-438, ISSN: 1542-9733

Pennell PB. (2003) Antiepileptic drug pharmacokinetics during pregnancy and lactation. *Neurology*. Vol.61, Suppl. 2, (September 2003), pp.S35-S42, ISSN: 0028-3878

Rating, D., Nau, H., Jäger-Roman, E., Göpfert-Geyer, I., Koch, S., Beck-Mannagetta, G., Schmidt, D., Helge, H. (1982). Teratogenic and pharmacokinetic studies of primidone during pregnancy and in the offspring of epileptic women. *Acta Pediatr Scand.* Vol.71, No.2, (Mar 1982), pp.301-311, ISSN: 0803-5253

Robert-Gnansia, E., Schaefer, C.(2007).Antiepileptics In: *Drugs during pregnancy and lactation*. Schaefer, C., Peters, P., Miller, R.K.(2nd edition). pp.255-287. Elsevier. ISBN 978-0-444-52072-2, London

Rochester, J.A., Kirchner, J.T. (1997). Epilepsy in pregnancy: *Am Fam Physician*.Vol.56, No.6, (October 1997), pp.1631-1638, ISSN: 0002-838X

Rosa, F.W. (1991). Spina bifida in infants of women treated with carbamazepine during pregnancy. *New England Journal of Medicine*. Vol.324, No.10, (March 1991), pp. 674-677. ISSN: 0028-4793

Saillenfait, A.M., Gallisot, F., Sabaté, J.P. (2007). Developmental toxic effects of N-ethyl-2-pyrrolidone administered orally to rats. *Journal of Applied Toxicology*. Vol.27, No.5, (September-October 2007), pp.491-497, ISSN 0260-437X

Selak, I. Pregabalin (Pfizer). (2001). *Curr Opin Investig Drugs*. Vol.2., No.6. (June 2001), pp. 828-834, ISSN: 1472-4472

Shepard, T.H., Lemire, R.J. (2004) Clonazepan In: *Catalog of teratogenic agents*. The John Hopkins University Press Baltimore, Maryland, USA. pp. 96 (11th ed.), ISBN 0-8018-7953-1

Shor, S., Koren, G., Nulman, I. (2007). Teratogenicity of lamotrigine. *Canadian Family Physician*.Vol.53, No.6, (June 2007), pp.1007 - 1009, ISSN: 0008-350X

Sorri, I., Herrgård, E., Viinikainen, K., Pääkkönen, A., Heikonen, S., Kälviäinen, R. (2005). Ophtalmologic and neurologic findings in two children exposed to vigabatrin in utero. *Epilepsy Research*. Vol.65, No.1-2, (June 2005), pp.117-120, ISSN: 0920-1211

Speigelstein, O., Chatterjie, N., Alexander, G., Finnell, R.H. (2003). Teratogenicity of valproate conjugates with anticonvulsant activity in mice. *Epilepsy Research*. Vol.57, No.2-3, (December 2003), pp.145-152, ISSN: 0920-1211

Steinlein, O.K. (2010). Gene polymorphism and their role in epilepsy treatment and prognosis. *Naunyn-Schmied Arch Pharmacol*. Vol.382, No.2 (August 2010), pp.109-118, ISSN: 0028-1298

Strickler, S.M., Dansky, L.V., Miller, M.A., Seni, M.H., Andermann, E., Spielberg, S.P. (1985). Genetic predisposition to phenytoin- induced birth defects. *Lancet*. Vol.326, No.8458, (October 1985), pp.746-749, ISSN: 0140-6736

Sullivan F.M., McElhatton, P.R. (1977). A comparison of the teratogenic activity of the antiepileptic drugs carbamazepine, clonazepam, ethosuximide, phenobarbital, phenytoin, and primidone in mice. *Toxicology and Applied Pharmacology*. Vol 40, No.2, (May 1977), pp. 365-378 ,ISSN 0041-008X

Sutcliffe, A.G., Jones, R.B., Woodruff, G. (1998). Eye Malformation associated with treatment with carbamazepine during pregnancy. *Ophthalmic Genet*. Vol.19, No.2, (June 1998), pp.59-62, ISSN: 1381-6810

ten Berg, K., Samren, E.B., van Oppen, A.C., Engelsman, M., Lindhout, D. Levetiracetam use and pregnancy outcome. (2005). *Reproductive Toxicology*. Vol.20, No.1, (May-June 2005), pp.175-178, ISSN: 0890-6238

Tomson, T. (2006). Seizure control and treatment in pregnancy: Observations from the EURAP Epilepsy Pregnancy Registry. *Neurology*. Vol. 66, No.3, (February 2006), pp.354 - 360, ISSN: 0028-3878

Tomson, T., Battino, D. (2009). Teratogenic effect of antiepileptic medications. *Neurol Clin.* Vol.27, No.4, (November 2009), pp. 993-1002, ISSN: 0733-8619

Tomson,T., Hiilesmaa, V. (2007). Epilepsy in pregnancy. *BJM* Vol.335, No.7623, (October 2007), pp. 769-773, ISSN: 0959-535X

Tripp, J.H., Hargreaves, T., Anthony, P.P., Searle, J.F., Miller, P., Leonard, J.V., Patrick, A.D., Oberholzer, V.G. (1981). Sodium valproate and ornithine carbamyl transferase deficiency. *Lancet.* Vol.317, No.8230 (May 1981), pp.1165-1166, ISSN: 0140-6736

Tung, E.W.Y., Winn, L.M. (2010). Epigenetic modification in valproic acid-induced teratogenesis. *Toxicology and Applied Pharmacology.* Vol. 248, No.3, (August 2010), pp.201-209, ISSN: 0041-008X

Vajda, F.J.E., Eadie, M.J. (2005). Maternal valproate dosage and foetal malformations. *Acta Neurol Scand.* Vol.112, No.3, (September 2005), pp.137-143, ISSN: 0001-6314

Vajda, F.J.E., Graham, J.E., Hitchcock, A.A., O´Brien, T.J., Lander, C.M., Eadie, M.J. (2010). Is lamotrigine a significant human teratogen? Observation from the Australia Pregnancy Register. *Seizure.* Vol.19, No.9, (August 2010), pp.558-561, ISSN: 1059-1311

Vajda, F.J.E., Lander, C.M., Hitchcock, A., Graham, J., Solinas, C., O´Brien, T.O., Eadie, M.J. (2007). Changing Australian prescribing pattern for antiepileptic drugs in pregnancy and their possible consequences. *Journal of Clinical Neuroscience.* Vol. 14, No.7, (July 2007), pp. 611-617, ISSN: 0967-5868. Avaible on www. elsevier. com/locate/jocn

Vajda, F.J.E., Hollingworth, S., Graham, J., Hichcock, A.A., O´Brien, T.J., Lander, C.M., Eadie, M.J. (2010) Changing patterns of antiepileptic drug use in pregnant Australian women. *Acta Neurologica Scandinavica* Vol. 121, No.2, (December 2010), pp.89-93, ISSN: 0001-6314

Verrotti, A., Tana, M., Pelliccia, P,. Chiarelli, F., Latini,G. (2006). Recent advances on neural tube defects with special reference to valproic acid. *Endocrine, metabolic and immune disorders – Drug target.* Vol.6, No.1, (March 2006), pp.25-31, ISSN: 1871-5303 31.5.2011. Available on www.benthamdirect.org/pages/b_viewarticle.php

Vila Cerén, C., Demestre Guasch, X., Raspall Torrent, F., Elizari Saco, M.J., Sala Castellví, P., Martínez Nadal, S. Topiramate and pregnancy. Neonate with bone anomalies. *An Pediatr (Barc).* Vol.63, No.4, (Oct 2005), pp.363-365. ISSN: 1695-4033

Wray, S.D., Hassel, T.M., Phillips, C., Johnston, M.C. (1982). Preliminary study of the effects of carbamazepine on congenital orofacial defects in offspring of A/J mice. *Epilepsia.* Vol.23, No.1, (February 1982), pp.101-110, ISSN: 0013-9580

Žižka J. (1994). Embryopathia hydantoinica In: *Diagnostika syndromů a malformací.* pp98-99. Galén, ISBN 80-85824-04-3, Prague, Czech Republic

11

Health Technology Assessment of Lacosamide as Adjunctive Therapy for Partial-Onset Epileptic Seizures

Steven Simoens
Katholieke Universiteit Leuven, Belgium

1. Introduction

Epilepsy is a neurological disorder that disrupts the normal transmission of electrical signals in the brain and is characterised by abnormal electrical neuronal activity resulting clinically in unprovoked recurring seizures. Partial-onset seizures are those that involve only a portion of the brain at seizure onset. The prevalence of epilepsy varies between 4 and 8 cases per 1,000 individuals in developed countries (Hauser, 1990), and partial seizures are the predominant type of epileptic seizures (Kotsopoulos et al., 2002).

Epileptic seizures are associated with significant morbidity, impaired quality of life, mortality, and are a primary driver of hospital admissions and health care costs. A literature review reported an increased mortality risk for people with epilepsy as compared with the general population (Hitiris et al., 2007). A bottom-up, prevalence-based, cost-of-illness analysis estimated the costs of epilepsy from a societal perspective in the 25 European Union member countries, plus Iceland, Norway, and Switzerland (Pugliatti et al., 2007). The estimated total cost of the disease in Europe was € 15.5 billion in 2004, indirect costs related to productivity loss being the single most important cost category (€ 8.6 billion). The total cost per case was € 2,000–11,500 and the estimated cost per European individual was € 33.

Treatment with anti-epileptic drugs (AEDs) is the mainstay of therapy for people with epilepsy and treatment tends to begin with monotherapy (Brodie & Dichter, 1997). First-generation AEDs available before 1980 (e.g. carbamazepine, phenytoin, phenobarbital, valproic acid) are used first-line as monotherapy (Perucca & Meador, 2005). Although many patients respond to their first treatment, more than 1 in 3 patients have seizures despite treatment with AEDs (Schmidt & Gram, 1995). Treatment of refractory epilepsy will move to polytherapy by adding second-generation AEDs available after 1993 (e.g. felbamate, gabapentin, lamotrigine, levetiracetam, oxcarbazepine, pregabalin, tiagabine, topiramate, vigabatrin, zonisamide) to monotherapy regimens (adjunctive therapy). A literature review of systematic reviews reported that second-generation AEDs were effective as adjunctive therapy for refractory epilepsy as compared with placebo (Wilby et al., 2005). Also, a literature review of economic evaluations of second-generation AEDs showed that adjunctive therapy of refractory epilepsy with AEDs appears to be cost-effective (Simoens, 2010).

Several factors inform the choice of the most appropriate treatment regimen in patients requiring adjunctive therapy. Of key importance is that adjunctive therapy for uncontrolled epilepsy is effective in achieving seizure freedom or reduction in a group of patients who have continued to experience a high seizure burden despite initial treatment for their epilepsy. Given the chronic nature of epilepsy and the requirement for life-long management in many cases, it is important that treatments are tolerable. The ease of use and convenience of the drug also need to be considered. Key positive attributes are treatments that do not require multiple administrations a day and those with flexible dosing options. Clinical guidance also states that the AED treatment strategy should be individualized according to the seizure type, epilepsy syndrome, co-medication and co-morbidity, the individual's lifestyle, and the preferences of the individual, their family and/or those who care for the patient as appropriate (National Institute for Health and Clinical Excellence, 2004).

Lacosamide (Vimpat®, UCB Pharma, Brussels, Belgium) is a second-generation AED which is indicated as adjunctive therapy for partial-onset seizures with or without secondary generalisation in patients from 16 years of age in Europe (European Medicines Agency, 2008). Lacosamide (R-2-acetamido-N-benzyl-3-methoxypropionamide) is a functionalised amino acid. Lacosamide is hypothesized to have a dual mode of action: it selectively enhances slow inactivation of voltage-gated sodium channels and binds to collapsin response mediator protein-2, a protein which is mainly expressed in the central nervous system.

Trials in healthy adults have shown that lacosamide is rapidly absorbed and is predominantly excreted as unchanged lacosamide (Ben-Menachem, 2008). It has an oral bioavailability of approximately 100% and an elimination half-life of around 13 hours. Lacosamide has a low potential for pharmacokinetic interaction. The protein binding is low (<15%), thus reducing the potential for displacement interactions. Also, lacosamide does not influence the pharmacokinetic profile or plasma concentrations of commonly-used AEDs such as carbamazepine or valproic acid. Pharmacokinetic parameters do not differ between genders or single or repeat dose administration (European Medicines Agency, 2008).

Lacosamide is available in five formulations in Europe, an oral tablet (50 mg, 100 mg, 150 mg and 200 mg) and a 15mg/ml syrup, and must be taken twice a day. The recommended starting dose is 50 mg twice a day which should be increased to an initial therapeutic dose of 100 mg twice a day after one week. Depending on response and tolerability, the maintenance dose can be further increased by 50 mg twice a day every week, to a maximum daily dose of 400 mg (200 mg twice a day). The recommended daily dose for lacosamide is 300 mg/day.

The aim of this chapter is to conduct a health technology assessment of adjunctive therapy with lacosamide for partial-onset seizures in adult patients by means of a review of the international literature. The literature study focuses specifically on the safety, tolerability, efficacy, costs, cost-effectiveness and budget impact of lacosamide. The findings may serve to aid local decision-makers in allocating scarce health care resources and to inform the prescribing behavior of physicians.

2. Methods

2.1 Search strategy

Studies were identified by searching PubMed, Centre for Reviews and Dissemination databases (Database of Abstracts of Reviews of Effects, National Health Service Economic

Evaluation Database, and Health Technology Assessments Database), Cochrane Database of Systematic Reviews, and EconLit from January 1999 to March 2011. Additionally, the bibliography of included studies was checked for other relevant studies. Search terms included 'epilepsy', 'refractory epilepsy', 'partial-onset seizures', 'adjunctive therapy', 'add-on therapy', 'anti-epileptic drugs', 'lacosamide', 'adult', 'safety', 'tolerability', 'efficacy', 'effectiveness', 'pharmaco-economics', 'cost', 'cost analysis', 'economic evaluation', 'cost-effectiveness', 'cost-minimisation', 'cost-consequence', 'cost-utility', 'cost-benefit', 'budget impact' alone and in combination with each other.

The literature search included articles published in peer-reviewed journals. Additionally, relevant congress abstracts were identified by searching the congress databases of the European Neurological Society, the American Academy of Neurology, and Outcomes Research Digest (an electronic database of abstracts presented at conferences of the International Society of Pharmacoeconomics and Outcomes Research). Finally, UCB Pharma was contacted for any unpublished studies.

2.2 Selection criteria

The literature review included clinical studies examining the safety, tolerability or efficacy of adjunctive therapy with lacosamide for partial-onset seizures in adult patients. The inclusion of clinical studies was restricted to randomized controlled trials or open-label extension trials. Other study designs (e.g. case studies) were not considered. Cost studies were included if they compared health care and/or other costs of lacosamide and an alternative treatment for partial-onset seizures. Evidence about cost-effectiveness was derived from economic evaluations. An economic evaluation was defined as a study comparing lacosamide with an alternative treatment in terms of both costs and consequences (Drummond et al., 2005) (see Figure 1). Economic evaluations were excluded if treatment of partial-onset seizures did not involve lacosamide or if studies analyzed a single intervention without a comparator.

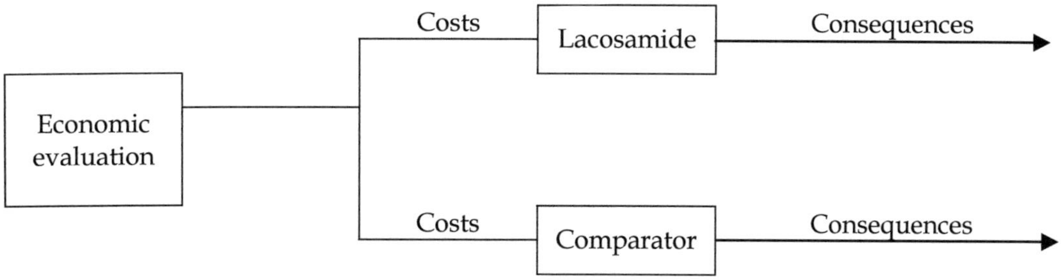

Fig. 1. Economic evaluation of lacosamide

A budget impact analysis explored how a change in the current mix of treatment strategies by the introduction of lacosamide would impact drug spending on partial-onset seizures (see Figure 2).

Studies evaluating intravenous lacosamide were excluded because this article focuses on chronic adjunctive therapy. Literature reviews were searched for original studies, but were not included as such. The review was limited to studies published in English, French, Dutch, or German for practical reasons.

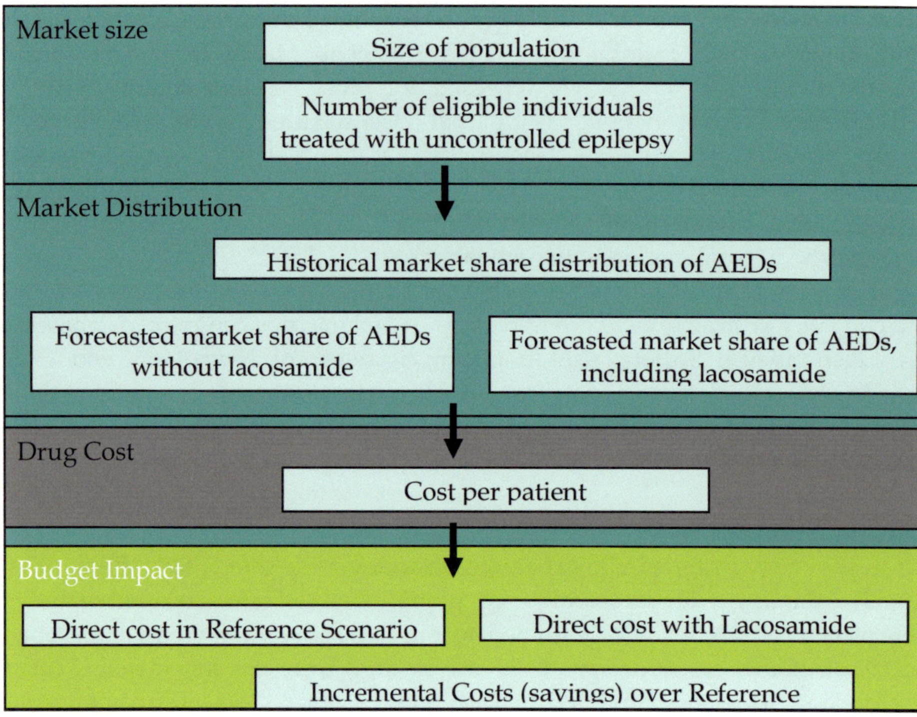

Fig. 2. Budget impact analysis of lacosamide

3. Results

3.1 Search results

Few studies have focused on adjunctive therapy with lacosamide for partial-onset seizures in adult patients: the researcher identified 32 citations, but only nine studies were included in the review: three randomized controlled trials published in peer-reviewed journals14-16, three open-label extension studies published as abstracts (Ben-Menachem et al., 2009; Rosenfeld et al., 2009; Faught et al., 2010; Husain et al., 2010), one economic evaluation published in a peer-reviewed journal (Bolin et al., 2010), and two economic evaluations published as abstracts (one of which also included a budget impact analysis) (Simoens et al., 2010; Soini et al., 2009). Studies were excluded because of one or more of the following reasons: disease other than refractory epilepsy; study not involving lacosamide; study of intravenous lacosamide; study of pharmacodynamic and/or pharmacokinetic profile of lacosamide; literature review rather than original study; case study.

3.2 Safety, tolerability and efficacy

Three randomised, multicentre, double-blind, placebo-controlled trials have been carried out on the efficacy of adjunctive therapy with lacosamide: phase IIb trial 667, phase III trial 754 and phase III trial 755 (Ben-Menachem et al., 2007; Chung et al., 2010; Halasz et al., 2009). The three trials were similar in design and patient baseline characteristics.

All patients included in these pivotal trials were patients who had uncontrolled epilepsy despite previous treatment with at least two other AEDs (concurrently or sequentially) and who were actively treated with concomitant AEDs as standard therapy. The most commonly used concomitant AEDs were carbamazepine, levetiracetam and lamotrigine. The primary objective of these trials was to evaluate the efficacy of lacosamide as adjunctive therapy following treatment failure with at least two other AEDs and co-administered with one or two other AEDs (trial 667) or up to three other AEDs (trials 754 and 755) in patients with uncontrolled partial-onset seizures. The secondary objective was to evaluate the safety of lacosamide. Patients were randomised to a 200 mg, 400 mg or 600 mg daily dose of lacosamide or placebo.

Outcomes were measured in terms of the reduction in seizure frequency, 50% responder rate and seizure-free status. Responder rate was assessed as a reduction in partial-onset seizure frequency of at least 50% from baseline to maintenance phase. Seizure-free status was determined for patients who completed the maintenance phase with zero seizures. Improvements in quality of life, patient function and health status were assessed via secondary endpoints including the Quality of Life Inventory In Epilepsy (QOLIE-31) scale, the Seizure Severity Scale (SSS) and the Patient Global Impression of Change (PGIC) scale.

Patients treated with lacosamide 400 mg/day and 600 mg/day in trial 667 showed a statistically significant reduction in seizure frequency at maintenance endpoint (after 18 weeks) as compared with placebo (400 mg/day: $p = 0.0023$; 600 mg/day: $p = 0.0084$). Patients in trial 754 and 755 also displayed a statistically significant reduction in seizure frequency when treated with lacosamide as compared with patients treated with placebo (Trial 754: 400 mg/day $p = 0.0078$, 600 mg/day $p = 0.0061$; Trial 755: 200 mg/day $p = 0.0223$, 400 mg/day $p = 0.0325$). Lacosamide was associated with a significantly greater median percent reduction in seizure frequency from baseline at a dose of 400 mg/day and 600 mg/day across trials. In trial 755, lacosamide 200 mg/day was associated with a significantly greater median seizure reduction as compared with placebo ($p = 0.04$). Treatment with lacosamide (200–600 mg/day) gave higher responder rates as compared with treatment with placebo. The differences were generally significant as compared with placebo for patients treated with lacosamide 400 mg/day and lacosamide 600 mg/day.

A pooled analysis of the trial data suggested that the median percent reduction in seizure frequency per 28 days from baseline to maintenance period amounted to 18.4% for placebo, 33.3% for lacosamide 200 mg/day ($p<0.01$), 36.8% for 400 mg/day ($p<0.001$), and 39.4% for 600 mg/day. The percentage of patients attaining a reduction in seizure frequency of at least 50% was 22.6% with placebo, 34.1% with lacosamide 200 mg/day ($p<0.05$), 39.7% with lacosamide 400 mg/day ($p<0.001$), 39.6% with lacosamide 600 mg/day. The median percent reduction in seizure frequency and the percentage of patients attaining a reduction in seizure frequency of at least 50% did not vary depending on the number of previously used AEDs. Patient responders with more than 50% seizure reduction in the lacosamide treatment groups experienced significant improvements in QOLIE-31 and SSS scores as compared to baseline ($p<0.05$ for all comparisons of responders to non-responders) (Cramer et al., 2010). The largest improvements were gained for quality-of-life scores including the QOLIE-31 subscales 'seizure worry' and 'social functioning', as well as the SSS overall score. With respect to PGIC, more than 80% of lacosamide responders reported an improved health status. Finally, there seemed to be a dose-responsive trend for seizure freedom rates: 2.7%, 3.3% and 4.8% for lacosamide 200, 400 or 600 mg/day as compared with 0.9% for placebo (French et al., 2009).

The most common drug-associated treatment-emergent adverse events in the lacosamide treatment arms of the pivotal trials were dizziness and nausea (Gil-Nagel et al., 2009). Headache was also commonly reported with lacosamide. The incidence of adverse events was generally higher in the forced titration phase as compared with the maintenance phase,

indicating a reduction in these adverse events over time. Forced titration does not reflect usual clinical practice. Adverse events were reported to be of mild or moderate intensity.
Three open-label extension studies of the pivotal trials explored the long-term safety, tolerability and efficacy of lacosamide (see Table 1) (Ben-Menachem et al., 2009; Rosenfeld et al., 2009; Faught et al., 2010; Husain et al., 2010). Long-term treatment with lacosamide produced a sustained efficacy in and was generally well tolerated by patients suffering from partial-onset seizures. The incidence of adverse events, as well as vital signs and clinical laboratory and ECG findings, among patients taking lacosamide were similar to those reported with short-term use (O'Brien, 2010).

3.3 Costs

No cost study comparing lacosamide with an alternative treatment for partial-onset seizures was identified in the literature. It is difficult to determine the cost implications of adjunctive therapy with lacosamide on patients, the health care system and society. Therefore, Table 1 proposes the major items that need to be considered when calculating costs from a societal perspective. With respect to direct health care costs, current treatment strategies include pharmacotherapy with AEDs throughout life, surgery, and alternative measures – usually palliative – such as vagus nerve stimulation. A study also needs to consider the cost (and clinical) implications of the fact that AED therapy may affect co-morbid disease, that drugs used to treat co-morbid diseases may influence the seizure threshold, that the toxicity of AEDs may be influenced by a co-morbid condition and that clinically relevant drug-drug interactions can arise from the co-administration of AEDs with drugs used to treat co-morbid diseases (Zaccara, 2009). In addition to direct health care costs, future studies need to elicit direct non-health care costs of transportation to health care professionals and indirect costs. With respect to the latter, attention needs to be paid to calculating the indirect costs of days lost to education, costs of reduced ability to carry out normal everyday activities, and the costs of productivity loss of patients and of family/friends who care for patients.

Direct health care costs			Direct non-health care costs	Indirect costs of patients and carers
Medication	Health care providers	Other		
Anti-epileptic drugs Antidepressants Antipsychotics Benzodiazepines Cardiovascular drugs Antineoplastic drugs Antibiotics Antiretroviral drugs Interferons	General practitioner Nurse Pharmacist Neurologist	Diagnostic tests Accident and Emergency visit Hospital stay Surgery Palliative care Home health care services Alternative medicine	Transportation to health care provider Child care costs Home adaptations	Absence from work Reduced productivity at work Time lost from education Reduced ability to carry out usual daily activities

Table 1. Items to be considered in cost studies of lacosamide

3.4 Cost-effectiveness

Three economic evaluations used a similar design to determine the cost-effectiveness of lacosamide from the health care payer perspective in Sweden, Finland and Belgium (Bolin et al., 2010; Simoens et al., 2010; Soini et al., 2009). These studies compared standard AED therapy plus lacosamide with standard AED therapy alone in treating partial-onset seizures with or without secondary generalization in epilepsy patients from 16 years who are uncontrolled on current treatment with at least two AEDs.

A decision-analytic model simulated the treatment pathway of a hypothetical patient cohort over two years. Data about health state probabilities, seizure frequency and utility values were taken from the pivotal trials or from the literature. For instance, the models used a probability of a seizure reduction of 0.368 and a probability of withdrawal due to non-response of 0.632 in patients treated with standard AED therapy plus lacosamide. Similarly, the probability of a 50% seizure reduction was 0.194 and the probability of withdrawal due to non-response was 0.806 in patients treated with standard AED therapy alone. Health care costs included costs of drugs, physician visits, laboratory tests, and hospitalization. The two consequence measures considered were the number of seizures and quality-adjusted life years because AED treatment primarily impacts seizure frequency and health-related quality of life. As the models did not take into account adverse events, the costs associated with adverse events associated with AED treatment was not considered when calculating the cost-effectiveness of lacosamide. Also, the models did not consider mortality. This is because the trials 754 and 755 did not report mortality rates in this specific population of uncontrolled epileptic patients and because of the limited time period of the models of two years (Chung et al., 2010; Halasz et al., 2009). The robustness of results was tested by means of deterministic and probabilistic sensitivity analyses.

The Swedish economic evaluation found that the incremental cost per seizure avoided amounted to € 156 and that the incremental cost per quality-adjusted life year gained was € 27,641 at 24 months (Bolin et al., 2010). If indirect costs of productivity loss would be considered, standard therapy plus lacosamide would be more effective and less expensive than standard therapy alone. According to the Finnish economic evaluation, standard therapy plus lacosamide led to a reduction of 8.92 seizures, an increase of 0.041 quality-adjusted life years, and a cost increase of € 831 per patient as compared with standard therapy alone over a 24-month period (Soini et al., 2009). Using a willingness to pay of € 30,000 and € 50,000 per quality-adjusted life year, the probability of standard therapy plus lacosamide being cost-effective was 74.4% and 87.7%, respectively. The Belgian economic evaluation observed that standard therapy plus lacosamide is more effective and less expensive than standard therapy alone under the two consequence measures considered and under the four time periods considered (6, 12, 18 and 24 months) (Simoens et al., 2010). Extensive sensitivity analyses demonstrated that these results were robust to changes in input parameters.

3.5 Budget impact

In addition to cost-effectiveness, the Finnish study calculated the budget impact of lacosamide from the health care payer perspective (Soini et al., 2009). The analysis compared the "world with lacosamide" to the "world without lacosamide" and calculated how a change in the mix of AEDs used to treat uncontrolled epilepsy would impact drug spending during 2008-2012. Data on the number of patients, AED market shares and unit costs were taken from Finnish sources. The authors applied the conservative assumption of using generic drug prices in the analysis. It should be noted that this analysis focused on drug costs only and did not consider the fact that lacosamide reduces costs of seizure management and withdrawal, as demonstrated by the economic evaluations (Bolin et al., 2010; Simoens et al., 2010; Soini et al., 2009). The results indicated that the expected annual drug budget increase due to the introduction of lacosamide would rise to € 232,600 in 2012. Expressed as a proportion of the annual epilepsy budget, the introduction of lacosamide would increase the budget by 2.23% in 2012.

4. Discussion

Insufficient epilepsy treatment in terms of seizure control may have a significant negative impact on patients' quality of life and represents a substantial economic burden for patients and society. There is an unmet need for treatment options for uncontrolled patients with partial-onset seizures. Lacosamide, a second-generation AED, is indicated for the treatment of such patients. This study has drawn on the international literature in order to provide a comprehensive review of various aspects of pharmacotherapy with lacosamide (i.e. safety, tolerability, efficacy, costs, cost-effectiveness and budget impact). Although the review considered both published articles and congress abstracts, the evidence on lacosamide was limited and studies suffered from a number of methodological limitations. The evidence, limitations and avenues for future research are discussed in the following paragraphs.

The safety, tolerability and efficacy of lacosamide as an adjunctive therapy in partial-onset seizures have been demonstrated across three randomised, placebo-controlled, double-blind, multicentre trials in over 1,300 adults with epilepsy. Patients receiving lacosamide demonstrated a significant reduction in seizure frequency and significantly higher 50% response rates in comparison with patients who received placebo. Furthermore, open-label extension studies showed that long-term treatment with lacosamide produced a sustained efficacy in and was generally well tolerated by patients.

The existing clinical evidence has investigated the efficacy of lacosamide under 'ideal conditions' rather than its effectiveness in real-life practice. Also, populations studied in clinical trials may not reflect populations observed in clinical practice. There is a need for post-marketing surveillance studies that conduct head-to-head comparisons of different combinations of AEDs including lacosamide. Although analyses based on cohort studies, case-control studies, or before-and-after studies may suffer from a number of biases and do not always establish a cause and effect relationship, such studies would provide information about the safety, tolerability, and effectiveness of lacosamide in real-life practice.

Existing economic evaluations have drawn on similar decision-analytic models to investigate the cost-effectiveness of lacosamide in three different countries. The evidence indicated that in patients who are difficult to treat with currently reimbursed treatment alternatives, standard AED therapy plus lacosamide is likely to constitute a cost-effective alternative. The budget impact of introducing adjunctive therapy with lacosamide is also likely to be limited. Uncertainty surrounds the cost-effectiveness of lacosamide because economic evaluations derived efficacy estimates from short-term trial data, thus necessitating extrapolation; there are few head-to-head comparisons of the efficacy of AEDs; and there are few data on utility values associated with epileptic health states.

There is a need for more economic evaluations of adjunctive therapy of partial-onset seizures with lacosamide. Studies need to be carried out that collect primary long-term data on effectiveness and cost-effectiveness of lacosamide as compared to other available AEDs.

Further research needs to assess quality of life, using preference-based measures of outcomes that generate appropriate utilities for economic evaluation.

5. Conclusion

Because of the complexity of epilepsy diagnosis and management, physicians should be presented with a wide choice of therapeutic options in order to individualize AED treatment to each patient. In light of the available evidence, lacosamide needs to be considered as a safe, efficacious and cost-effective option as adjunctive therapy for patients with partial-onset epilepsy with or without secondary generalization who are uncontrolled having previously used at least three AEDs. However, these results need to be validated by studies that explore the impact of lacosamide in real-life clinical practice.

6. References

Ben-Menachem, E. (2008). Lacosamide: an investigational drug for adjunctive treatment of partial-onset seizures. *Drugs of Today*, Vol.44, pp. 35-40

Ben-Menachem, E.; Biton, V.; Jatuzis, D.; Bou-Khalil, B.; Doty, P. & Rudd, G.D. (2007). Efficacy and safety of oral lacosamide as adjunctive therapy in adults with partial-onset seizures. *Epilepsia*, Vol.48, pp. 1308-1317

Ben-Menachem, E.; French, J.; Isojarvi, J.; Hebert, D. & Doty, P. (2009). *Long-term efficacy of lacosamide for partial-onset seizures: an interim evaluation of completer cohorts exposed to lacosamide for up to 36 months*, Available from http://www.aesnet.org/go/publications/aes-abstracts/abstract-search/mode/display/st/lacosamide/sy/ all /sb/All/id/9936

Bolin, K.; Berggren, F. & Forsgren, L. (2010). Lacosamide as treatment of epileptic seizures - cost utility results for Sweden. *Acta Neurologica Scandinavica*, Vol.121, pp. 406-412

Brodie, M.J. & Dichter, M.A. (1997). Established antiepileptic drugs. *Seizure*, Vol.6, pp. 159-174

Chung, S.; Sperling, M.R. & Biton, V. (2010). Lacosamide as adjunctive therapy for partial-onset seizures: a randomized controlled trial. *Epilepsia*, Vol.51, 958-967

Cramer, J.; De La Loge, C. & Borghs, S. (2010). *Improvement in patient-reported outcomes seen in patients responding to lacosamide: pooled QOLIE-31, SSQ and PGIC data from Phase II/III clinical trials*. American Academy of Neurology, Toronto

Drummond, M.; Sculpher, M.J. & Torrance, G.W. (2005). *Methods for the economic evaluation of health care programmes*. Oxford University Press, Oxford

European Medicines Agency. (2008). *Assessment report for Vimpat (lacosamide)*. European Medicines Agency, London

Faught, E.; Chung, S. & Husain, A. (2010). *Long-term efficacy of lacosamide as adjunctive therapy in patients with uncontrolled POS: results from a phase III open-label extension trial*, Available from http://www.aesnet.org/go/publications/aes-abstracts/abstract-search/mode/display?st=1%2E263&sy=2010&sb=All&id=12463

French, J.; Brodie, M.J.; Hebert, D.; Isojarvi, J. & Doty, P. (2009). Evaluation of Seizure Freedom and 75% Responder Rates with Lacosamide in Subjects with Partial-Onset Seizures in Phase II/III Clinical Trials. *Epilepsia*, Vol.50, pp. 112

Gil-Nagel, A.; Biton, V.; Fountain, N.; Rosenow, F.; Hebert, D. & Doty, P. (2009). The Safety and Tolerability of Lacosamide in Randomized, Double-Blind, Placebo-Controlled Phase II/III Trials. *Epilepsia*, Vol.50, pp. 110

Halasz, P.; Kalviainen, R.; Mazurkiewicz-Beldzinska, M.; Rosenow, F.; Doty, P.; Hebert, D.; Sullivan, T. & SP755 Study Group. (2009). Adjunctive lacosamide for partial-onset seizures: efficacy and safety results from a randomized controlled trial. *Epilepsia*, Vol.50, pp. 443-453

Hauser, W. (1990). *Epilepsy: frequency, causes, and consequences*. Demos Press, New York

Hitiris, N.; Mohanraj, R. & Norrie, J. Mortality in epilepsy. (2007). *Epilepsy Behaviour*, Vol.10, pp. 363-376

Husain, A.; Faught, E. & Chung, S. (2010). *Long-term safety of lacosamide as adjunctive therapy in patients with uncontrolled partial-onset seizures: results from a phase III open-label extension trial*, Available from http://www.aesnet.org/go/publications/aes-abstracts/abstract-search/mode/display?st=1%2E265&sy=2010&sb=All&id=12465

Kotsopoulos, I.A.; van Merode, T.; Kessels, F.G.; de Krom, M.C. & Knottnerus, J.A. (2002). Systematic review and meta-analysis of incidence studies of epilepsy and unprovoked seizures. *Epilepsia*, Vol.43, pp. 1402-1409

National Institute for Health and Clinical Excellence. (2004). *Newer drugs for epilepsy in adults*. National Institute for Health and Clinical Excellence, London

O'Brien, E. (2010). *Data presented at the American Academy of Neurology Meeting demonstrated long-term efficacy and tolerability of Vimpat® (lacosamide)*, Available from http://www.ucb.com

Perucca, E. & Meador, K.J. (2005). Adverse effects of antiepileptic drugs. *Acta Neurologica Scandinavica*, Vol.181, pp. 30-35

Pugliatti, M.; Beghi, E.; Forsgren, L.; Ekman, M. & Sobocki, P. (2007). Estimating the cost of epilepsy in Europe: a review with economic modeling. *Epilepsia*, Vol.48, pp. 2224-2233

Rosenfeld, W.; Rosenow, F. & Isojarvi, J. (2009). Long-term safety and tolerability of lacosamide for partial-onset seizures: an interim evaluation of patients exposed to lacosamide in double-blind and open-label trials. *Epilepsia*, Vol.50, pp. 453

Schmidt, D. & Gram, L. (1995). Monotherapy versus polytherapy in epilepsy: a reappraisal. *Drug Therapy CNS Drugs*, Vol.3, pp. 194-208

Simoens, S. (2010). Pharmacoeconomics of anti-epileptic drugs as adjunctive therapy for refractory epilepsy. *Expert Review of Pharmacoeconomics and Outcomes Research*, Vol.10, pp. 309-315

Simoens, S.; Dedeken, P. & Benhaddi, H. (2010). Cost-utility analysis of lacosamide adjunctive therapy in the treatment of partial-onset seizures in epileptic patients in Belgium. *Value in Health*, Vol.13, pp. A393

Soini, E.; Martikainen, J. & Vanoli, A. (2009). Cost-effectiveness and budget impact modelling of lacosamide in the treatment of partial-onset seizures in Finland. *Value in Health*, Vol.12, pp. A367

Wilby, J.; Kainth, A.; Hawkins, N.; Epstein, D.; McIntosh, H.; McDaid, C.; Mason, A.; Golder, S.; O'Meara, S.; Sculpher, M.; Drummond, M. & Forbes, C. (2005). Clinical effectiveness, tolerability and cost-effectiveness of newer drugs for epilepsy in adults: a systematic review and economic evaluation. *Health Technology Assessment*, Vol.9(15)

Zaccara, G. (2009). Neurological comorbidity and epilepsy: implications for treatment. *Acta Neurologica Scandinavica*, Vol.120, pp. 1-15

12

Treatment of Epilepsy Secondary to Neurocysticercosis

Humberto Foyaca-Sibat and Lourdes de Fátima Ibañez-Valdés
Walter Sisulu University, Faculty of Health Sciences,
Nelson Mandela Academic Hospital, Division of Neurology,
South Africa

1. Introduction

Lack of curative treatment in most of neurological disorder has been a permanent frustration for almost all of us. Fortunately, good news about novel therapeutic approaches and its excellent responses are gradually arriving and today we can celebrate some therapeutic advances such as: cytokines-based therapies for immune-mediated inflammatory myopathies; myoclonal antibodies for the treatment of certain types of immune-mediated inflammatory neuropathies, myopathies, and T-cell mediated disorders; enzyme replacement therapy for Pompe's disease. Non-ergoline dopamine agonist and deep-brain stimulation of subthalamic nucleus and the globus pallidus internus in Parkinson disease, and immunomodulatory agents for multiple sclerosis among others and some exciting therapeutic approaches will come very soon for example: antisense oligonucleotides in Duchenne muscular dystrophy. Stem-cell therapy and gene therapy for inherited neuromuscular disorders, up-regulation of fetal isoforms in hereditary disorders such as: myophophorylase deficiency, and novel forms of neuromodulation. Unfortunately, for treatment of epilepsy secondary to neurocysticercosis (NC) no therapeutic advances has been reported and apart from carbamazepine (CBZ) and valproic acid (VA) no other antiepileptic drug (AED) has proven better efficacy. Although, levetiracitam seems to be as well as CBZ and VA it is not available in rural clinics and in most of the public hospitals from developing countries where NC is endemic. Therefore, several millions of epileptic patients cannot reach levetiracitam worldwide.

Pharmacoresistance in developed countries, lack of AED or poor access to the AED in developing countries continue playing an important role in the high prevalence of difficult-to-control adult epilepsy and are even more 45% of the epileptic population continue experience regular seizures then the only choice that we have is to improve treatment approaches to NC hoping that it may contribute to a better control of epilepsy.

Neurocysticercosis is the leading cause of epilepsy in developing countries and it is becoming one of the most common causes of epilepsy in developed countries due to globalization. It is a preventable and potentially eradicable neurological disorder. [Roman 2000]. At the present moment, treatment of NC in patients presenting epilepsy still has some controversial aspects (Goldberg, 1984; Moodley & Moosa, 1989; Kramer, 1990; Rajshekhar, 1991; Carpio et al. 1995). Apart from dosages of anti-parasitic drugs and its duration; whether or not to use albendazole or praziquantel and how to use it, as part of the treatment for NC, is not certain. Based on findings from other researchers and our results, we will establish a clear-cut guideline for the best management of this problem in this chapter.

Tenia solium is transmitted among humans and between humans and pigs. Taeniosis is acquired only by humans after eating raw or undercooked pork meat contaminated with cysticerci, the larval form of parasite. When ingested, the cysticerci migrate to the intestine of humans where they establish and become adults. These adult worms shed eggs in human feces that can infect other humans and pigs by direct contact or by indirect contamination of water or food. In developing countries, pigs are often allowed to roam freely and they can easily eat human feces. Ingested eggs result in larvae migrating to different parts of the pig or the human and forming cysts. A principle site of migration in humans is the CNS. Human NC occurs when the cysts develop in the brain or spinal cord. Seizures are the most common clinical presentation of NC, affecting from 66% to 90% of cases (Carpio & Hauser, 2002; Wallin & Kurtzke; 2004). In addition to acute seizures and epilepsy, NC can manifest with severe headaches, obstructive hydrocephalus, chronic meningitis, symptoms intracranial hypertension, and dementia (Prabhakar & Singh, 2002). Based on the stage of the intracerebral parasite on CT/MRI, then NC can be classified as "active": when scolex of parasite is visible within a cyst on imagenology, colloidal stage: when the cyst is filled with turbid fluid and there is an intense inflammatory response in the surrounding parenchyma also in imagenology, and calcified or "inactive": when parasite remnants form a mineralized granuloma (Bhigjee & Rosemberg, 2006).

The manner in which NC presents clinically and the severity of the symptoms (from asymptomatic to severe) are thought to depend both on the location of the cysts in the brain (e.g., intraventricular, parenchymal, subarachnoid), their developmental stage and the types and degree of immune response stimulated by the cysts (Garcia & Del Brutto, 2000, 2005; Chavarria *et al.*, 2005; Uddin *et al*, 2005; Bhigjee & Rosemberg, 2006). The initial vesicular stage is usually not associated with an inflammatory response as you can see in Figure 1, which typically occurs later when the cyst degenerates (colloidal stage) by natural causes or due to antiparasitic effect. Astrocytes would play an important role in initiating the immune response to a degenerating cysterci by secreting chemokine in response to TNF-α from monocytes stimulated by larval antigen (Uddin *et al.*, 2005). Over-expression of the immune response stimulated by degenerating cysterci, which is characterized primarily by a Th1-type cytokine profile, can result in chronic inflammation and granuloma formation of the type seen in NC patients with calcified lesions (Uddin *et al.*, 2005). More severe symptoms were shown to be associated with an increased number of inflammatory cells in the CNS of patients with NC (Chavarria *et al.*, 2005). Acute seizures can be seen associated with vesicular or colloidal cysts whereas epilepsy is often found in association with calcified cysts (Bhigjee & Rosemberg, 2006). The incubation period of cysticercosis is extremely variable (Prabhakar & Singh, 2002), and the proportion of infected cases who develop NC is unknown (Bern *et al.*, 1999; Carpio & Hauser, 2002).

The duration of NC-associated symptoms and the proportion of cases with full recovery from symptoms with or without treatment remain ill-defined (Bern *et al.*, 1999; Prabhakar & Singh, 2002). The prevalence of epilepsy in Sub-Saharan Africa has been estimated to be two to three times higher than that found in industrialized countries, a difference that may be attributed, in part, to NC (Preux & Druet-Cabanac, 2005).

Diagnostic criteria for NC have been well-established based on Imagenology. Categories of absolute criteria (patognomonic) are acceptable when the histological demonstration of the parasite from a biopsy of the brain or spinal cord lesion is made, or cystic lesion showing the head of the parasite (scolex) on CT or MRI is seen, or when sub retinal parasites can be visualized by fundoscopy examination. In places where a CT scan is not available, plain X rays of muscular tissues in the limbs showing "cigar shape" calcifications or plain skull X rays with intracranial calcifications (between 1 to 10 mm of diameter) can be useful to support the diagnosis; other options such as Major, Minor or Epidemiological criteria's can be reviewed in the original article (Del Brutto et al., 2001).

1.1 Should be treated neurocysticercosis in epileptic patients?

Neurocysticercosis is a zoonotic infection of central nervous system (CNS) caused by the larval stage (Cysticercus cellulose) of the pig tapeworm *Taenia Solium* and it is the most common helminth to produce CNS infection in human beings. Some authors consider anti-parasitic treatment as a cause epilepsy and recommend do not use it. Researches supporting the theory of "non-antiparasitic drugs" basically defend four hypotheses: First, the sudden destruction of parasites may trigger an inflammatory reaction that precipitates seizures and transient neurologic effects, mostly headache and vomiting. Second, in a considerable number of patients, neurocysticercosis is clinically silent, producing only occasional seizures that are easy to manage with anticonvulsive therapy; thus, exposing these patients to the risk of adverse reactions to cysticidal therapy may be unnecessary. Third, in some cases, the cysticerci will be adequately eliminated either by the host's immune response or by spontaneous regression. Finally, the physical elimination of a parasite, objectively confirmed by neuroimaging studies, does not in itself mean that the patient's neurologic dysfunction will improve. (Sotelo, 2004).
Serum levels of phenytoin and carbamazepine may also be lowered as the result of simultaneous praziquantel administration (Bettencourt et al., 1992). It is also true that T *solium* may remain asymptomatic from months to years until a diagnosis is made incidentally when neuroimaging study is performed. Symptoms and signs are related both to the parasite which can show a different biological pattern from one place to another and to the inflammatory-immunological response of the host (Foyaca-Sibat & Ibañez-Valdés, 2002, 2008).
The introduction of praziquantel (PZQ) by Robles, (1979) and albendazole (ABZ) by Escobedo, (1987) as specific antiparasitic agents was enthusiastically adopted by most of our medical community; it's represented the beginning of a revolutionary process to eradicate NC. Nevertheless, some authors reported cases series where they noted that some types of parenchymal NCC can resolve on imaging studies without being treated with antiparasitic drugs soon after the initial descriptions of successful use of praziquantel and albendazole in neurocysticercosis were done (Miller, 1983; Mitchell, 1988)
We studied 3 762 epileptic patients from rural areas with well documented NC during the past 14 years and our experience clearly indicates that anti-parasitic medication can be prescribed in most of epileptic patients.

1.1.1 From our previous studies

From June 1999 to July 2001, one hundred eighty nine patients fulfilling the clinical criteria of uncontrolled epileptic seizures due to NC were identified prospectively for the study among patients referred to neurology clinic at Umtata General Hospital (South Africa) from rural clinics. Most of those patients presented with an associated HIV infection, pulmonary tuberculosis and some of them a history of haematuria probably due to schistosomiasis.
After the CT scan of the brain, eligible patients (n=163) had active and/or chronic forms of NC and uncontrolled tonic-clonic generalized seizures in spite of taking the regular antiepileptic treatment (phenytoin 300 mg orally at night). After neurological evaluation of all participants, nobody had previous history of neurological disorder apart from epilepsy and those with concomitant disorders such: metabolic disorders, cerebrovascular diseases, meningoenchephalitis, and head injuries were excluded. No patients receiving treatment for

any other disease requiring immunomodulatory agents within the past six months were admitted to the study.

Other exclusion criteria included alternative cause for intracranial calcifications or suspicion of tuberculomas, pyogenic brain abscesses, mycotic granulomas, and primary or metastatic brain tumors. Apart from antiepileptic drugs, steroids medications and anti-parasite treatment, other concomitant treatment was prohibited for patient while participating in the study. The study was designed as: a randomized, placebo-controlled double blind clinical trial over a redesigned 1-years period. Patients were assigned to receive 400 mg of phenytoin every night, 40 mg of prednisone orally during five days, and one day treatment with 100 mg/Kg of praziquantel divided in four doses to be given every two hours (group 1) or only 400 mg of phenytoin at night during the same period of time (group 2) according to block-randomization procedure.

1.1.2 Outcomes measures

Response to antiepileptic medication and an associated anti-parasite treatment were assessed with the neurology UGH scale in which 0 is the lowest: no change, I: equivalent to decreased frequency of seizures II: diminished frequency and duration of seizures III: the highest free of seizures Each patient received the same supporting treatment and was encouraged to eat a rich carbohydrate meal and were evaluated throughout the study by the same personnel. Two-side t. Test was used to analyses the primary outcome measure between baseline and the end of the treatment.

1.1.3 Results and comments

Absolute criteria for NC based on neuroimaging studies were present in all selected patients considering the cystic lesion with scolex as pathognomonic.

The efficacy analysis included 71 patients (36 males and 35 females, mean age 38,27, years, range 13 to 59) treated with phenytoin/praziquantel/prednisone (PPP) and 72 (32 women and 40 men, mean age 49,28 years, range 13 to 62) with phenytoin (P) only. A mild improvement in both groups at the beginning was observed but at baseline no difference in UGH scale was found between groups treated with PPP and a group treated with P (PPP 0.06 ±1. 02 versus P 0.02 ±0. 09, p=0. 56). One month after the treatment with praziquantel, improvement was seen when comparing UGH scale results between two different groups (mean SE, 0,74 ± 0.14 versus -0.2 ± 0.2, 0.63 ± 0.25, mean difference ± SE; *p=0. 005*). In the PPP group 73 % improved in frequency and duration of epileptic attacks. We found that odds ratio of 0. 74 in P group, and 0.43 in PPP with 82 % of the confidence interval (See table I)

In 2001 we have not a clear idea about HIV/AIDS and its role in the pathogenesis of epilepsy and that conclusion was not 100% confident. Therefore, years later we designed another study to investigate this factor and our finding will be discussed later in this chapter.

2. Approach to patients presenting epileptic seizures and neurocysticercosis

Some colleagues still have problems with differentiated epileptic seizures from epilepsy. Remember that epilepsy is a chronic brain disorders characterized by epileptic seizures while seizures can be caused or triggered by other causes no related to chronic brain pathology and they are not recurrent in absent of those causes. Hypoglycemia is a good example as a cause of epileptic seizures. Seizures respond well to a single antiepileptic, and the seizure recurrence rate is low in cases with single lesions; those with multiple, persistent or calcified lesions usually have recurrent seizures. (Singhi, 2011)

After the seizure of whatever cause finish, patients are probably groggy, tired, experiencing local or generalized headache, muscle pains, and cognitive dysfunction.
General guidelines for immediate care of patients presenting tonic-clonic generalized seizures (TCGS) due to NC does not differ from general guidelines to approach patients with TCGS seizures due to other cause. Below, please find 15 valuable recommendations for the general population to support epileptic patients:

1.	Stay calm and protect the person experiencing the seizure
2.	Make sure he/she is breathing normally and keep the person's airway open
3.	Remove dangerous objects that the person might hit during the seizure
4.	Check his/her awareness by asking questions
5.	Turn the person onto his/her side. Do not hold down
6.	Inform to the patient, family, relatives or friends about what happened
7.	Loosen tight neckwear to ease breathing.
8.	Do not shake the person or shout and cushion the person's head
9.	Please describe to the doctor the ictal event.
10.	Do not insert any object in the person's mouth.
11.	Stay with the person until the seizure ends and he or she is completely alert.
12.	Offer to call a taxi, a friend, or a relative to help the person get home safely
13.	Do not restrain a person during a seizure unless there is a danger
14.	Allow them to do what they want to do
15.	Talk to patient in a soft voice to reassure them

In patients presenting seizures lasting more than 20 minutes or recurrent fits without regaining their normal level of conscious in between, a diagnosis of status epilepticus should be considered. Below, please find a list of 11 medications that can be used to control seizures from most of etiologies.

1.	**Lorazepam** (Ativan): 0.1 mg/kg at 2 mg/min
2.	**Diazepam** (Valium), 10–20mg at 2-5 mg/min (Alt)
3.	**Clonazepam** (Klonopin) 0.5-1.0 mg three times a day up to 0.025 mg/kg; 1 mg/5 min (Alt)
4.	**Phenytoin** (Dilantin): 15–20 mg/kg not exceeding 50 mg/min in adults. Slow infusion rate if hypotension occurs
5.	**Valproic acid** (Epilim; Episenta): 20–25 mg/kg over 5–10 min followed by 2 mg/kg/h
6.	**Phosphenytoin**: 15–20 mg/kg of phenytoin equivalents at 100–150 mg/min
7.	**Phenobarbital**: 10–20 mg/kg at 100 mg/min (Re)
8.	**Midazolam**: Loading dosage 0.15–0.2 mg/kg. Maintenance dosage: 0.1–0.4 mg/kg/h (Alt)
9.	**Thiopental**: 100–250mg bolus over 20 seconds then further 50mg boluses every 2-3 min until seizure control, followed by infusion to maintain burst suppression, usually at 3–5 mg/kg/h (Re)
10.	**Propofol**: LD: 2 mg/kg, MD: 6–12 mg/kg/h (Alt)
11.	**Pentobarbital** (LD: 12 mg/kg, MD: 5 mg/kg/h (Re)
12.	*LD: loading dose; MD: maintenance dose; Alt: alternative; Re: Refractory*

Note how long the seizure lasts and symptoms that occurred so you can get a diagnosis.
If you see someone having a non-convulsive seizure, remember that the person's behavior is not intentional. The person may wander aimlessly or unusual gestures. In some epileptic patients you should consider some alarming signals for saving lives. Below find another 15 recommendations.

2.1 When do I be alarmed?

1.	When there are signs of cardiac or respiratory disturbances
2.	When the person does not begin breathing again
3.	When a patient does not return to consciousness after the seizure stops.
4.	When another seizure starts before the person regains consciousness.
5.	When the person is pregnant, or ethanol abused, or has diabetes mellitus.
6.	When the seizure happened in water or other dangerous situation
7.	When the seizure lasts more than five minutes (Most seizures last less than three minutes)
8.	When a patient has hypoglycaemia and electrolytes imbalance
9.	When the person has two or more seizures in a row.
10.	When the person has injuries from the seizure.
11.	When seizures are accompanied by progressive worsening headache
12.	When there is associate nausea, vomiting and diplopia
13.	When there is prolonged post ictal manifestations
14.	When seizures are characterized by laryngeal constrictions, dysphagia and perioral paresthesia.
15.	When a patient presents comorbid mental health disorders

This is a first seizure or you think it might be. If in doubt, check to see if the person has a medical identification card or jewelry stating that they have epilepsy or a seizure disorder. Timing the seizure using a watch is helpful because a brief seizure may seem longer than it is, so by the time an emergency medication is ready to be administered; chances are the seizure is over.

2.2 Epilepsy diagnosis and treatment

Epilepsy is a chronic brain disorder characterized by recurrent seizures with or without associate abnormal behavioral and other neuropsychiatric manifestations.
About 80% of these cases can be easily treated with medication or surgery, while the remaining patients currently intractable. In some cases, usually involving children and adolescents, symptoms may simply end.
Before diagnosing epilepsy, a thorough review of medical records of past seizures is consulted and blood tests are run to ensure that epilepsy is indeed the reason the seizures are occurring.
Epilepsy is diagnosed by clinical assessment and its can be supported by:

- Brain imaging
- Electroencephalogram.

Brain imaging is the most useful tool for clinically assessing epilepsy. When combined with symptom observation epilepsy experts are able to confidently diagnosis the type of epilepsy and make a recommendation about how to treat the condition. The imaging techniques used to assess brain function vary but include CT (computed tomography) scans, fMRI (functional magnetic resonance imaging), or the non-visual EEG which yields graphs of electrical activity.

3. Approach to patients with epilepsy and neurocysticercosis

As mentioned in the introduction, the first line of defense against epilepsy is a pharmaceutical option as prescribed by their doctor. This is the least imposing on the patient and more often than not proves effective. Treatment approaches to epilepsy secondary to NC is almost the same used in epilepsy due to other conditions. Below, are listed all medications more and less commonly used. We included a brand and a generic name because the generic usually is cheaper, sometimes by quite a lot.

3.1 Pharmacological treatment

Treatment of epilepsy secondary to NC differs from treatment of other causes only for the management of the underlying aetiology therefore we prescribe same anti-epileptic drugs (AED). List of medications used you can see as follow:

Narrow-spectrum AEDs	**Broad-spectrum AEDs**
phenytoin (Epanutin) ++	valproic acid (Epilim) +
carbamazapine (Tegretol) (Degranol) (Carbatrol) +	lamotrigine (Lamictal) ++
phenobarbital (Luminal) ++	topiramate (Topamax) +++
oxcarbazepine (Trileptal) +++	zonisamide (Zonegran) +++
gabapentin (Neurontin) ++	clonazepam (Klonopin) ++
pregabalin (Lyrica) +++	levetiracetam (Keppra) +++
lacosamide (Vimpat) +++	rufinamide (Banzel) +++
vigabatrin (Sabril) +++	

AED commonly used+ AED used from time to time++ Drugs never used+++ (In our setting)

In our experience carbamazepine (Tegretol,) is a favorite partial seizure medicine. It affects sodium channels, and inhibits rapid firing of brain cells. Long-acting forms such as Carbatrol or Tegretol-XR can be given once a day while valproic acid is the ideal one for every type of motor seizures and seems to be that sodium valproate is safe and effective in HIV-positive patients on concurrent HAART (Yacoob, 2010). In our experience, generic medicine (CBZ for example) usually works well, but it may not generate the same blood levels as do the brand name or an alternative generic medicine and many patients are able to identified different effect and their seizures are not well controlled. We do recommend to epileptic patients to refill their medications form the same manufacturer and to our health professionals to educate their patient about this knowledge's.

When AED has approval for monotherapy or its benefit seems to exceed the risk, it is the best way of treatment. Side effects seen more often are: blurred vision, stomach upset, headaches, fatigue, dizziness, unsteadiness, and cognitive dysfunction. If valproic acid increases replication of the HIV virus or not it is not certain. Therefore, we recommend do not prescribe valproic acid in HIV-positive patients until this problem be completely clarified.

Weight gain tends to occur with	Weight loss tends to occur with
valproic acid (Depakote)	topiramate (Topamax),
gabapentin (Neurontin)	zonisamide (Zonegran)
pregabalin (Lyrica)	felbamate (Felbatol).
carbamazepine (Tegretol, Carbatrol).	

In endemic areas for NC once the drug has kept the patient seizure-free no less than five years then we recommend that the patient cease its use.

3.2 Surgery

The second option for treating epilepsy due to NC is usually surgery to remove giant subarachnoid cysts, to perform ventricular-peritoneal shunts in IV-NC or to remove the part or parts of the brain malfunctioning that are causing the uncontrolled seizures which is a very uncommon situation.

Patients presenting uncontrolled fits and focal neurological signs due to associate stroke secondary to infective vasculitis are unsuitable for surgery.

3.3 Implantation

A third treatment for epilepsy due to NC is device implantation. For patients from rural places with high level of poverty, where local government and health authorities have other health priorities this procedure is practically unreachable. A vagus nerve stimulator is a fairly recent biomedical technology to help control seizures. Once implanted, the device stimulates the vagus nerve which can reduce the frequency of seizures by 30% on average if patients continue taking their antiepileptic medication post-implantation.
Also from our personal experience, most of epileptic patients with NC respond very well to phenytoin, valproic acid or carbamazepine for control of their seizures and that is fully enough. We prefer valproic acid as a drug of choice for focal or generalized motor or myoclonic seizures in HIV-negative patients and carbamazepine for patients presenting focal complex seizures. Most of our general practitioner prescribes phenytoin more than other AED because it is inexpensive and is almost always available.

3.4 Comments

In our study the total scores at baseline in both groups were similar securing adequacy of randomization and the mild improvement observed was in relation with increased dosage of phenytoin. Our report provides documentation that PZQ, prednisone (PRED) and phenytoin (PPP) were effective in patients with NC and recurrent seizures. Using an UGH score as the primary outcome variable, we found a statistically significant difference between PPP and P. Therefore we have hypothesized about the advantages to combine the antiepileptic drug and antiparasitic medication for patients with recurrent seizures and NC mainly in endemic areas for cysticercosis; clinical manifestation of NC is related to the inflammatory-immunological response of the patient when the parasite is degenerating or dying as result of cysticidal therapy influenced by the number of viable cysts, size and stage of the lesions, site of the cyst in the intracranial region, and the amount of re-infections along the time. However many patients remain asymptomatic and the risk of intracranial infection after T solium egg or proglotides ingestion depend on the combination of immunological status of the patient, the biological characteristic of the parasite, geographical and atmospherically conditions. It also serves to explain clinical differences and different results with the same treatment from one place to another. In places where NC is endemic, other parasitic zoonoses of the brain and retroviral infections co-exist, then regular cycles of praziquantel and/or albendazole and prednisone should be done precede by CT scan/MRI of the brain and fundoscopy. If patients presenting more than cysts, fundoscopy shows intraocular parasite, or patient present signs of meningoenchephalitis treatment should be evaluated by a specialized health professional. This cycle should be repeated until that region will be covered by a good primary health care system, adequate level of employment and cash income, safe and clean water, proper toilet facilities, proper refuse disposal, electricity, telecommunication, good health education program, reform of animal husbandry technique, vaccination of pigs against Taenia Solium and poverty eradicated. (Foyaca-Sibat & Del Rio, 2007)

The main measure to prevent Taeniosis from measly pork meat could be summarized as follows:

Cook meat until the juices run clear or to an internal temperature of 60º C.
Freeze pork less than 15 cm thick for 20 days at -15oC to kill any worms.
Do not allow hogs to eat uncooked carcasses of other pigs.
Clean meat grinders thoroughly if you prepare your own ground meats.
Make people aware that braai, curing (salting), drying, smoking, or microwaving pork meat does not consistently kill parasites.

Studies about treatment of NC in human beings have shown an increased level of IgG, interleukin-2, and neopterin in the CSF of these patients after being treated with praziquantel. Elevate eotaxin and interleukin-5 in serum and elevated interleukin-5 and interleukin-6 concentration in the CSF has been reported as well (Foyaca & Ibañez, 2003).

In inmunodepressed patients by HIV infections or any other similar condition the parasite can produce more damage on the nervous tissue because there can remain viable for a longer period of time compared with non-inmunodepressed patient. About 10 years ago he has hypothesized that in those patients there is one particular stage of the parasite called "critical stage" (Foyaca-Sibat et al., 2001) which is between its vesicular stage and colloid stage, where the releasing of taeniaestatin (serine proteinase inhibitor) is increased or is less destroyed, and the prostaglandins and cytokines production from the glial cells are importantly affected therefore a global cortical neuronal dysfunction is present affecting the mitochondrial activity and its ATP production, disturbance of neuronal membrane metabolism leading to recurrent paroxysmal activity but whether or not the parasite is affected by other condition needs further research.

In pigs affected by NC there is no evidence of seizure disorder probable because their neuronal membrane works differently and their mitochondrial system and supporting cell play a different role or simply because sodium and potassium pump works differently, we do not know. Therefore, deeper investigations on porcine cysticercosis probably help to know more about the human brain and the pathophysiology of epilepsy secondary to NC.

In patients with insular epilepsy (laryngeal constriction, dysphagia, and peribucal paresthesiae) and viable cysts on the insular lobe anti-parasitic medication can cause local insult dysfunction leading to neurogenic heart and sudden unexpected death of epilepsy.

Therefore it should give with extreme caution. (Foyaca-Sibat & Ibañez-Valdés, 2006). In epileptic patients due to disseminate cysticercosis with cardiac involvement, cysticidal drugs should be used with caution because the risk of associate cardiac dysfunction; presence of subcutaneous cysticercosis may help suspecting that condition. (See figure 1)

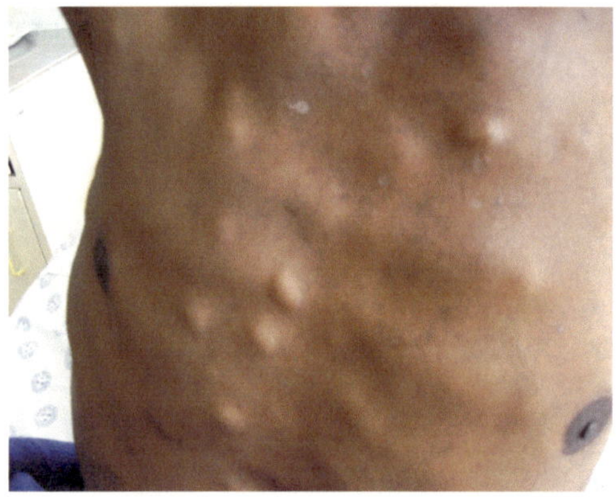

Fig. 1. Shows disseminate subcutaneous cysticercosis

4. Conclusion

Although treatment of NC continues to be debated, in epileptic patients should be treated with cysticidal medicines which are inexpensive and no complications have been reported (Foyaca, Ibañez & Mashiyi 2004). Below, you can see our recommendations:

ABZ: 800mg daily (up to 30mg/kg) plus 40mg of prednisone daily for no less than a week for IV-NC and SA-NC. With extreme caution if cysts at least 50 mm in diameter and hydrocephalus is present (*)	PZQ: 100mg/kg plus 40 mg of prednisone during two weeks or more for intraperanchymal-NC and failure to ABZ (**)	PRED: 60-100 mg (***) daily for insular-NC, ocular-NC, disseminate-NC with cardiac involvement, more than 50 cysts (****) SA-NC, and meningoenchephalitis follow by ABZ/PZQ after improvement.	In refractory NC, ABZ and PZQ should be combined and can be used for a longer period of time until Imagenology does not show active cysts

(*) Intensive medical treatment can be effective in patients with neurocysticercosis characterized by giant cysts. Neurosurgery may be required only when there is an imminent risk of death (Proaño, 2001; Göngora-Rivera, 2006).

(**) A combination therapy for albendazole and praziquantel was statistically comparable to sole therapy with albendazole in eradicating lesions and preventing seizures. (Kaur et al., 2009)

(***) Using corticosteroids at higher dosages bring the inconvenience that destruction of the parasite is delayed probable because most of necessary immunocomponents to participate are affected.

(****) The combination of albendazole and surgical maneuvers to reduce intracranial pressure is a safe and effective method for treating severe NC (more than 100 cysticerci) proceed by higher doses of PRED; CT scans of the brain can be useful for its differential diagnosis. (See figure 2). The fatal prognosis is reported when more than 1 000 viable cysts are present (Yuan et al., 2004).

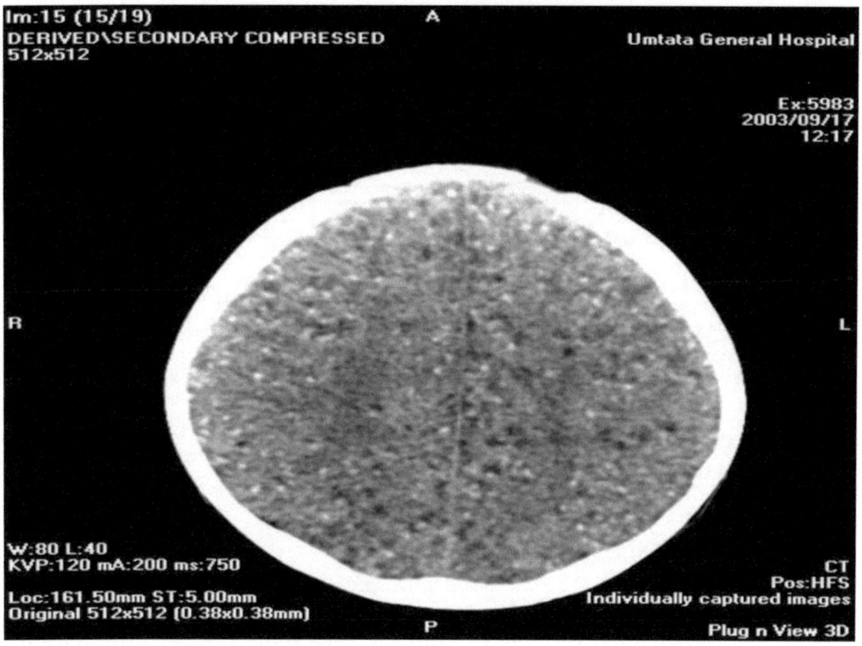

Fig. 2. CT scans of the brain show severe NC.

Both drugs (PZQ/ABZ) have similar equivalent efficacy and greatly improve the therapeutics of cysticercosis. (Sotelo, 1988)

If patients from endemic areas, whom have not well control of epileptic fits but not active cyst are seen on Imagenology, despite calcified-NCC with peripheral edema could explain the presence of seizure disorder, we personally recommend:

> One day treatment with praziquantel at doses of 100mg/kg/day divided in four dosages at 2/3 hours interval plus 40 mg of prednisone for three days every three to six months, for epileptic patients living in the endemic areas if there is not contraindication but fundoscopy looking for ocular cysticercosis should be performed before treatment.

5. Treatment of refractory epilepsy secondary to neurocysticercosis

Refractory epilepsy is uncommon in patients with intraperanchymal NC and when these patients do not respond to the first line anti-epileptic drugs other causes should be investigated. (Ibañez-Valdés & Foyaca-Sibat, 2006). Looking into other causes of refractory epilepsy we studied the first 100 consecutive patients attending to Epilepsy and NC clinic at Nelson Mandela Academic Hospital in South Africa presenting more than eight epileptic seizures per month were confirmed by neuroimaging techniques (CT and/or MRI), EEG and ELISA for the detection of antibody to cysticerci of Taenia solium. Selecting criteria and criteria for exclusion were established as follows:

5.1 Subject inclusion criteria

Step 1.	Patients suffering from focal seizures (FS) or tonic-clonic generalized seizures (TCGS) according to the ILAE classification of epileptic seizures, whether or not secondarily generalized.
Step 2.	Diagnosed with epilepsy for no less than one year prior to be selected for this study
Step 3.	Epilepsy documented clinically and by paroxysmal activity on EEG.
Step 4.	Multiple 2-10 mm intracranial calcifications with or without peripheral edema on imagenology
Step 5.	Patient under regular treatment and good compliance for at least two months before the selection
Step 6.	Presenting at least eight FS with or without generalization or six TCGS per month
Step 7.	Patients between 13 to 75 years old, weighed more than 50 kg
Step 8.	Signed and dated written informed consent.

5.2 Subject exclusion criteria

Pregnant patients or who are lactating.
Subjects whose seizures cannot reliably be counted on a regular basis due to their fast and repetitive occurrence, severe or moderate mental retardation and illiterate peoples unable to report seizures.
History of stroke, cerebral schistosomiasis, current intracranial mass, progressive cerebral disease or any other progressive neurodegenerative disease.
History of poor compliance, pseudo seizures, neuropsychiatric problems.
Normal CT scans of the brain.

5.3 Results and comments

Eleven patients with NC, uncontrolled epilepsy and intracranial structural lesions were identified. Three had arachnoids cysts. Schizencephaly was confirmed in two, six patients presented SA-NC (Figure 3) and in four radiological signs of neuro-AIDS were documented (Figure 4). NC and associated neuron-AIDS was the commonest cause of uncontrolled epilepsy in this series (Table I). Arachnoids cysts often are an incidental finding on imaging and, usually, patients are asymptomatic even if the cyst is quite large. The most commonly associated clinical features are headache, calvarial bulging, and seizures, with focal neurological signs occurring less frequently.

The so-called racemose variety occurs in the ventricles or basal cisterns and is characterized by abnormal growth of cystic membranes with degeneration of the parasite's head (scolex) (Bickerstaff, 1952; Rabiela, 1989). Diagnosis is based on imagenology (See figure 3). These cases follow a progressive course, and even after ventricular shunting, the membranes or inflammatory cells and proteins frequently block the shunt.

Controversy surrounds the treatment of arachnoids cysts. Some clinicians advocate treating only patients with symptomatic cysts while others believe that even in asymptomatic patients, cysts should be decompressed to avoid future complications. The most effective surgical treatment appears to be excision of the outer cyst membrane and cystoperitoneal shunting.

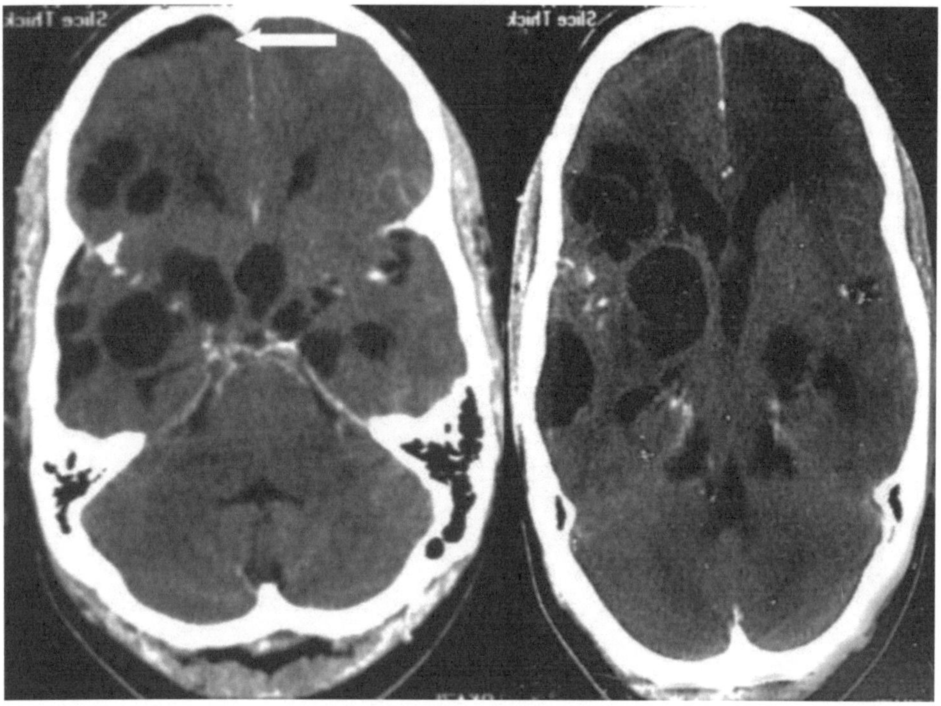

Fig. 3. CT scans of the brain show SA-NC (Racemose's presentation)

Since the cyst membrane is thin and the fluid is isodense with the cerebrospinal fluid, uninflamed extraparenchymal cysticerci are usually not visible on CT and may only reveal subtle, indirect findings on MRI. Between 60% and 85% of parenchyma brain cysticerci are killed after standard courses of treatment, with most trials showing a higher parasiticidal effect of albendazole. (García, 2002). Cysts of the middle cranial fossa (50%) may compress the tip of the temporal lobe, displacing it in the occipital direction. This has been described as temporal lobe agenesis, although there is doubt as to the existence of a true temporal lobe agenesis. Pathologists believe that a malformation of the brain causing selective agenesis of the temporal does not exist. However, middle cranial fossa cysts are linked to ipsilateral chronic subdural hematomas. Rarely, they may communicate with the subdural space, forming a slight extension over the hemispheric surface. At the present moment, information about refractory epilepsy and SA-NC in HIV/AIDS patients is not available in the medical literature.

5.4 Conclusions

In absent of ischemic stroke or other intracranial infection:	**SA-NC in HIV/AIDS patients should be considered as an important cause of refractory epilepsy.**

6. Treatment failure and its consequences

Albendazole has better penetration into cerebrospinal fluid; its concentration is not affected when given with steroids (Jung, 1990; Kim, 1999) and it is cheaper than praziquantel.

In our experience most of epileptic patients with active NC respond very well to first course of PZQ (two weeks) or ABZ (one week) if they have less than 10 cystic lesions (sometimes less than 20) in the parenchyma tissue (Foyaca-Sibat & Ibañez-Valdés, 2002). Single small enhancing computer tomography lesions (SSECTL) of the brain with or without peripheral edema, as a solitary cysticercus granuloma can be a benign form of parenchymal neurocysticercosis (P-NC) and it is considered to be the most common etiology for SSECTL. (See figure 4)

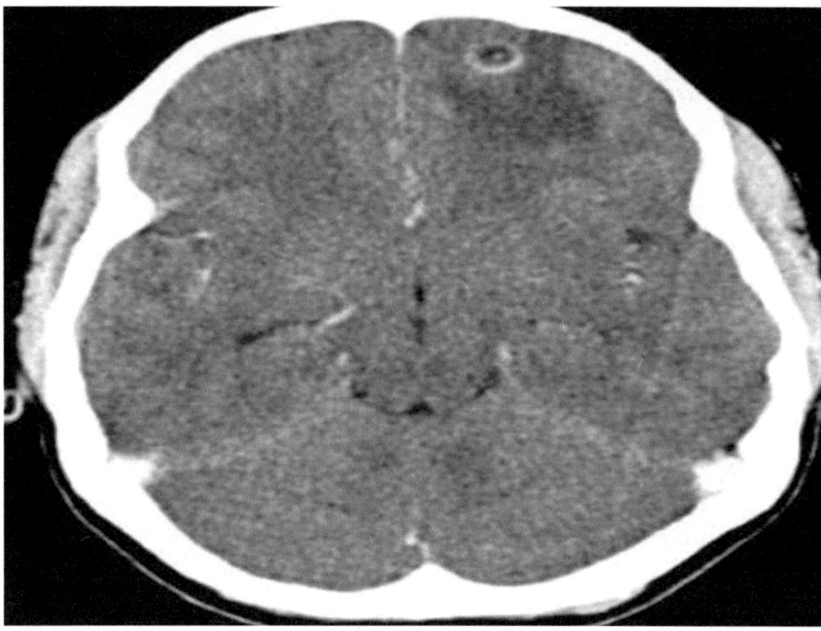

Fig. 4. CT scans of the brain show SSECTL on the left frontal lobe with perilesional oedema

In patients presenting with seizures due to single viable parenchymal neurocysticercosis, albendazole hastens the resolution of SSECTL if treatment is given in the early phase of the illness (Thussu, 2008). For patients with intraventricular NC (IV-NV) the medication of choice is ABZ even in HIV-positive patients (Foyaca-Sibat & Ibañez-Valdés, 2003). However subarachnoid neurocysticercosis (SA-NC) shows a poor response to anti-parasitic medication and some authors reported not adequate response to ABZ, at all (Bandres et al., 1992; White et al., 1992; Del Brutto, 1997; Cardenas et al., 2010). Cysts in the basal cisterns can cause an inflammatory reaction, fibrosis and progressive thickening of the leptomeninges at the base of the brain. In approximately 75% of the cases, there is a progressive obstacle that impedes the normal CSF circulation; resulting in obstructive hydrocephalus therefore we consider ventricular and basal cisternal locations as malignant forms of NC.

The stages of NC before cited, are not seen in the IV-NV or SA-NC (multilocular cyst resembling a bunch of grapes or racemose) at the suprasellar, Sylvan and quadrigeminal cisterns where ABZ or PZQ does not show a good efficacy. Although resistance of cysticerci to ABZ in humans has never been reported, it may occur as it has been observed in other related parasites (Bannur, 2001). Unfortunately, a well-designed clinical trial for SA-NC has not been published and the cause of the parasite's resistance to treatment, despite the ABZ treatment, remains unknown. We also have hypothesized about the immunological condition of the host, biology of the *T solium,* pharmacological limitation of the anti-parasitic drugs at subarachnoid space, and even environmental factors. These non-responsive cases are not the most often but their severity should encourage controlled studies to evaluate new forms of medical intervention and management. Therefore, new therapeutic approaches should be developed. Perhaps, combining ABZ/PZQ with ivermectine, nitazoxanide or tizoxanide will bring better results but because no evidence has been delivered, to perform a well-designed randomized, double-blind placebo clinical trial is mandatory, before to deliver this recommendation. Seven recommendations should be considered in all cases:

1.	Guidelines for treatment of NC must be individualized in terms of the number and location of viable cysts.
2.	Growth of a parenchymal cysticercus is not a common event and may be life-threatening.
3.	Active cystic lesions deserves active management, either with antiparasitic drugs or by surgical excision and epilepsy must be controlled
4.	In epileptic patients with intracranial hypertension secondary to NC, the priority is to manage the raised intracranial pressure before considering any other form of therapy.
5.	Antiparasitic drug treatment is never the main priority in the setting of elevated intracranial pressure
6.	Antiepileptic drugs are the principal therapy for seizures in NC.
7.	Prophylaxis of recurrent infection based on the adequate primary health care system and good health education is mandatory.

6.1 Current situation

Conspicuously absent in the case reports available in the current medical literature are the following research questions: What is the prevalence of SA-NC in epileptic patients? Is SA-NC a risk factor for ischemic stroke (IS) in epileptic population? Does HIV comorbidity increases the stroke frequency in patients infected with NC? These questions were not answered before, therefore the main aim of this study is to explore this inquiry and propose new hypotheses for future study.

6.2 Material and method

We did a cross-sectional study of patients diagnosed with NC from January 1999 to December 2003 at Umtata General Hospital and from January 2004 to January 2010 at Nelson Mandela Academic Hospital from the rural areas selected for a case control-study under the project: "Epilepsy and Neurocysticercosis" All patients were classified into one of the two respective sample groups according to presence and type of NC, all cases presented focal or generalized recurrent motor seizures and were grouped in A= (SA-NC), B= (P-NC) or C= (chronic headache).

6.2.1 Inclusion criteria

All patients from group A met the following selection criteria:

1.	A positive serology ELISA test for cysticercosis
2.	CT/MRI images of the brain with intravenous contrast or gadolinium enhancement consistent with definitive evidence of cystic lesion (isolate or racemose) in the subarachnoid space without hydrocephalus and suitable to evaluate: • Focal arachnoiditis, when there was contrast enhancement in only one cerebral basal cistern. • Bilateral cystic lesions with diffuse arachnoiditis, in which contrast enhancement involved several basal cisterns. • Ischemic infarction, in which the number and location of cerebral lesions were analyzed and classified as superficial, deep no lacunar (>16 mm), and deep lacunar (<15 mm) at the basal ganglia, without an associate cardiac-embolic disease.
3.	Demographic, and associated stroke was analyzed in accordance with the presence of SA-NC.
4.	Recurrent epileptic motor seizures with good compliance

From the large number of patients with NC in our database we selected only a number of patients in group B similar to group A regarding age and gender to assure a better statistical analysis and under an absolute diagnosis of intraperanchymal NC (both active and calcified at the same time) and epilepsy.
All patients received 800 mg of ABZ and 40 mg of PRED per os daily during the ten days as part of the routine treatment for NC and 600 mg of carbamazepine daily.

6.2.2 Exclusion criteria

•	Gross modifiable risk factors for stroke.
•	Heart problems or signs of infective vasculitis.
•	Suspicion of primary or secondary vascular disease
•	Cognitive or sensory deterioration
•	Lack of check-ups (NC/SA-NC/Stroke) for more than eleven months
•	IV-NC and/or associate hydrocephalus
•	Terminal illnesses, serious psychological illnesses
•	Active addictions to psychoactive substances
•	Younger than 13 years old
•	Pregnancy
•	Lived more than six months outside of our territory.
•	HIV/AIDS in stage IV
•	No written consent

6.2.3 Ethical aspects

Written informed consent forms were administered in the first contact with the eligible patients following verbal agreement for participation. All patients were provided information on the study's purpose and procedures in addition to ethical considerations, including and the participant's right to intimacy, anonymity, confidentiality, withdrawal, and information. Due to the large proportion of illiteracy among our population, oral consent observed and confirmed by an impartial witness were necessary in some cases. For patients selected between 1999 and 2002 only oral informed consent was taken.

All investigators completed the CITI training - course on the Protection of Human Research. All are sworn to the Hippocratic Oath and committed to respecting the norms of good clinical practice, as well as the requirements of the Helsinki Declaration.

Methods for patient selection and information processing was approved by clinical governance at Umtata General Hospital, and the research protocol was evaluated and approved by Mthatha Hospital Complex, University of Transkei, and Walter Sisulu University IRB and the respective Ethical Committees (UGH:0001/99, UNITRA:0018/05, and WSU:0068/09).

6.2.4 Data analysis

All statistical analyses were conducted using Statistical Package for the Social Sciences (SPSS) version 16.0 for Windows (SPSS Inc., Chicago, Ill). Analyses were performed using an intention to treat bias. A descriptive analysis and an analysis of baseline comparison between the studies groups were performed for all study variables. To investigate the potential associations between ischemic stroke outcomes and the variability of NC group-type, prevalence odds ratios at 95% confidence intervals were calculated.

6.2.5 Results

Out of a total of 280 eligible patients asked to participate, six patients refused to participate at the baseline evaluation. Two out of the six patients agreed to participate during their follow-up appointment, and their data are included here (n=276).

Group A (n=133), 70 males (52.6%) and 63 females (47.4%). Group B (n=143), 67 males (46.9%) and 76 females (53.1%). In total: 137 males (49.6%) and 139 females (50.4%).

Mean age of group A: 38.63 years (13-82, SD 16.93) and group B: 37.27 years (13-80. SD 15.43). In total, 153 serial CT/MR scans with at least 1 scan (range = 1 to 2) per subject were available in group A and 167 CT/MRI scans in group B, over the 10-years study period.

In total, six patients (3.2%) with good clinical response anti-parasitic treatment developed an ischemic stroke (IS) while 31 (36.0%) patients with poor response developed an IS (OR: 16.11) (6.57-39.47, IC: 95%). See table 1

Response to ABZ			Stroke Yes	Stroke No	Total
Clinical Response	Yes	Count	6	184	190
		% within Clinical Response	3.2%	96.8%	100.0%
	No	Count	31	55	86
		% within Clinical Response	**36.0%**	64.0%	100.0%
Total		Count	37	239	276
		% within Clinical Response	**13.4%**	86.6%	100.0%

Table 1. Clinical response

The risk to develop stroke was 2.82 times more in group A compared with group B. This suggests that although co-infection with HIV increases the risk of IS, the location of NC in the brain is a better predictor of IS risk than comorbidity status when there is not a good response to anthelmintic medicine. Taking into consideration the HIV status of patients by groups we found 40% of patients presented ischemic stroke (group A) and the risk to develop an IS among groups A and B is almost three times more.
In group A, 19 (44.2%) patients responded poorly to anti-parasite treatment and developed an ischemic stroke. OR: 15.29, (4.99-46.83 IC 95%) while 12 (27.9%) from group B presented similar situation. OR: 15.63, (3.79-64.42, IC 95%). (See table 2 and 3)

Response to ABZ			Stroke Yes	Stroke No	Total
Clinical Response	Yes	Count	4	86	90
		% within Clinical Response	4.4%	95.6%	100.0%
	No	Count	19	24	43
		% within Clinical Response	**44.2**%	55.8%	100.0%
Total		Count	23	110	133
		% within Clinical Response	17.3%	82.7%	100.0%

Table 2. Group A

Response to ABZ			Stroke Yes	Stroke No	Total
Clinical Response	Yes	Count	2	98	100
		% within Clinical Response	2.0%	98.0%	100.0%
	No	Count	12	31	43
		% within Clinical Response	**27.9**%	72.1%	100.0%
Total		Count	14	129	143
		% within Clinical Response	9.8%	90.2%	100.0%

Table 3. Group B

After comparing all groups with similar age, gender and HIV-positive status the risk to develop an IS increase to more than seven times in patients presenting SA-NC over the control group and almost four times in patients presenting intraperanchymal NCC.

6.2.6 Imagenological changes after cysticidal treatment

Twenty nine (31.9%) patients from both groups did not present imagenological changes after treatment and developed ischemic stroke. OR: 9.85 (4.36-22.28, IC 95%). See table 4.
Only eight (4.3%) patients with SA-NC (Group A) presenting unequivocal imagenological changes after treatment and IS while 29 (31.9%) patients from the same group did not present changes and developed IS. In this group we found: OR= 13.15 (4.32-40.00, IC 95%).
In group B, 10 (22.2%) patients did not present imagenological changes after treatment and developed IS and OR= 6.21 (1.92-20.00, IC 95%).

Response to ABZ			Stroke Yes	Stroke No	Total
Imagenology Changes	Yes	Count	8	177	185
		% within Imagenology Changes	4.3%	95.7%	100.0%
	No	Count	29	62	91
		% within Imagenology Changes	**31.9**%	68.1%	100.0%
Total		Count	37	239	276
		% within Imagenology Changes	13.4%	86.6%	100.0%

Table 4. Imagenology changes. Group A

6.2.7 Discussion and conclusion

Commodity of *T solium* and HIV in epileptic patients would be expected to occur more frequently because of the increasing frequency of HIV infection in endemic areas of cysticercosis. However, little is known about the influence of HIV infection on the frequency of epileptic seizures and the clinical course of cysticercosis. Giant cysts and racemose forms of neurocysticercosis seem to be more frequent in HIV-infected patients and may be secondary to an uncontrolled parasitic growth because of an impaired cell-mediated immune response. At present we believe that toxins released by the cysticercus cause inflammatory changes on the perforating arteries (toxic vasculitis) at the subarachnoid space rather than as a direct effect on the parasite (mechanical compression). In our study, only one patient died from Group A and that low mortality rate may be related to the exclusion of patients with subarachnoid cysticercosis growing to giant size causing mass effect and obstructive hydrocephalus with mechanical compression. The disease course in SA-NC has been often long in duration and cysticerci continue to grow and proliferate through tissue and epilepsy control was diminished in HIV patient with an associated SA-NC and cerebrovascular complication as we expected. Strengths of this study include the large sample size, geographically distinct locations of the participating clinics, and potential feasibility of its replication. Weaknesses of this study include the omission of a number of variables that may have contributed to the analysis, especially CD-4 level and MR images.

Epileptic patients with an associated SA-NC and HIV infection have a higher risk to develop ischemic stroke if antiparasitic treatment is not effective enough.

7. Way forward

At the present moment, we are investigating the effect modification of HIV-associated CNS diseases by parasitic zoonoses in the Eastern Cape Province; South Africa (Carabin & Foyaca-Sibat, 2011) and a clinical trial on cerebral toxocariasis and NC will be performed.

8. Acknowledgment and source of funding

We like to thanks to all veterinarian researches working on this field.
We also want to thank to all radiologists and radiographers from Nelson Mandela Academic Hospital and Inkhosi Albert Luthuli Central Hospital in South Africa for their contribution to this study.

Special thanks are due to the Cuban Ministry of Health and Institute of Tropical Medicine "Pedro Kouri", and authorities of Nelson Mandela Academic Hospital, School of Medicine, Faculty of Health Sciences and Directorate: Research Development from Walter Sisulu University for their kind support. Finally, we wish to declare publicly our eternal and deepest gratitude to Lorna María Foyaca García, Fátima Susana Foyaca Ibañez and Thabo Humberto Foyaca Ibañez for their delight support.
Hereby, we acknowledge financial support from the Directorate of Research Development, Walter Sisulu University in South Africa, University of Oklahoma, and South African Medical Research Council. The founder had no role in study design, data collection and analysis, decision to publish, or preparation of the manuscript.

9. References

Arpino C, Castelli Gattinara G, Piergili D, et al. (1990) *Toxocara* infection and epilepsy in children: a case-control study. Epilepsia 31:33-36.

Bandres JC, White AC Jr, Samo T, Murphy EC, Harris RL. (1992) Extraparenchymal neurocysticercosis: report of five cases and review of management. Clin Infect Dis. 15:799–811.

Bannur U, Rajshekhar V. (2001) Cisternal cysticercosis: a diagnostic problem, short report. Neurol India. 49(2):206-20

Bittencourt, P. R. M., C. M. Gracia, R. Martins, A. G. Fernandes, H. W. Diekmann, and W. Jung. (1992) Phenytoin and carbamazepine decrease oral bioavailability of praziquantel. Neurology 42:492-495

Bickerstaff C, Hughes B, Smith W. (1952) The racemose form of cerebral cysticercosis. Brain 75:1-18.

Bern C, Garcia HH, Evans C, Gonzalez AE, Verastegui M, Tsang VC, Gilman RH. (1999) Magnitude of the disease burden from neurocysticercosis in a developing country. Clin Infect Dis. 29:1203-1209.

Bhigjee AI and Rosemberg S. (2006) Optimizing therapy of seizures in patients with HIV and cysticercosis. Neurol 67(Suppl 4):S19-S22.

Carabin H, Krecek RC, Cowan LD, Michael L, Foyaca-Sibat H, Nash T, Willingham AL(2006)Estimation of the monetary burden of *Taenia solium* cysticercosis in the Eastern Cape, South Africa". Trop. Med. Int. Health.(ISSN: 1360-2276).11: 906-916.

Cárdenas C, Carrillo-Mezo R, Jung H, Sciutto E, Soto Hernandez JL, Fleury A. (2010) Subarachnoidal Neurocysticercosis non-responsive to cysticidal drugs: a case series. BMC Neurol. 10: 16.

Carpio, A., F. Santillan, P. Leon, C. Flores, and W. A. Hauser. (1995). Is the course of neurocysticercosis modified by treatment with antihelminthic agents? Arch. Intern. MED 155:1982-1988

Carpio A and Hauser WA. (2002) Neurocysticercosis and epilepsy. *In*: Singh G and Prabhakar S. *Taenia solium* cysticercosis. From basic to clinical science. New York: CAB International. 211-20pp

Chavarria A, Fleury A, Garcia E, Marquez C, Frogoso G, Sciutto E. (1997) Relationship between the clinical heterogeneity of neurocysticercosis and the immune-inflammatory profiles. Analysis of 17 patients. J Neurol Neurosurg Psychiatry. 62:659–661

Del Brutto OH. (1998) Albendazole therapy for subarachnoid cysticerci: clinical and neuroimaging.

Del Brutto OH, Rajshekhar V, White AC, Tsang VCW, et al (2001) Proposed diagnosis criteria for neurocysticercosis. Neurology 57:177-181

Escobedo F, Penagos P, Rodriguez J, and J. Sotelo. (1987) Albendazole therapy for neurocysticercosis. Arch. Intern. Med. 147:738-741.

Evans CWE, Garcia HH, Hartnell A, et al. Elevated concentrations of eotaxin and interleukin-5 in human neurocysticercosis. Infect Immun 1998;66:4522-4525.

Foyaca-Sibat H, Ibañez-Valdés LdeF, Fernandez-Mena C. "Neurocysticercosis in Critical Stage". Third International Congress of Critical Care Medicine on Internet. IBSN 0007-A5342-XL2001 Available online from: http://www.uninet.edu/cimc2001/comunicaciones/foyaca.html

Foyaca-Sibat H, "Tapeworm and the brain" Journal of Sciences of Africa 2002;1:5-12 http://www.scienceofafrica.co.za/2002/june.worn.htm

Foyaca-Sibat H, Ibañez-Valdés LdeF. Clinical trial of praziquantel and prednisone in rural patients with neurocysticercosis presenting recurrent epileptic attacks" The Internet Journal of Neurology 2002; 2:41-50. Full article available at the URL: http://www.ispub.com/journal/the_internet_journal_of_neurology/volume_1_number_2_39/article/clinical_trial_of_praziquantel_and_prednisone_in_rural_patients_with_neurocysticercosis_presenting_with_recurrent_epileptic_attacks.html (Last review Jan 13, 2011)

Foyaca Sibat H, Ibañez-Valdés L de F, Vascular dementia type Binswanger's disease in patients with active neurocysticercosis. Electron Biomed / Electron J Biomed 2003;1(1):32-42. Full article available at the URL: http://biomed.uninet.edu/2003/n1/foyaca.html

Foyaca-Sibat H, Ibañez-Valdés LdeF "Intraventricular neurocysticercosis in HIV patients" The Internet Journal of Neurology 2003;2 (1): 23-31 Full article available at the URL: http://www.ispub.com/journal/the_internet_journal_of_neurology/volume_2_number_1_37/article/intraventricular_neurocysticercosis_in_hiv_positive_patients.html. (Last review on January 25, 2011)

Foyaca-Sibat H, Ibañez-Valdés LdeF."Pseudoseizures and Epilepsy in neurocysticercosis" Electron J Biomed 2003;2(2):20-29. Full article available at the URL: http://www.uninet.edu/reb/2003/n2/2foyaca.html

Foyaca-Sibat H, Ibañez-Valdés LdeF "Neurocysticercosis in HIV-positive patients" The Internet Journal of Infectious Diseases. 2003:2(2):15-23. Full article available at the URL: http://www.ispub.com/ostia/index.php?xmlFilePath=journals/ijn/current.xml

Foyaca-Sibat H, Ibañez-Valdés LdeF, Mashiyi MK. Disseminate cysticercosis. One-day treatment in a case. Rev Electron Biomed / Electron J Biomed 2004;3:39-43. Full text available at URL: http://biomed.uninet.edu/2004/n3/foyaca-n.html

Foyaca-Sibat H, Ibañez-Valdés LdeF. "Pseudoseizures and Epilepsy in neurocysticercosis: some advices to Family Doctors" The Internet Journal of Neurology. 2004:2(2):4-17. Full article available at the URL: http://www.ispub.com/journal/the_internet_journal_of_neurology/volume_2_number_2_h34/article/pseudoseizures_and_epilepsy_in_neurocysiticercosis_some_advice_for_family_doctors.html

Foyaca-Sibat H, Ibañez-Valdés LdeF" Clinical trial of praziquantel and prednisone in rural patients with neurocysticercosis presenting recurrent epileptic attacks" The Internet Journal of Neurology 2002;2:41-50 Full article is available at the URL:http://www.ispub.com/journal/the_internet_journal_of_neurology/volume

_1_number_2_39/article/clinical_trial_of_praziquantel_and_prednisone_in_rural_patients_with_neurocysticercosis_presenting_with_recurrent_epileptic_attacks.html [last review done on February 3, 2011]

Ibañez-Valdés LdeF, Foyaca-Sibat H. Refractory epilepsy in neurocysticercosis. The Internet Journal of Neurology 2006;5(2):34-41. Full article available at the URL: http://www.ispub.com/journal/the_internet_journal_of_neurology/volume_5_number_2_19/article/refractory_epilepsy_in_neurocysticercosis.html

Foyaca-Sibat H, Ibañez-Valdés LdeF : Occipital Lobe Syndrome Due To Giant Intraperanchymal Neurocysticercosis . The Internet Journal of Neurology. 2006; volume 5 number 2. Full text is available at the URL: http://www.ispub.com/journal/the_internet_journal_of_neurology/volume_5_number_2_19/article/occipital_lobe_syndrome_due_to_giant_intraparenchymal_neurocysticercosis.html

Foyaca-Sibat H. Ibañez-Valdés LdeF. Insular Neurocysticercosis: Our Finding and Review of the Medical Literature. The Internet Journal of Neurology 2006 volumen 5 number 2. Full article available at the URL: http://www.ispub.com/journal/the_internet_journal_of_neurology/volume_5_number_2_19/article/insular_neurocysticercosis_our_findings_and_review_of_the_medical_literature.html

Foyaca-Sibat H, RIA Del Rio: "Epilepsy, Neurocysticercosis and, Poverty at Mphumaze and Marhambeni Locations, in South Africa". The Internet Journal of Neurology (ISSN: 1531-295X). 2007;7(1):8-14. Full article available at the URL: http://www.ispub.com/journal/the_internet_journal_of_neurology/volume_7_number_1_7/article/epilepsy_neurocysticercosis_and_poverty_at_mphumaze_and_marhambeni_locations_in_south_africa.html

Foyaca-Sibat H, Del Rio- Romero AI: "Prevalence of Epilepsy in an endemic area for neurocysticercosis in South Africa". The Internet Journal of Neurology. (ISSN: 1531-295X). 2008;9(1):8-18. Full article available at the URL: http://www.ispub.com/journal/the_internet_journal_of_neurology/volume_9_number_1_6/article/prevalence_of_epilepsy_in_an_endemic_area_for_neurocysticercosis_in_south_africa.html

Foyaca-Sibat H Cowan LD, Carabin H, Serrano-Ocaña G, , Krecek RC, Willingham A. "Accuracy of serological exam for the diagnosis of neurocysticercosis in outpatients with epilepsy, Eastern Cape Province, South Africa" PLOS Negleted Trop.Dis.Dec.2009; 3 (3): 1-7

Foyaca-Sibat H, Ibañez-Valdés LdeF. "Pseudoseizures and Epilepsy in neurocysticercosis" Electron J Biomed 2003;2(2):20-29. Full article available at the URL: http://www.uninet.edu/reb/2003/n2/2foyaca.html

Foyaca-Sibat H, Ibañez-Valdés LdeF "Neurocysticercosis in HIV-positive patients" The Internet Journal of Infectious Diseases 2003:2(2):15-23. Full article available at the URL: http://www.ispub.com/ostia/index.php?xmlFilePath=journals/ijn/current.xml

Foyaca-Sibat H, Ibañez-Valdés LdeF. "Pseudoseizures and Epilepsy in neurocysticercosis: some advices to Family Doctors" The Internet Journal of Neurology 2004:2(2):4-17. Full article available at the URL: http://www.ispub.com/ostia.index.xmlFilePath=journals/ijn/current.xml

Garcia HH and Del Brutto OH. Taenia solium cysticercosis. Infect Dis Clin North Amer 2000; 14:97-119.

García HH, Evans C, Nash T, Takayanagui O, Clinton White A et al. Current Consensus Guidelines for Treatment of Neurocysticercosis Clinical Microbiology Reviews 2002; 15(4):747-756

Garcia HH and Del Brutto OH. Neurocysticercosis: updated concepts about an old disease. Lancet Neurol 2005;4:653-661.

Goldberg, M. A. 1984. Praziquantel for cysticercosis of the brain parenchyma. N. Engl. J. Med. 311:732-734

Göngora-Rivera F, Soto-Hernández JL, González Esquivel D, Cook HJ, Márquez-Caraveo C, Hernández Dávila R, Santos-Zambrano J. Albendazole trial at 15 or 30 mg/kg/day for subarachnoid and intraventricular cysticercosis. Neurology. 2006;66:436–438.

Jung H, Hurtado M, Medina M, Sanchez M, and Sotelo J. Dexamethasone increases plasma levels of albendazole. J. Neurol.1990; 237:279-280

Jung H, Hurtado M, Medina M, Sanchez M, and Sotelo J. Plasma and cerebrospinal fluid levels of albendazole and praziquantel in patients with neurocysticercosis. Clin. Neuropharmacol. 1990;13:559-564

Kaur S, Singhi P, Singhi S, Khandelwal N. Combination therapy with albendazole and praziquantel versus albendazole alone in children with seizures and single lesion neurocysticercosis: a randomized, placebo-controlled double blind trial. Pediatr Infect Dis J. 2009 May;28(5):403-6.

Kim, S. K., K. C. Wang, S. H. Paek, K. S. Hong, and B. K. Cho. 1999. Outcomes of medical treatment of neurocysticercosis: a study of 65 cases in Cheju Island, Korea. Surg. Neurol. 1999;52:563-569

Kramer, L. D. 1990. Antihelminthic therapy for neurocysticercosis. Arch. Neurol. 47:1059-1060

Little SE. Parasitic zoonoses: parasites transmitted from cats and dogs to children. Contemporary Pediatrics 2003;5:1-21

Miller B, Grinnell V, Goldberg MA, and Heiner D. Spontaneous radiographic disappearance of cerebral cysticercosis: three cases. Neurology 1983;33:1377-1379.

Mitchell W G and Crawford TO Intraparenchymal cerebral cysticercosis in children: diagnosis and treatment. Pediatrics 1988; 82:76-82.

Moodley, M., and A. Moosa. 1989. Treatment of neurocysticercosis: is praziquantel the new hope? Lancet i:262-263

Nicoletti A, Bartoloini A, Reggio A, et al. Epilepsy, cysticercosis, and toxocariasis. A population-based case-control study in rural Bolivia. Neurology 2002;58:1256-1261.

Nicoletti A, Bartolini A, Sofia V, Mantella A, Nsengiyumva G, Frescaline G, Preux P-M. Epilepsy and toxocariasis : a case-control study in Burundi. Epilepsia 2007;48 :894-899.

Nicoletti A, Sofia V, Mantella A, Vitale G, Contrafatto D, Sorbello V, Biondi R, Preux P-M, Garcia HH, Zappia M, Bartolini A. Epilepsy and toxocariasis: a case-control study in Italy. Epilepsia 2008;49:594-599.

Prabhakar S, Singh G. Neurocysticercosis: an overview of clinical presentations. *In*: Singh G and Prabhakar S. (eds.) *Taenia solium* cysticercosis. From basic to clinical science. New York: CAB International; 2002 : pp. 169-176.

Preux P-M and Druet-Cabanac M. Epidemiology and aetiology of epilepsy in sub-Saharan Africa. Lancet Neurol 2005; 4:21-31.

Proaño JV, Madrazo I, Avelar F, López-Félix B, Díaz G, Grijalva I. Medical treatment for neurocysticercosis characterized by giant subarachnoid cysts. N Engl J Med. 2001 Sep 20;345(12):879-85.

Rabiela T, Rivas A, Flisser A. Morphological types of Taenia solium cysticerci. Parasitol. Today 1989;5:357-359.

Rajshekhar, V. 1991. Etiology and management of single small CT lesions in patients with seizures: understanding a controversy. Acta Neurol. Scand. 84:465-470

Robles C and Chavarría M. Presentación de un caso clínico de cisticercosis cerebral tratado medicamente con un nuevo fármaco: praziquantel. Salud Pública Mex. 1979;21:603-618

Roman G, Sotelo J, Del Brutto O, Flisser A, Dumas M, Wadia N, Botero D, Cruz M, Garcia H, de Bittencourt PRM, Trelles L, Arriaga C, Lorenzana P, Nash TE, Spina-Franca A. A proposal to declare neurocysticercosis and international reportable disease. Bull WHO 2000; 78:399-406.

Singhi P. Neurocysticercosis. Therapeutic Advances in Neurological Disorders January 26, 2011 1756285610395654. Full text available at URL: http://tan.sagepub.com/content/early/2011/01/23/1756285610395654 (last review on February 13, 2011)

Sotelo J, Escobedo F, Penagos P. Albendazole vs Praziquantel for Therapy of Neurocysticercosis. A Controlled Trial. Arch Neurol. 1988;45(5):532-534.

Sotelo J. Neurocysticercosis — Is the Elimination of Parasites Beneficial? N Engl J Med 2004; 350:280-282

Thussu A, A Chattopadhyay A, I M S Sawhney I, Khandelwal N. Albendazole therapy for single small enhancing CT lesions (SSECTL) in the brain in epilepsy. J Neurol Neurosurg Psychiatry 2008;79:272-275

Uddin J, Garcia HH, Gilman RH, Gonzalez AE, Friedland JS. Monocyte-astrocyte networks and the regulation of chemokine secretion in neurocysticercosis. J Immunol 2005; 175:3273-3281.

Yacoob Y, et al. Sodium valproate and highly active antiretroviral therapy in HIV positive patients who develop new onset seizures. Seizure: Eur J Epilepsy (2010), doi;10.1016/j.seizures.2010.09.09 (In press)

Yuan Z, Ren HJ, Ding YZ, Zhang JS, Wang WP, Wu XL, Qiu MD. Clinical study about treatment of severe neurocysticercosis. Sheng Chong Bing Za Zhi. 2004;22(4):213-7.

Wallin MY and Kurtzke JF. Neurocysticercosis in the United States: review of an important emerging infection. Neurology 2004; 63:1559-1564.

White AC Jr, Samo T, Murphy EC, Harris RL. Extraparenchymal neurocysticercosis: report of five cases and review of management. Clin Infect Dis. 1992;15:799–811.

Part 2

Non-Pharmacological Treatment of Epilepsy

13

Brain Stimulation for Seizure Control: Considerations and Potential Mechanisms

Benedict C. Albensi
University of Manitoba,
Dept. of Pharmacology & Therapeutics, Faculty of Medicine,
Division of Neurodegenerative Disorders, St. Boniface Research Ctr.,
Dept. of Electrical & Computer Engineering, Faculty of Engineering,
Canada

1. Introduction

Attempts at nervous system electrical stimulation (a.k.a., brain stimulation, neurostimulation, electrical stimulation, neuromodulation, or deep brain stimulation (DBS)) have been made to treat drug-resistant forms of movement disorders and other conditions such as chronic pain, major depression, and more recently, seizure disorders (Theodore and Fisher 2004; Theodore 2005). Experimental results in some cases have been promising and DBS, a form of electrical stimulation, has been approved (2002) by the Food and Drug Administration (FDA) as a treatment for Parkinson's Disease.

Recent lab and clinical data also suggest that electrical brain stimulation in central and peripheral nervous system targets reduces seizure frequency in epileptic patients and in animal models of recurrent seizures (Cooper, Upton et al. 1982; Engbaek, Ostergaard et al. 1989; Benabid, Pollak et al. 1991; Brusa, Pierantozzi et al. 2001; Benabid, Minotti et al. 2002; Vitek 2002; Lang, Kleiner-Fisman et al. 2003; Vonck, Boon et al. 2003; Benabid, Wallace et al. 2005; Boon, Vonck et al. 2007; Velasco, Velasco et al. 2007; Arai, Yokochi et al. 2008; Montgomery and Gale 2008; Aybek, Lazeyras et al. 2009; Baumer, Hidding et al. 2009; Berweck 2009; Boon, Raedt et al. 2009; Rezai 2009). These findings may seem counter intuitive given the fact that electrical stimulation in the nervous system has been used in many cases to excite neurons, or to replace a lost function following injury. Nevertheless, electrical stimulation under certain conditions has been shown to reduce seizure activity. For example, in the peripheral nervous system, vagus nerve stimulation (VNS) has been performed in humans for many years (FDA approved 1997) where clinical studies show reductions in seizure frequency (Woodbury and Woodbury 1990; Vonck, De Herdt et al. 2009). More recently electrical stimulation of the central nervous system has been attempted to treat epilepsy in both animals and humans where animal studies have varied in efficacy and human studies, although very promising, have not always been well designed or controlled.

Neurostimulation for seizure control typically involves the stimulation of brain structures that can be conceptually divided into three groups. These include structures that are: 1)

directly involved in epileptic activity, such as the hippocampal formation, 2) white matter tracks, which are connected to epileptogenic regions, or 3) deep brain structures, such as the subthalamic nucleus.
However, in spite of the fact that brain stimulation has been utilized in clinical settings in humans, no mechanism for neurostimulation has yet been substantiated with sufficient evidence. In addition, more work is needed to elucidate targets and electrical parameters for optimal delivery, such as stimulation frequency and mode, etc.
This chapter will cover the key points of neurostimulation and also some of the unresolved aspects of neurostimulation in epilepsy, namely targets for stimulation, parameters of stimulation, and potential mechanisms associated with stimulation. It will primarily focus on aspects of CNS neuromodulation. It will conclude with interesting highlights from two clinical trials, both of which are currently ongoing and to date have shown positive results. Finally, some brief discussion will be made concerning future directions of neurostimulation.

2. Targets for stimulation

Electrical stimulation has been attempted in several regions of the brain and includes the hippocampal formation, cerebellum, caudate nucleus, centromedian thalamus, anterior thalamus, subthalamus, and neocortical regions, to name a few (Table 1). However, the best structures to stimulate and the most effective stimulation protocols to use in each target are still a matter of debate and are under investigation (Theodore and Fisher 2004). As mentioned above, these targets can be subdivided conceptually into several categories including: direct focal targets (ie., epileptogenic zone), deep brain nuclei, and white matter tracts.
More specifically, one approach that has been taken with white matter tract stimulation is to stimulate a white matter tract that is connected to the majority of the neurons in the epileptic zone. For example, stimulation of the corpus callosum or the fornix has been accomplished with the hope that by applying supramaximal stimulation intensity to these tracts that epileptogenic activity can be completely blocked (a.k.a., overdrive stimulation) (Luders, Najm et al. 2004). The rationale for using supramaximal intensities is that at this level of intensity it appears unlikely to elicit additional epileptic seizures. Pilot animal studies thus far using bilateral stimulation of the fornix have been encouraging, but are limited in number.
With regard to direct stimulation of the epileptic zone, cortical and hippocampal targets have been the most common targets explored thus far. In particular, hippocampal sclerosis is one of the most common forms of epilepsy where these patients are frequently not surgical candidates due to concerns about potential memory deficits following surgery. Therefore, it is hoped that electrical stimulation of the hippocampus might be developed as a viable therapeutic alternative for these individuals. To date, small clinical trials by Velasco et al. (Velasco, Velasco et al. 2000; Velasco, Velasco et al. 2000; Velasco, Velasco et al. 2007) have been performed and have showed promising results, however these studies were not double-blinded in design and so more work is needed in this area.
Several deep brain structures have also been targeted. These include the caudate nucleus, the posterior hypothalamus, the thalamic nuclei, and the subthalamic nuclei. Among these targets, recent studies appear to favor the thalamic and subthalamic nuclei (STN). Interestingly, in the early 1980s the nigral control of epilepsy system (NCES) was described

(Iadarola and Gale 1982) where the STN seems to play major role in this system. Past studies indicated that abnormal activity in the STN was a main feature in the pathology of movement disorders. However, more recently the role of the STN in epilepsy has been investigated and targeted with DBS stimulation protocols.

3. Parameters of stimulation

There are a number of variables that are important to consider when attempting to understand the parameters associated with neurostimulation. These include the basic physical properties and relationships such as *energy sources, voltage, current, resistance, capacitance, and fields*, etc. An exhaustive discussion of these properties and relationships is not the focus of this chapter and there are many excellent references that can be examined in this regard (see (Feyman, Leighton et al. 1977)). Our consideration will be qualitative for the most part. One fundamental relationship to briefly present in this context is of course, Ohm's law, $V = IR$ or $R = V/I$. In this relationship, *resistance (R)* measures the magnitude of *voltage (V)* across an element when passing the circuit *current (I)*. We introduce this concept since neurons and glial cells of the brain have resistive properties. Similar to resistance we can think of another property, that of *resistivity* (ρ), which takes into account a current flowing through a cross-sectional area (such as a fiber tract). The reciprocal of resistivity or $1/\rho$ is the *conductivity* (σ). It is often more intuitive to think in terms of conductivity when analyzing ion channel function in the nervous system.

In addition, one needs to consider the location of the stimulation electrodes, the strength and duration of a stimulus, the geometry of the target being stimulated, and other electrical characteristics of the target tissue. When analyzing the geometry of potential nervous system targets, there are two shapes that are typically used as models, that is, a spherical cell and a cylindrical fiber. For a quantitative description of these models several resources are suggested for additional reading (Plonsey 2008). In actual biological systems, cells and tissues are considerably more complex than simple spheres or cylinders, but this geometry serves as a useful starting point for our discussion.

For example, an external device such as a stimulator delivers current to the target cells and creates a rising transmembrane voltage, which at first is subthreshold (ie., a graded potential) when delivered at low intensities. In this simplistic model, the transmembrane potential will be nearly uniform at all points on the cell membrane and the entire membrane will respond in a similar manner. However, fibers are evaluated using stimuli placed in different locations along the length of the fiber and require additional considerations. Another perspective that is helpful is to think of action potentials propagating along a cylindrical nerve fiber, which has an excitable membrane. In this scenario, each patch of excitable membrane initiates the transfer of a packet of energy to adjacent patches of excitable membrane. Classic cable theory has been applied to nerve fibers to mathematically describe the propagation process (Plonsey 2008) more precisely. In addition, the reader is referred to standard neurophysiology texts (Kandel, Schwartz et al. 2000) that discuss the well documented permeability changes that involve sodium and potassium flux, etc. One other noteworthy point regarding geometry is that the orientation of nerve cells relative to the voltage field (ie., voltage gradient) is important since those cells in the direction of the voltage gradient will more likely be activated than those cells lying along an isopotential line.

In addition, neurostimulators are either monopolar or bipolar in configuration. Depending on which type is used will determine the current density around the electrode, how easily some cells are activated, and which population of cells is activated. In general, nerve cells that are nearer the electrode will more likely be stimulated. However, axons will be stimulated at lower stimulation intensities than nerve cell bodies. In addition, larger axons will respond to lower stimulus intensities than will smaller axons. Also, axons with multiple branches will be more easily activated than axons without branching processes.

Other programmable parameters that neurostimulators utilize for neuromodulation include voltage, pulse width, cycle on and off times, ramping, duration, and frequency. The combination of these parameters is critical for maximum efficacy. For example, both low and high frequency stimulation protocols have been attempted for seizure control. Historically, low frequency protocols (1 Hz), have been used in neurophysiological experiments involving synaptic plasticity and memory. In particular, 1 Hz stimulation in many circumstances resulted in so-called, long-term depression (LTD), a molecular correlate of memory associated with amnesia and forgetting. Because, LTD also leads to decreases in neuronal excitability, it has been postulated that low frequency protocols around 1 Hz should be effective in reducing seizure frequency. However, the evidence to date shows mixed results in this regard. For example, Weiss et al. demonstrated that the application of 1 Hz (15 min.) to the hippocampus or amygdala following a so-called kindling stimulus (60 Hz for 1 sec once daily) produced a long lasting suppressive effect on seizure activity (Weiss, Li et al. 1995). However, in a follow-up study by the same lab, it was reported that the stimulators that were used in the original study emitted an unexpected low level (i.e., 5 - 15 μA) direct current, which was suspected to have a significant effect on the inhibition on seizure activity (Weiss, Eidsath et al. 1998). Substantially more experimental work has actually been accomplished to date in both animal models and in human trials using higher frequencies of stimulation (ie., around 130 Hz) for seizure control. Overall, frequencies from 0.1 to 450 Hz have been tried in both animals and humans with various results (Rise 2004; Albensi, Oliver et al. 2007).

One other aspect is worth mentioning. Stimulation can be applied using either open loop or closed loop systems (Li and Mogul 2007; Pollo and Villemure 2007). Closed loop is defined as the delivery of electric current to a target, exclusively in response to a prompt. This type of delivery would be defined by a computer algorithm, whose onset is triggered by a seizure detection device. An example of open loop stimulation would be any stimulation protocol that is delivered independently of the time of occurrence between seizures.

Finally, a mention of safety issues is also appropriate. Early attempts in electrical stimulation resulted in some deleterious results. For example, repeated applications of direct current caused tissue injury, which was reversed if one used charge-balanced pulses instead. In other words, a stimulus protocol that utilizes two phases of current flow (positive and negative phases) resulting in a net charge flow of zero proved optimal and is now the standard method for pulse delivery. Other experimental attempts have resulted in the realization that only delivering limited levels of charge density per phase are essential so that the overall risk of injuring tissue is minimized. Some infections near the site of electrode implantation have also been reported, however, these occurrences are quite low and have not been serious. There are also some concerns when using DBS in a MRI context and some cases have been where excessive heating of the implanted electrodes has been an issue (Sharan, Rezai et al. 2003; Coffey 2004; Rezai, Phillips et al. 2004)

4. Mechanisms of stimulation

As of this writing, mechanisms for DBS or VNS are not known. Several theories have been put forward for nervous system studies involving electrical stimulation in general, and for DBS and VNS in particular. For example, some speculate that prolonged electrical stimulation "jams" neuronal circuits (Greenberg 2002); however, this explanation is vague from a neurophysiological point of view. Slightly more developed theories (Pollo and Villemure 2007; Shapiro, Vaillancourt et al. 2007; Montgomery and Gale 2008) have proposed mechanisms involving "inhibition of synaptic transmission", a.k.a. the neurochemical hypothesis, or "depolarization blockade", a.k.a. the electrical hypothesis, but substantial evidence is lacking in both regards and these ideas have not yet been thoroughly substantiated in experimental models.

Interestingly, the effects of neurostimulation are known to change with the frequency of stimulation and also with the duration of the pulse or train of stimulation. This implies that stimulation at any particular target may attenuate seizures with some electrical parameters and induce seizures with other parameters. Evidence to date also supports this notion; for example, it is well known that kindling protocols (Fisher 1989; Weiss and Post 1998; Albensi, Oliver et al. 2007) are used to indirectly induce epilelptiform activity in intact animals. It should also be realized that there may be several mechanisms responsible for efficacy - not just one, which makes the investigation of mechanisms more complex than perhaps originally thought.

There is also one other concept that is often brought up when one discusses potential mechanisms of action and that is the idea of remote control versus direct control (Pollo and Villemure 2007). Central to this idea, electrical stimulation of specific circuits in cortical and basal ganglia networks appear to result in different levels of control depending on which brain region network is being targeted. In other words, targeting the area of epileptiogenesis (ie., seizure focus) with neurostimulation is called direct control. Whereas, electrically stimulating one of the intermediate relays or fibers in some circuit that connects to the epileptic zone is considered remote control. Examples of remote control include neurostimulation of the dorsal midbrain anticonvulsant zone (DMAZ), anterior thalamic nuclei, white matter tracts, and the centromedial thalamic nuclei. An example of direct control would be electrical stimulation of the hippocampus. Both approaches have shown efficacy and are active areas of investigation to determine which approach may be more effective.

5. Recent studies

Over the last several months promising human data has been published by Fisher et al. showing that electrical stimulation of the anterior nucleus of the thalamus reduced seizure frequency in individuals with refractory epilepsy (Fisher, Salanova et al. 2010). This ongoing study was prospective, randomized, parallel, and double-blinded in design. One hundred and ten patients were randomized at the start of the trial. Those treated were adults with refractory partial seizures, including subjects with secondarily generalized seizures. In this study, at least three anti-seizure drugs must have failed to produce seizure control prior to baseline in order to be eligible for inclusion. At baseline seizure frequency was approximately 19.5%. At the time of this writing the study is over two years old. During months 1-4 of the trial, all participants were blinded where one-half received stimulation (typically using 145 Hz) and the other one-half received no stimulation. In the last month of the blinded phase (ie., month 4) the stimulated group had a 29% greater reduction in seizures compared with the control group (p=0.002). By two years, there was a 56% median percent reduction in seizure frequency. Interestingly, participants showed no group differences in mood or cognition, but those in the stimulated group were more likely to report problems with memory or depression. Overall, it was concluded that bilateral stimulation of the anterior thalamus was effective at reducing partial and secondarily generalized seizures.

In yet another recent study, a multi-center, prospective, randomized, double-blinded, sham controlled trial of individuals 18 to 70 years of age with medically intractable seizures for 3 months or more and localized to one or two foci is underway (Spencer, Gwinn et al. ; Skarpaas and Morrell 2009). In this trial, one-hundred and ninety-one subjects were recruited in order to test a cranially implanted programmable responsive neurostimulator (NeuroPace, Inc.). This device was used for treating partial onset seizures with or without secondary generalization. To be eligible for inclusion, subjects had to have failed 2 or more antiepileptic medications. One month following implantation, subjects were randomized 1:1 to receive sham or active responsive stimulation. In this study, the neurostimulator was programmed to acquire data on seizure detection. Stimulation was then delivered at the time and site of detection (eg., mesial temporal structures - hippocampus), before seizure spread or before any overt symptoms appeared. In other words, the system is designed to detect abnormal electrical activity in the brain and to deliver electrical stimulation to suppress seizures before there are overt seizure symptoms. Subjects were blinded to their treatment for 3 months. During this blinded period, neurostimulation was shown to significantly (p=0.012) reduce the number of seizures per day by 37.9% as compared to 17% in the untreated arm. After three months of blinded treatment the individuals were allowed to continue in the study in an open label manner. Some complications were seen from treatment, such as implant site infections and intracranial hemorrhage, but these side effects were relatively low in frequency.

6. Future directions

The use of neurostimulation for nervous system modulation is rapidly increasing. The success of this therapy, however, is far ahead of our understanding of the mechanism(s) associated with neurostimulation. It is also important to remember that early success using neurostimulation techniques occurred with technology that was not specifically fabricated for the current applications. In other words, only recently have the medical devices used for neurostimulation been designed and tailored for their present use and so it is possible the field may soon witness unprecedented growth given improved technology in the future.

One past limiting factor has been the ability to predict and detect seizure onset. Much work is still needed in this regard, but some very recent advances have been made (see discussion above concerning the NeuroPace trial). How to determine when a seizure will begin remains one of the great unanswered questions in epilepsy. Without a doubt, this limitation is a serious one, but once overcome, we will greatly advance the implementation of technology for responsive forms of neurostimulation. Advances in signal processing and detection devices will most certainly help in this regard.

It should also be noted that other technologies are being developed in parallel and may profoundly influence the field of neuromodulation therapy in epilepsy and other CNS disorders. For example, transcranial magnetic stimulation is also under development and has been shown to noninvasively interfere with neural activity. In particular, low frequency repetitive transcranial magnetic stimulation appears to temporarily improve intractable epilepsy. At this time, it is hard to predict if and how this technology may or may not advance in unison with techniques that involve the chronic implantation of electrodes.

From a neurobiological point of view it is hard to believe that repetitive stimulation has no effect on the genome. The truth is we do not know if it does or does not and to date very little research has been accomplished to explore this possibility. Future studies are warranted that would profile gene expression at various frequencies and other conditions to determine the long term effects of electrical stimulation on cell physiology.

Interestingly, attempts at using DBS in obesity have resulted in some unexpected results. In a recent study by Lozano et al. (Hamani, McAndrews et al. 2008), physicians were attempting to treat a morbidly obese man using DBS and found that electrical stimulation of the hypothalamus/fornix caused the patient to experience vivid memories. The individual suffered from type 2 diabetes and also sleeping disorders and failed to respond to other forms of treatment for these conditions. DBS for treating obesity is very new and only a few attempts have been made in this regard. Following surgery the patient recovered for two months, and later when the implanted electrodes were stimulated once again, he experienced the recollection of more memories. These results suggest that DBS might be a viable alternative for those with memory disorders; in particular, for those with Alzheimer's disease (AD). To this end, Lozano and colleagues are currently conducting a pilot study in AD patients (Laxton, Tang-Wai et al.) where 6 patients are being treated with this therapy. Data from this study suggested that DBS treatment in hippocampal areas resulted in an early and striking reversal of impaired glucose utilization in temporal and parietal lobes (as measured by PET scans) that was maintained after 12 months of continuous stimulation. These data are so new and unexpected and the sample sizes are so low, that it is important to add a note of caution in association with these studies. Regardless of the studies' limitations, further work is warranted to investigate these very preliminary, but exciting findings.

It is also expected that scientists and physicians from a variety of disciplines, such as bioengineering, computer science, neurophysiology, neurology, and psychiatry, etc. will work together more cohesively than in the past in order to advance the field of neurostimulation; this will be important with regard to understanding mechanisms of action, advancing technology, and improving the quality of life of epilepsy patients and others with serious CNS disorders.

In any case, it should be obvious that we are witnessing a new horizon with promising results thus far and unimaginable rewards and outcomes yet to come.

Target Stimulated	Proposed Pathway and/or Mechanism	Efficacy
Cerebellum	Direct anterograde cortical inhibition or stimulation	Significant seizure reduction in uncontrolled human studies, but no significant change in controlled human trials (Walker 1938; Moruzzi and Magoun 1949; Cooper, Upton et al. 1982)
Caudate	Direct anterograde cortical stimulation	Significant seizure reduction in uncontrolled human studies (Sramka, Fritz et al. 1976; Chkhenkeli 1978)
Posterior hypothalamus	Direct anterograde cortical stimulation	Significant increase in seizure threshold in pentylenetetrazol (PTZ) rat model (Mirski and Fisher 1994)
Anterior thalamic nucleus	Direct anterograde cortical stimulation	One uncontrolled human study showing seizure reduction in 3 out of 5 patients (Cooper, Upton et al. 1980)
Centromedian thalamic nucleus	Direct anterograde cortical stimulation	Significant seizure reduction in uncontrolled human trials, but no significant change in controlled human trials (Velasco, Velasco et al. 1987)
Subthalmic nucleus	Nigral control of epilepsy system or antidromic cortical stimulation	Significant seizure reduction in uncontrolled human trials, but no controlled human trials performed (Vercueil, Benazzouz et al. 1998; Benabid, Minotti et al. 2002)
Cortical stimulation	Direct stimulation of epileptogenic focus	Brief bursts of pulse stimulation reported to terminate afterdischarges caused by cortical stimulation (Lesser, Kim et al. 1999; Luders, Najm et al. 2004)
Hippocampal stimulation	Direct stimulation of epileptogenic focus	Significant seizure reduction rats and in uncontrolled and controlled human studies (Velasco, Velasco et al. 2000; Albensi, Ata et al. 2004; Velasco, Velasco et al. 2007; Albensi, Toupin et al. 2008)
Vagal nerve stimulation	Direct anterograde cortical stimulation via activation of thalamic, brainstem, and limbic structures	Significant seizure reduction in rats and controlled human trials (Penry and Dean 1990; Woodbury and Woodbury 1990)
Trigeminal nerve stimulation	Direct anterograde cortical stimulation via desychronization of cortical and thalamic structures	Significant seizure reduction in rats, but no human studies to date (Fanselow, Reid et al. 2000)
White matter tract stimulation	Direct anterograde and retrograde stimulation of epileptogenic focus	Significant seizure reduction in rats, but no human studies to date (Luders, Najm et al. 2004)

*Modified from, Luders et al., (Luders, Najm et al. 2004)

Table 1. Summary of Electrical Stimulation Studies in Epilepsy in Humans and Animal Models*

7. Acknowledgements

This work was supported by: the Natural Sciences and Engineering Research Council of Canada (NSERC), Canadian Institutes of Health Research (CIHR), Heart and Stroke Foundation of Canada (HSFC), the St. Boniface General Hospital Research Foundation, and the Honourable Douglas Everett, Patricia Everett and the Royal Canadian Properties Endowment Fund. Dr. Ben Albensi holds the Honourable Douglas Everett, Patricia Everett and the Royal Canadian Properties Endowment Fund Chair. He is an Associate Professor of Pharmacology and Therapeutics at the University of Manitoba, a Principle Investigator at the St. Boniface Research Centre, a Research Affiliate at the University of Manitoba's Centre on Aging, and a Scientist at the Manitoba Institute of Child Health (MICH).

8. References

Albensi, B. C., G. Ata, et al. (2004). "Activation of long-term synaptic plasticity causes suppression of epileptiform activity in rat hippocampal slices." Brain Res 998(1): 56-64.

Albensi, B. C., D. R. Oliver, et al. (2007). "Electrical stimulation protocols for hippocampal synaptic plasticity and neuronal hyper-excitability: are they effective or relevant?" Exp Neurol 204(1): 1-13.

Albensi, B. C., J. D. Toupin, et al. (2008). "Controlled pulse delivery of electrical stimulation differentially reduces epileptiform activity in Mg(2+)-free-treated hippocampal slices." Brain Res 1226C: 163-172.

Arai, N., F. Yokochi, et al. (2008). "Mechanisms of unilateral STN-DBS in patients with Parkinson's disease : a PET study." J Neurol 255(8): 1236-43.

Aybek, S., F. Lazeyras, et al. (2009). "Hippocampal atrophy predicts conversion to dementia after STN-DBS in Parkinson's disease." Parkinsonism Relat Disord 15(7): 521-4.

Baumer, T., U. Hidding, et al. (2009). "Effects of DBS, premotor rTMS, and levodopa on motor function and silent period in advanced Parkinson's disease." Mov Disord 24(5): 672-6.

Benabid, A. L., L. Minotti, et al. (2002). "Antiepileptic effect of high-frequency stimulation of the subthalamic nucleus (corpus luysi) in a case of medically intractable epilepsy caused by focal dysplasia: a 30-month follow-up: technical case report." Neurosurgery 50(6): 1385-91; discussion 1391-2.

Benabid, A. L., P. Pollak, et al. (1991). "Long-term suppression of tremor by chronic stimulation of the ventral intermediate thalamic nucleus." Lancet 337(8738): 403-6.

Benabid, A. L., B. Wallace, et al. (2005). "Therapeutic electrical stimulation of the central nervous system." C R Biol 328(2): 177-86.

Berweck, S. (2009). "BP-DBS for dystonia-choreoathetosis cerebral palsy." Lancet Neurol 8(8): 692-3.

Boon, P., R. Raedt, et al. (2009). "Electrical stimulation for the treatment of epilepsy." Neurotherapeutics 6(2): 218-27.

Boon, P., K. Vonck, et al. (2007). "Deep brain stimulation in patients with refractory temporal lobe epilepsy." Epilepsia 48(8): 1551-60.

Brusa, L., M. Pierantozzi, et al. (2001). "Deep brain stimulation (DBS) attentional effects parallel those of l-dopa treatment." J Neural Transm 108(8-9): 1021-7.

Chkhenkeli, S. (1978). "Inhibitory influences of caudate stimulation on the epileptic activity of human amygdala and hippocampus during temporal lobe epilpesy." Physiol Hum Anim 4: 406-411.

Coffey, R. J. (2004). "Re: Neurostimulation system used for deep brain stimulation (DBS): MR safety issues and implications of failing to follow safety recommendations." Invest Radiol 39(5): 304.

Cooper, I. S., A. R. Upton, et al. (1980). "Some effects of electrical stimulation of the thalamus and internal capsule in man." Appl Neurophysiol 43: 244-258.

Cooper, I. S., A. R. Upton, et al. (1982). "Chronic cerebellar stimulation (CCS) and deep brain stimulation (DBS) in involuntary movement disorders." Appl Neurophysiol 45(3): 209-17.

Engbaek, J., D. Ostergaard, et al. (1989). "Double burst stimulation (DBS): a new pattern of nerve stimulation to identify residual neuromuscular block." Br J Anaesth 62(3): 274-8.

Fanselow, E. E., A. P. Reid, et al. (2000). "Reduction of pentylenetetrazole-induced seizure activity in awake rats by seizure-triggered trigeminal nerve stimulation." J Neurosci 20(21): 8160-8.

Feyman, R. P., R. B. Leighton, et al. (1977). The Feyman Lectures on Physics. Reading, Massachusetts, Addison-Wesley Publishing.

Fisher, R., V. Salanova, et al. (2010). "Electrical stimulation of the anterior nucleus of thalamus for treatment of refractory epilepsy." Epilepsia 51(5): 899-908.

Fisher, R. S. (1989). "Animal models of the epilepsies." Brain Res Brain Res Rev 14(3): 245-78.

Greenberg, B. D. (2002). "Update on deep brain stimulation." J ECT 18(4): 193-6.

Hamani, C., M. P. McAndrews, et al. (2008). "Memory enhancement induced by hypothalamic/fornix deep brain stimulation." Ann Neurol 63(1): 119-23.

Iadarola, M. J. and K. Gale (1982). "Substantia nigra: site of anticonvulsant activity mediated by gamma-aminobutyric acid." Science 218(4578): 1237-40.

Kandel, E. R., J. H. Schwartz, et al. (2000). Principles of Neural Science. New York, McGraw-Hill.

Lang, A. E., G. Kleiner-Fisman, et al. (2003). "Subthalamic DBS replaces levodopa in Parkinson's disease: two-year follow-up." Neurology 60(1): 154-5; author reply 154-5.

Laxton, A. W., D. F. Tang-Wai, et al. "A phase I trial of deep brain stimulation of memory circuits in Alzheimer's disease." Ann Neurol 68(4): 521-34.

Lesser, R. P., S. H. Kim, et al. (1999). "Brief bursts of pulse stimulation terminate afterdischarges caused by cortical stimulation." Neurology 53(9): 2073-81.

Li, Y. and D. J. Mogul (2007). "Electrical control of epileptic seizures." J Clin Neurophysiol 24(2): 197-204.

Luders, J., I. M. Najm, et al. (2004). Brain stimulation and epilepsy: basic overview and novel approaches. Deep Brain Stimulation and Epilepsy. H. O. Luders. London, Martin Dunitz: 3-17.

Mirski, M. A. and R. S. Fisher (1994). "Electrical stimulation of the mammillary nuclei increases seizure threshold to pentylenetetrazol in rats." Epilepsia 35(6): 1309-16.

Montgomery, E. B., Jr. and J. T. Gale (2008). "Mechanisms of action of deep brain stimulation(DBS)." Neurosci Biobehav Rev 32(3): 388-407.

Moruzzi, G. and H. W. Magoun (1949). "Brain stem reticular formation and activation of the EEG." Electroencephalogr Clin Neurophysiol 1(4): 455-73.

Penry, J. K. and J. C. Dean (1990). "Prevention of intractable partial seizures by intermittent vagal stimulation in humans: preliminary results." Epilepsia 31 Suppl 2: S40-3.

Plonsey, R. (2008). Bioelectricity: A Quantitative Approach New York, Springer.

Pollo, C. and J. G. Villemure (2007). "Rationale, mechanisms of efficacy, anatomical targets and future prospects of electrical deep brain stimulation for epilepsy." Acta Neurochir Suppl 97(Pt 2): 311-20.

Rezai, A. (2009). "DBS for neurobehavioral disorders." Stereotact Funct Neurosurg 87(4): 267.

Rezai, A. R., M. Phillips, et al. (2004). "Neurostimulation system used for deep brain stimulation (DBS): MR safety issues and implications of failing to follow safety recommendations." Invest Radiol 39(5): 300-3.

Rise, M. T. (2004). Brain stimulation and epilepsy: electrical stimulus characteristics. Deep Brain Stimulation and Epilepsy. H. O. Luders. London, Martin Dunitz: 45-54.

Shapiro, M. B., D. E. Vaillancourt, et al. (2007). "Effects of STN DBS on rigidity in Parkinson's disease." IEEE Trans Neural Syst Rehabil Eng 15(2): 173-81.

Sharan, A., A. R. Rezai, et al. (2003). "MR safety in patients with implanted deep brain stimulation systems (DBS)." Acta Neurochir Suppl 87: 141-5.

Skarpaas, T. L. and M. J. Morrell (2009). "Intracranial stimulation therapy for epilepsy." Neurotherapeutics 6(2): 238-43.

Spencer, D., R. Gwinn, et al. "Laterality and temporal distribution of seizures in patients with bitemporal independent seizures during a trial of responsive neurostimulation." Epilepsy Res 93(2-3): 221-5.

Sramka, M., G. Fritz, et al. (1976). "Some observations in treatment stimulation of epilepsy." Acta Neurochir (Wien): 257-262.

Theodore, W. H. (2005). "Brain stimulation for epilepsy." Nat Clin Pract Neurol 1(2): 64-5.

Theodore, W. H. and R. S. Fisher (2004). "Brain stimulation for epilepsy." Lancet Neurol 3(2): 111-8.

Velasco, A. L., F. Velasco, et al. (2007). "Electrical stimulation of the hippocampal epileptic foci for seizure control: a double-blind, long-term follow-up study." Epilepsia 48(10): 1895-903.

Velasco, A. L., M. Velasco, et al. (2000). "Subacute and chronic electrical stimulation of the hippocampus on intractable temporal lobe seizures: preliminary report." Arch Med Res 31(3): 316-28.

Velasco, F., A. L. Velasco, et al. (2007). "Deep brain stimulation for treatment of the epilepsies: the centromedian thalamic target." Acta Neurochir Suppl 97(Pt 2): 337-42.

Velasco, F., M. Velasco, et al. (1987). "Electrical stimulation of the centromedian thalamic nucleus in the treatment of convulsive seizures: a preliminary report." Epilepsia 28(4): 421-30.

Velasco, M., F. Velasco, et al. (2000). "Subacute electrical stimulation of the hippocampus blocks intractable temporal lobe seizures and paroxysmal EEG activities." Epilepsia 41(2): 158-69.

Vercueil, L., A. Benazzouz, et al. (1998). "High-frequency stimulation of the subthalamic nucleus suppresses absence seizures in the rat: comparison with neurotoxic lesions." Epilepsy Res 31(1): 39-46.

Vitek, J. L. (2002). "Deep brain stimulation for Parkinson's disease. A critical re-evaluation of STN versus GPi DBS." Stereotact Funct Neurosurg 78(3-4): 119-31.

Vonck, K., P. Boon, et al. (2003). "Neurostimulation for refractory epilepsy." Acta Neurol Belg 103(4): 213-7.

Vonck, K., V. De Herdt, et al. (2009). "Vagal nerve stimulation--a 15-year survey of an established treatment modality in epilepsy surgery." Adv Tech Stand Neurosurg 34: 111-46.

Walker, A. (1938). "Electricity in Medicine." J Neurophysiol 1: 16-23.

Weiss, S. R., A. Eidsath, et al. (1998). "Quenching revisited: low level direct current inhibits amygdala-kindled seizures." Exp Neurol 154(1): 185-92.

Weiss, S. R., X. L. Li, et al. (1995). "Quenching: inhibition of development and expression of amygdala kindled seizures with low frequency stimulation." Neuroreport 6(16): 2171-6.

Weiss, S. R. and R. M. Post (1998). "Kindling: separate vs. shared mechanisms in affective disorders and epilepsy." Neuropsychobiology 38(3): 167-80.

Woodbury, D. M. and J. W. Woodbury (1990). "Effects of vagal stimulation on experimentally induced seizures in rats." Epilepsia 31 Suppl 2: S7-19.

14

Presurgical Assessment of Patients with Refractory Temporal Lobe Epilepsy

Hector Jaramillo et al.*
Instituto Neurológico de Antioquia, Colombia

1. Introduction

The consideration of temporal lobe epilepsy (TLE) surgery for those with medically refractory seizure disorders requires a well-functioning multidisciplinary team and a systematic approach to the candidates, with the aim of advising patients of their chances of being seizure free following surgery, and the risks of any procedure. It is crucial that patients and their families are given realistic expectations of what may and may not be achieved with surgical treatment, and that long-term follow-up is maintained post-operatively.

Complex partial seizure (CPS) of temporal lobe is the most common type of seizure disorder, and approximately 70% of patients are referred for surgical treatment.

In this chapter we want to discuss the different forms of presurgical evaluation and patient selection. The patients that are considered as possible candidates for epilepsy surgery, need to have a detailed clinical history and demonstration of drug resistant-epilepsy.

We assume that the issues about clinical history have been mentioned in previous chapters, so our approach will start from the identification of the epileptogenic zone (I. Irritative zone, II. Seizure-onset zone, III. Symptomatogenic zone, IV. Epileptogenic lesion and V. Functional deficit zone) and patient selection using different diagnostic techniques, that include:

- Semiology
- Neurophysiological criteria
- Neuropsychological evaluation
- Intracarotid Amobarbital Procedure (IAP), and
- Neuroimaging

2. Semiology

In assessing the clinical semiology of the syndrome of TLE, in medical literature, the first thing to take into account, is that symptoms originate from different areas of propagation of the discharge located in other lobes, rather than the temporal lobe itself.

---

* Mónica Massaro, José Luis Ascencio, Juan Felipe Álvarez, René Andrade, José Fernando Zapata, Luz Marina Galeano, Vanessa Benjumea, Esteban Jaramillo, Marta Jiménez and Refractory Epilepsy Group

Many of the symptoms observed in ictal and postictal mesial temporal sclerosis (MTS) can be attributed to typical patterns of propagation from the mesial regions (automatisms possibly caused by activation of cingulate gyrus, postictal aphasia due to Todd paralysis from the temporal basal area and/or Wernicke's area, etc.) and lateralizing signs seen in the mesial temporal seizure on-set zone are also an expression of the propagation of adjacent brain regions [basal ganglia for contralateral dystonia, areas of language for postictal aphasia, ipsilateral motor area for contralateral version and clonic seizures, etc.] (Lüders, 1999). These manifestations do not reflect per se the cause. That is why this chapter will not mention the propagated symptoms, which help in the clinical context of the lateralization and location of the seizure, but are not part of typical semiology of TLE.

The symptomatogenic area (cortical area that generates symptoms) will be mentioned, but not the epileptogenic area or the preictal and postictal symptoms, which are another semiological feature of TLE (Andrade, 2011).

TLE in children represents a different scenario and a less homogeneous syndrome when compared with its manifestations in adults, and also the process of brain maturation modifies the ictal semiology in both groups. In children under 6 years of age the manifestations are predominantly motor, resembling frontal lobe seizures (Ray, 2005). In adults the auras and automatisms are the most frequent semiological expressions. That is why the signs found in the adult TLE syndrome will be discussed and studied more profoundly in this chapter.

It is important to remember that the diagnostic value of the waking semiology of seizures of TLE is similar to dream semiology (Rodriguez, 2007).

Ictal behavior is sporadic, and an anatomo-clinical correlation is difficult to establish, as opposed to when there is a neurological injury which leaves a persistent deficit.

In the adult population, the temporal lobe seizures are the most commonly presented, and the ones involving mesial structures, representing the classic complex partial seizures (CPS), dominate in the clinical setting. Many of them are preceded by auras (interpreted as seizures), but these may frequently be presented independently.

The temporal lobe can be divided anatomically and functionally in structures:

- Mesiobasal limbic area: The mesial (union of "medial" and "basal" regions) comprise the anterior amygdala to the hippocampus, hippocampus, uncus and parahippocampal gyrus.
- Basal and lateral neocortical area: Lateral temporal cortex includes the gyrus of Heschl's as the primary auditory area and the area of Wernicke´s which is responsible for speech perception.
- Insular area: This region is usually not accessible to epilepsy surgery, for which its manifestations are less defined than the mesial or lateral semiology. The insula is essential for gustatory and autonomic functions.

The manifestations of the TLE may vary in presentation and behavior in relation to the ictal on-set zone and the symptomatogenic zone (Chiosa, 2010).

Taking into consideration the information above, we can divide TLE symptoms as subjective and objective.

2.1 Subjective symptoms or "epileptic auras"

Auras are part of the onset of seizures, occurring in up to 80% of the TLE cases and they can provide a high value to locate and lateralize the epileptogenic zone. However, the aura may

only represent a part of the propagation of the discharge. Within the phenomenology of the aura symptoms are psychic, autonomic, sensory and sensory special.
According to its most frequent anatomical location, they can be divided into 3 groups:

- Mesio-temporal auras, including psychic symptoms such as dysmnesic, affective and cognitive auras.
- Mesio-lateral auras are originated in the mesial temporal-insular network and include autonomic auras as epigastric sensations, with or without other autonomic signs or symptoms.
- Neocortical auras, in which its commitment suggests a temporal and extratemporal neocortical compromise. Include auditory, somatosensory, visual and dizzy auras (Castilho Garcia, 2010).

2.2 Subjective phenomenon

Psychic or experiential auras can be subdivided into dysmnesic, affective and cognitive. It can generate different phenomena: deja vu (already seen), jamais vu (never lived), pleasure, anger, fear, living in another dimension or being transported to another place, structured visual hallucinations associated with pleasure or displeasure, depersonalization, state of "reverie", distortions of time, forced thinking (although these may occur more frequently in frontal seizures) (Andrade, 2011).
The psychic auras can be divided into the "experiential" or "interpretive" phenomena.
Gloor (1990) summarized the characteristics of the "experiential" responses as follows: (a) Can be experienced or intrusive from the past; (b) There is a sense of familiarity or reminiscence (déjà vu, déjà vécu); (c) sense of living a dream; (d) the patient says he is always aware of the incongruity and illusory experience; (e) affective states like fear, anger, sexual arousal are common; (f) these responses have some lack of features such as absence of progression over time and scenes that do not evolve; and (g) auditory hallucinations are said to be felt without semantic content (Kasper, 2010).

2.2.1 Dysmnesic auras

Amnesia of the event can be found with the phenomena of déjà vu and Jamais vú (feeling of familiarity and unfamiliarity) or déjá entendú o Jamais entendú. "Deja vu" refers to a feeling of familiarity associated with the present context; jamais vu is a rare symptom and is a false sense of unfamiliarity.

2.2.2 Affective auras

Patients may have different emotional symptoms, including anger, hatred, contempt, shame, joy, love, excitement, fear. Fear occurs frequently in TLE, but it is also described in frontal onset epilepsy (Biraben, 2001; Manford, 1996).
Ictal fear can easily be confused with a psychiatric disorder, and a definite link with panic disorder may not be fully defined. It has been identified that patients with TLE have an increased incidence of panic disorders (Mintzer, 2002).
Panic attacks with autonomic and behavioral changes (agitation, paralysis, thinking terror, asking for help) have been described, and recordings of deeper EEG electrodes have shown that the areas involved are located in the orbital-prefrontal regions, anterior cingulate gyrus and limbic temporal cortex, and more frequently in the nondominant hemisphere (Biranben, 2001).

2.2.3 Cognitive auras

These are situations in which the perception of internal or external reality is altered. The main cognitive auras are: distortion of the appreciation of time, sense of unreality, depersonalization, changes in body image and forced thinking, which consists of imposed and intrusive thoughts at the beginning of the seizure (Parra, 1999; Fernádez-Torre, 2002).

2.2.4 Interpretative auras: hallucinations and illusions

Based on new studies with stereoelectroencephalography it is clear that there are specific anatomical locations for many hallucinatory states. Specific anatomical areas cause elementary hallucinations that begin in the visual and auditory cortex. For the occurrence of complex hallucinatory states to occur, the involvement of the limbic cortex is a prerequisite.

Generally, elementary hallucinations correspond to the activation of primary sensory areas (eg buzzing, with the involvement of the activation of the Heschl's gyrus, and if unilateral it indicates a contralateral origin) and complex hallucinations (such as music, voices) have a more extensive tracking and seem to correspond to the activation of association areas. For example we can see visual changes in shape, size (macro and mycropsia), color (acromatopsy), movement and distance, hearing impairment in the perception and understanding of volume, tone and character of sounds.

Sensations that are less frequent include gustatory and olfactory auras and unilateral headache. Olfactory sensations can be pleasant or unpleasant, which is thought to be originated in the amygdala. The gustatory auras are rare and are usually described as an unpleasant taste and are associated with insular onset (Chiosa, 2010; Hausser-Hauw, 1987; Fried, 1995).

The olfactory auras are known as ´´uncinate crisis´´ and its origin seems to be in the mesial region close to the amygdala or orbitofrontal regions. The most common underlying diseases are tumors in the temporal region (Archarya, 1998).

2.2.5 Autonomic phenomena

They are produced by a compromise of the amygdala, insula and spread to the hypothalamus.

The seizures originating from the mesial area characteristically begin with a “limbic” aura characterized by epigastric discomfort or abdominal auras, which can be described as a rising sensation, nausea, "butterflies in the stomach," or the feeling of being in an elevator. Although this type of aura is correlated with onset mesial temporal crisis, its exact location between the mesial temporal structures is still controversial (Wieser, 1983; Gloor, 1990; French, 1993; Van Buren, 1963; Henkel, 2002).

The epigastric aura is more common in the mesial TLE subtype that in the lateral TLE, but is not exclusively of the temporal lobe. In all patients with an abdominal aura followed by automatisms, epilepsy is located in the temporal regions (Henkel, 2002).

These auras can be associated with autonomic characteristics (skin color, heart rate, blood pressure, pupil diameter, piloerection, sweating) or perceptual manifestations such as anxiety (amygdala commitment). Extreme bradycardia and even atrioventricular block has been described when compromising autonomic control centers at the temporal lobe. As a general rule, the autonomic manifestations of temporal lobe seizures such as ictal vomiting, urinary urgency, spitting, tend to lateralize to the non-dominant hemisphere for language (Ostrowsky, 2000). Ictal vomiting may be the only manifestation of simple partial seizures, and has been linked to temporal lobe seizures in the non-dominant hemisphere (Kotagal, 1995; Devinsky, 1995).

2.3 Objective phenomenon

2.3.1 Awareness commitment

This is the phenomenon most frequently found. It is considered as the individual's inability to interact appropriately with the environment, with confusion or amnesia of the event, activity inhibition and automatic behavior. CPS could last from seconds to minutes, but in the limbic status from hours to days, where a patient walks around with an automatic behavior, and then not remembering the event. Over 50% of seizures with impaired consciousness were associated with motor events, purposeless, stopping the activity that the individual was carrying out, and this crisis can be unilateral or bilateral (Andrade, 2011).

2.3.2 Automatisms

They occur in 40% to 80% of patients with TLE. They are stereotyped, as involuntary oral and manual movements during the crisis. They can be oroalimentary (swallowing, chewing, tasting, pressing the lips, spitting, drinking water, etc.), gestures (touching, scratching, manipulating objects in the environment surrounding it or touching people), simple or complex (recall a human action, such as unbutton, rub your fingers, cross themselves, pray, clap, walk, etc.), or mimicking (crying, laughing, etc.) (Serrano-Castro, 1998; Ebner, 1995).
Oral automatisms originate more frequently in the amygdala and anterior temporal region. It is an involuntary motor activity where only in 10% of cases, awareness, is not affected. When the right hemisphere is involved the patient is usually amnesic. These automatisms are less violent than those evidenced in frontal lobe seizures. Unilateral dystonic postures may occur, reflecting a compromise of the basal ganglia and can help to lateralize the onset to the contralateral hemisphere. A typical association of ipsilateral hand automatisms and contralateral dystonic posture is often found in temporal lobe seizures.

2.3.2.1 Complex automatisms with unique characteristics for their localizer or lateralizing value

- Spitting: It is associated with right temporal lobe seizures, although there are documented cases with an origin in the left temporal lobe. There are reports with coughing up, an automatism with right temporal lobe onset. Until 1999 the literature reported 17 cases, 12 of which began in the non-dominant temporal lobe (Kaplan, 1999).
- Sex Auras: It is pleasant erotic thoughts or feelings. May be accompanied by orgasm. Occur predominantly in women, are most frequently associated with right compromise in TLE (Aull-Watschinger, S., 2008)
- Sign of the Cross: A rare sign of presentation. The patient touches his forehead, chest and hands crossed back and forth touching the shoulders; described in right TLE (Lin, 2009).
- Speech automatism: The patient says phrases, words or verses (automatic language). Can be verbal or nonverbal. (Andriani Rahal, 2006).
- The postictal yawn can occur in up to 2% of patients with TLE and always in the postictal period (Kuba, 2010).
- Gestural automatisms directed to the cephalic portion of the body: movements directed to the nose, face, cheek and head displayed during the crisis, to separate them of the most common, occurring in the interictal and postictal periods, usually seen in patients with temporal seizures (Meletti, 2003).

- Postictal dysphasia, and "nose-wiping": The postictal dysphasia lateralizes the focus to the language dominant hemisphere and the classic sign of "nose-wiping" to the ipsilateral focus in 90% of cases when it is present (Loddenkemper, 2005).

2.3.3 Disorders characterized by non-automatic movements

In TLE, when it involves the posterior and superior temporal gyrus, the patient displays a horizontal motion and sudden eye movement, with its fast phase directed toward the side contralateral to the epileptogenic zone (epileptic nystagmus), although they can also be seen in front crisis.

The insula seizures deserve special mention. It has been shown that in this area there is a major somatosensory, language and movement integration.

By stimulating the insula, patients may describe sensations such as numbness, pins and needles, electricity, heat, feel that they have air inside them. The areas most frequently involved are the naso-pharyngeal, cervical region and limbs.

Most of the time the sensations are evoked contralaterally to the site of stimulation but they may also be bilateral. According to the frequency of symptoms reported, there is involvement with the viscera; causing nausea, vomiting, hot ascending feeling, gustatory sensations and facial flushing. Other symptoms may occur as the elevation of contralateral limb and eye movements that impede fixation of an object in the visual field, as well as bimanual and hyperdrive automatisms.

Stimulation can evoke an auditory response referred to as sound going away, hearing an echo, or having their ears plugged. There is sometimes vertigo and sudden loss of speech.

It is interesting to note that in the insula exists a somatotopic, tonotopic and viscerotopic map: In the anterior insula there appears to be a visceral integration, somatotopic to the area of the face (eyes, nose, mouth and neck) and partial integration of eye movements, while the posterior region integrates related somatic sensations with foot and leg movements and the antero-superior region exists proprioceptive, vestibular and language integration in the dominant hemisphere (Ostrowsky, 2000).

2.4 Differentiation between mesial and neocortical onset of the seizure

Making this differentiation is essential to find the epileptogenic zone, necessary for surgical decision making in the case of drug resistance. There are several studies that attempt to find such differences that are named as followed: complex partial seizures with secondary generalization are more frequently of cortical origin, but simple partial seizures may also occur.

Temporal lobe seizures may have a more gradual onset, gradually developing during the course of a minute and at the same time having a longer duration of the ictal and postictal period compared to extratemporal seizures (particularly frontal onset).

3. Neurophysiological criteria: ictal EEG and interictal EEG

3.1 EEG-video monitoring and technical considerations

The continuous, non-invasive EEG-video monitoring is a technique that uses both electroencephalographic and video features for electroclinical correlation. This diagnostic tool has been used by most authors as the gold standard for the study of patients with refractory epilepsy. For the temporospatial analysis of the electroencephalographic activity, an arrangement of electrodes is placed on the patients scalp, following the standard method known as the international 10-20 system (Jasper, 1958). To increase the sensitivity of the diagnosis, and to analyze certain EEG abnormalities it is necessary to use non standard locations such as sphenoidals, foramen ovale, anterior temporal (T1/T2), nasopharyngeal, zygomatic and mandibulary electrodes. (Morris, 1987; Silverman, 1960). When surface EEG shows non-conclusive results, the ictal semiology is atypical or the neuroimaging studies are normal, it is necessary to use invasive recording techniques, using subdural electrodes or intracerebral depth electrodes. (Dubeau, 2000; Noachtar, 2009).

3.2 Interictal abnormalities in temporal lobe epilepsy

It´s possible to observe focal temporal or regional persistent slowing, if it´s associated with structural alteration or intermittent when it´s associated with a ´´functional´´ alteration, which can indicate a subjacent epileptic zone (Mohammed, 2010). Temporal intermittent rhythmic delta activity (TIRDA) is a good interictal indicator of temporal lobe crisis. It´s arrhythmic variant can also be present even thought is less specific. TIRDA has had more association with MTLE (Geyer, 1999; Koutroumanidis, 2004). Spikes or sharp waves with an electronegative peak over the anterior temporal region (F7/F8) are the main interictal abnormality in TLE. For surgical purposes, it is necessary to establish the difference between mesial origin (MTLE) and a neocortical origin (NTLE).

In MTLE the surface recordings show spikes and localized sharp waves mainly in sphenoidal electrodes or in the anterior temporal region, while in NTLE discharges are observed more frequently in the mediotemporal (T3/T4) or posterior electrodes (T5/T6). There are studies that try to establish differences in the irritative epileptogenic activity between MTLE and NTLE showing overlapping results of both entities. Pfander et al., and O'Brien et al. Couldn´t find differences in the interictal EEG in patients with MTLE or NTLE (Lüders, 2008).

Similarly, there haven't been any differences found between both epilepsies subtypes of the temporal lobe with respect to the lateralization of the irritative epileptogenic activity.

3.3 Ictal abnormalities in temporal lobe epilepsy

Multiple ictal patterns exists, the ones that stand out are irregular 2-5 Hz lateralized activity, background attenuation, start-stop-start phenomenon, 5-10 Hz sinusoidal waves and repetitive epileptiform potentials. Similarly is not possible to observe an EEG change, being minimum or presenting an increase in heart rate just before the onset of ictal EEG discharges, the latter associated with an origin at mesial temporal structures (Ebersole, 1996; Vossler, 1998; Walczak, 1992; Di Gennaro, 2004).

Multiple studies have investigated the differences between the patterns found in MTLE and NTLE. For example, Lüders (2008) describes an increase in frequency of rapid sharp rhythmic waves (>4Hz) in the ictal EEG of patients with MTLE, while patients with NTLE develop bilateral ictal EEG changes more frequently and rapidly. Dantas (1998) demostrated that the EEG is important to lateralize the epileptogenic lobe, considering the rythmic ictal activity and the postictal findings. Nevertheless, is not possible to determine with certainty the difference between MTLE and NTLE. Dericioglu (2008) found in patients with MTLE thirteen different ictal onsets, being the most frequent the cessation of interictal discharges followed by ipsilateral delta-theta temporal rythmic activities.

Ebersole (1996) showed that the rhythmic waves of 5–9 Hz that are first seen in the temporal region during seizures, are specific to MTLE, but he also found rhythmic waves of various frequencies from the delta to beta band in both MTLE and NTLE, indicating that these are not specific to MTLE.
Sakai (2002) concludes that scalp EEG activity during the ictal period could provide information with which differentiation between MTLE and NTLE can be deduced with high accuracy. However, they provide an incomplete assessment of laterality in MTLE. Others have also reported that EEG seizure patterns of MTLE and NTLE patients showed no differences (Gil-Nagel, 1997; Saygi, 1994; Gates, 1990).

3.4 Invasion for temporal lobe epilepsy

There is debate in the epilepsy group around the world about the risk of the use of depth electrodes located in both hippocampus, to lateralize the ictal-onset zone in patients with medial TLE and previous discordant results. The reason is that while it provides greater accuracy for lateralizing the epileptogenic zone, this would generate a potential damage to the healthy hippocampus, which may lead the patient to have consequences from the neuropsychological and / or neurophysiological points of view. However there are studies that conclude the safety of both, postoperative and in the long-term monitoring. When there is reasonable evidence that the patient has a resectable epileptogenic focus, but the information obtained non-invasively is imprecise and requires more specific data, it is necessary intracranial electrode implantation. In MTLE, surface video-EEG does not give a definitive lateralization in all cases and some of them lead to a false lateralization (Alssadi, 2001; Sammaritano, 1987; Napolitano, 2010; McIntyre, 2008; Napolitano, 2008). Therefore it is necessary for some patients with TLE on surface video-EEG to require intracranial recording, particularly when neuroimaging does not help to locate (Engel, 1993; Immonen, 2010).
In conclusion, surface video-EEG allows interictal and ictal patterns in patients with TLE to manifest. There are numerous electroclinical differences between patients with MTLE and NTLE, but none of them are sufficient to arrive to a clear distinction between both types of epilepsies. It is possible to differentiate lesional NTLE from MTLE based on features of the history of the crisis, sintomatology of the crisis and surface ictal EEG recordings. Nevertheless, many of the overlapping electroclinical findings make it necessary to realize invasive studies for the correct localization and lateralization of the epileptogenic zone.

4. Neuropsychological evaluation

For Kochen, Oddo and Solís (2003), the neuropsychological evaluation allows characterizing the cognitive aspects of patients with epilepsy, and in humans it confronts us with an in vivo model of the study of brain plasticity, making it an almost ideal model for the study of cognitive functions. Neuropsychological evaluation provides relevant information for the diagnosis, prognosis and rehabilitation of patients undergoing surgery for epilepsy (Drake, 2002). It allows:

- Assessing the current cognitive status, knowing the possible effects of epilepsy and/or consumption of long-standing AEDs on cognitive function. In the case of patients with TLE, the prevalent cognitive functions are memory and language in particular the denomination.

- Obtain data to draw conclusions about lateralization (right hemisphere, left hemisphere) and the location of the neuropsychological symptoms and their possible correlation with ictal onset zone.
- Predicting cognitive potential risks of surgery. In the case of temporal lobe epilepsy might be, first, a memory deficit that may range from a global amnesia, to amnesia for specific material, or a reduction of premorbid performance level. On the other hand a deficit in language, more specifically an anomia with varying degrees of severity. The compromise is explained by the structural and functional relationship of the hippocampus with memory system, and that is functionally lateralized, the left hippocampus related with memory for verbal material (the decrease or loss is well documented in cases of left temporal lobectomy) and the right for visuospatial memory (the decline is not so consistently documented as the previous one). This point has an important predictive value in surgical decision and should be part of the information given to the patient and the family, which also will help in surgery related decisions. Another important consideration, and well documented, is related to the preoperative level of memory performance and magnitude of the possible postoperative amnesia. Thus, patients with adequate preoperative performance on tests of verbal memory (left temporal), are at increased risk of amnesia after surgery when resection was performed in the dominant temporal lobe.
- To establish current and future needs of rehabilitation. Current because the cognitive status might now draw cognitive symptoms that are affecting the performance level of the patient and future because the characteristics of the surgery or any of its possible complications could cause sequelae susceptible of rehabilitation.
- To compare the neuropsychological performance before and after surgery, determining what functions remain intact, which have been improved and which have been deteriorated and then required to redirect the rehabilitation.

The evaluation protocol must be general and specific, covering if not all, the majority of cognitive functioning; it must also contain more specific and concrete tests for dysfunctional issues. This implies the need for an extensive protocol that meets the characteristics specified, including assessment of intellectual capacity, attention, memory, gnosis, praxis, language and executive functions.

Certainly, the neuropsychologist must have an extensive knowledge of cognitive activity, its development and its different forms of alteration, so that you can, from the patient's history and performances in the different tests, make a reading beyond quantitative psychometric data. In this regard, and to maximize the results of neuropsychological assessment it is necessary to manage a variety of knowledge related to: 1) functional brain asymmetry, 2) asymmetry in case of the injury, 3) performances suggestive hemispheric damage, and 4) brain plasticity.

First, in terms of functional brain asymmetry, according with Ardila & Rosselli (1992) indicate that for the majority of people, regardless of whether they are right or left handed, the dominant hemisphere for logical linguistic aspects is the left hemisphere. Thus, interhemispheric differences exist not only in the type of information processing, but how it is done. While the left hemisphere processes logical, linguistic, and temporal information, the right hemisphere does so with emotional information, rhythm, image, color and Spatial. The first processing (left hemisphere) is sequential, serial, symbolic and analytical; the second (right hemisphere) is simultaneous, parallel, rhythmic, melodic and emotional.

Given this, each hemisphere is involved in cognitive function in an unequal manner, each one performs different cognitive tasks but are complementary, thus, no function seems to be completely independent of the activity of a single cerebral hemisphere, and then the interaction of the both hemispheres is essential for proper operation. In addition, hemispheric specialization grades vary from one person to another and interact with variables such as sex, education, training, age at which the patient suffered the injury, characteristics of the crisis and extent of the injury.

Second, asymmetries in case of brain injury. The above information essentially leads to understanding how an injury to the left or right hemisphere leads to different changes, even within the same cognitive activity. Therefore, if there is a language disturbance found, the left injury would cause aphasia, with varying degrees of alteration in phonological, morphological, syntactic, semantic aspects corresponding with their reading, writing and arithmetic alterations. In a right injury it would be aprosodia, with the possibility of finding agraphia, alexia and acalculia, moreover, changes in paralinguistic aspects may be found. If praxis are affected, in left lesions ideomotor apraxia will be found and in right lesions visoconstructional apraxia; if it alters the corporal perception, in left lesions will find autotopoagnosia and in right lesions hemisomatoagnosia; if it alters the memory, in left lesions will encounter verbal amnesia and in right lesions nonverbal amnesia; in terms of affection, if the injury is left, the patient will have a catastrophic reaction, by their awareness of the defect, but if there is a right injury the reaction will be of indifference, which is closely related with their anosognosia.

Third, executions suggesting hemispheric dysfunction. In this case, for example, behavioral and emotional changes, emotional mutism as apathy, disinterest, concrete thinking, lack of spontaneity and initiative, adynamia and catastrophic reaction against the deficit suggest left frontal lesions, whereas symptoms like behavioral disinhibition , hyperreactivity, childish behavior, pseudo-psychopathy, inability to judge emotions, behavioral inadequacy and indifference reactions to the deficit would be indicative of right lesions.

Also associative agnosia, right - left disorientation and finger agnosia involve left lesions, but apperceptive agnosia, a non verbal auditory agnosia, unilateral Spatial agnosia and hemisomatoagnosia would be indicative of right lesions, visoconstructional apraxia with features like: scheduling problems, simplification of the drawing, lack of internal details, microforms, copy from left to right, would suggest a left side injury.

By contrast, features such as visuospatial problems (rotations, inversions), complexity of design, lack of perspective, better picture to the right side macroreproduction and copy from right to left, would suggest a right injury. Corporal apraxias would be indicative of left lesions, while the dressing apraxia would be right. Problems in thinking processes as: concrete, nominalism, syncretism, animism, alterations in solving verbal problems and poor verbal fluency, indicate left lesion, whereas failure in visuospatial problems and poor design flow, would point to right side injury.

Fourth, the concepts of brain plasticity. According with Aoki & Stekevitz (1988), brain plasticity is the ability to renew or reconnect neural networks in order to perform new tasks and adapting, recovering lost function after an accident or an injury, in some degree, the brain is constantly changing. The recovery of function does not occur all of a sudden, it is a slow change following a logical sequence. According with this, the brain can continue to develop in adulthood. Brain plasticity has physiological and biochemical bases, which explains why when a brain injury occurs during the first years of life, the opposite hemisphere and healthy adjacent areas can assume the functions involved. According with this, patients with epilepsy with early brain damage can have reorganization of functions by brain plasticity.

Neuropsychological evaluation provides the differential diagnosis of temporal and extratemporal epilepsies (Maestu, 2000), from cognitive deficits, which also is a differential predictive value. Patients with extra-temporal neuropsychological signs or diffuse brain disorder, have a worse prognosis for seizure control after surgery, but on the contrary patients with cognitive alterations lateralized and localized, have a greater predictor of seizure control, if it includes the existence of a single focus, such as medial temporal discharges restricted to one hemisphere would have a positive predictive value of seizure control (Jones-Gottman, 2000; Rausch, 2001). It is also important to consider that in patients with TLE there can be frontal functions affected, which can be explained by the connections between the two lobes (Orozco-Giménez, 2002).

Another fact that becomes important is the multifactorial nature of cognitive impairments. There are different variables, such as the etiology of seizures, drug treatment, age of onset, seizure type, duration of illness, seizure frequency and academic and cultural limitations, therefore, the cognitive impairment in this disease is variable and may be, from very severe, or not identify significant changes. Thus, in people with mental retardation there can be found immature development of certain cognitive domains, whereas in patients where the epilepsy is the manifestation of a focal brain disease, defects in memory may be the only evidence of cognitive alterations. All these turns the neuropsychological evaluation in a multivariate process that requires several hours to complete, but it is essential to know the patient's mental status (Oddo, 2000; Drake, 2002).

5. Intracarotid Amobarbital Procedure (IAP)

The Intracarotid Amobarbital Procedure (IAP) or Wada Test is considered the gold standard for lateralization of language and memory functions in patients who are candidates for epilepsy surgery (Sharan, 2010; Baxendale, 2009; Spencer, 2000; Trenerry, 2006). The interpretation of the IAP results is presented in terms of hemispheric dominance: right, left or bilateral / mixed, taking into account that the cerebral organization of cognitive functions is complex and that this complexity can be increased even further in refractory epilepsy, due to the effects of brain plasticity and atypical cognitive organization presented in focal brain lesions. Additionally, they must take into consideration the individual and gender differences that may occur in the hemispheric lateralization of functions.

Given its invasive nature, frequency of complications of the IAP ranges from 0 to 10.9%, those are mainly related to the angiography and not to the Amobarbital injection (including: encephalopathy, seizures, stroke or transient cerebral ischemia and hemorrhage at the catheter insertion site), but most centers report rates below 1% per year and only 0.36% of permanent morbidity (Sharan, 2010).

All the above considerations require a solid theorical knowledge and clinical experience of the neuropsychologist, neurologist and neuroradiologist involved in the IAP.

The importance of the IAP in the presurgical evaluation of patients with temporal lobe epilepsy lies in: 1) determining the cerebral representation of language, 2) identify patients at risk of decline in memory or amnesia after surgery and 3) provide information about lateralization and localization of the epileptogenic zone (Trenerry, 2006).

5.1 Intracarotid Amobarbital Procedure and cerebral representation of language

The value of the language test during the IAP depends in first instance of the concept we have of language. This is a universal competition which implies the existence of symbols and signs, represented mentally; this is a cortical process, expressed through speech. During the IAP, when injected into the dominant hemisphere for language, it could produce an alteration of language that can range from global aphasia to a complete expressive and partial receptive aphasia, or vice versa, or only partially one of the two.

The interpretation of the results can be affected by cross-dominance or right hemispheric dominance for language. It is unclear the effect of atypical dominance in neuropsychological tests, as there are no pathognomonic indicators of this one in traditional batteries. Almost 6% of healthy people may have an atypical language representation; condition even more evident in people with developmental disabilities or chronic illnesses such as epilepsy. In fact, nearly 30% of people with epilepsy have altered language lateralization (bilateral hemispheric representation or variability in dominance). This atypical representation for language is more common in left-handed patients with epilepsy and those with: extrahipocampal structural or functional compromise, early onset of epilepsy, short latency period between the initial precipitating injury and the onset of the seizures, and the presence of epileptiform discharges interictal temporal bilateral and extratemporal in the EEG (Sharan, 2010; Trenerry, 2006).

5.2 Intracarotid Amobarbital Procedure and cerebral representation of memory

The IAP as a technique for assessing cerebral representation of memory was introduced by Milner in the fifties, to predict whether the contralateral hemisphere to the epileptogenic area could support memory functions after temporal lobectomy. If after unilateral anesthesia, ipsilateral to the focus, the patient could remember the events immediately following, it could be concluded that the contralateral hemisphere could support memory function, and consequently, surgery does not involve risk of postoperative amnesia (Milner, 1966).

One of the main applications of the IAP is that the asymmetric execution of the memory can predict postoperative memory impairment. This prediction is based on the concepts of "functional reserve" and "functional adaptation" (Chelune, 1995; Chelune, 2001; Loring, 2001). Although several studies report that the results of the asymmetry of memory on the IAP are associated with the postoperative prognosis of crisis management, the results are not consistent and this could be explained by additional clinical factors, differences in the interpretation of the asymmetry in the procedure and dissimilar postoperative follow-up times (Yu, 2010; Trenerry, 2006).

5.3 Lateralization and localization of epileptogenic zone with the Intracarotid Amobarbital Procedure

The hemispheric asymmetry scores in language and memory in the IAP has a close relationship with the side of seizure onset in patients with TLE, especially with structural abnormalities in MRI´s. Its diagnostic accuracy for identifying the epileptogenic area is 80-98%. Thus patients show a poor performance on the IAP during injection into the contralateral hemisphere to the focus.

By contrast, the ipsilateral injection to the focus, being functional the opposite hemisphere, will not produce more deficits than that reported in the baseline. It should be mentioned that, while it is true that the lateralized value of the IAP is not one of its major applications, it is particularly important when other presurgical evaluations are not conclusive, providing information that may even obviate the need of more invasive intracranial EEG records (Sharan, 2010; Trenerry, 2006).

5.4 Non-Invasive alternative to the Intracarotid Amobarbital Procedure: Functional Magnetic Resonance Imaging (fMRI)

Among the new imaging techniques available for the preoperative evaluation of patients with refractory epilepsy, who are candidates for surgery, Functional Magnetic Resonance Imaging (fMRI) is perhaps the most promising alternative in our scenario. Unlike the IAP which is a test of inactivation, fMRI is an activation test to visualize areas of regional brain activity in response to cognitive paradigms. fMRI is a noninvasive alternative to electrocorticography and the IAP for mapping of eloquent cortex and language lateralization. With regard to language lateralization, studies report nearly 90% concordance between fMRI and the IAP. Although less widely studied, it is also in the process of validating the role of fMRI in predicting postoperative memory outcome and the localization of ictal activity (Paolicchi, 2008; Abou-Khalil, 2007; Kesavadas, 2008; Dupont, 2010).

5.5 Present and future of Intracarotid Amobarbital Procedure

In recent years, it has been proposed that fMRI is a noninvasive alternative to the IAP, however, this technique cannot answer the question of how a task could be executed if part of a particular hemisphere is resected, which itself is done by IAP. People question the validity and reliability of the IAP, and although there is no standard procedure for the IAP and fMRI, when addressing memory paradigms.

Predictive models of postoperative memory changes have major implications for preoperative counseling of patients. The amnesic risk cannot be neglected specially after surgery of TLE. For example, the ability to predict the development of an amnesic syndrome differs from the ability to identify patients at risk of significant impairment of memory for specific material, verbal or nonverbal, that although amnesic syndrome is not considered fully established, has the sufficient severity to limit vocational options and other aspects of quality of life for patients, that deserve the neuro-rehabilitation plan.

In our experience, the IAP provides valuable information not only for hemispheric dominance of functions, but also because in conjunction with other diagnostic evaluations can support the surgical decision regarding: lateralization, localization, cognitive risk, surgical planning, extent of resection, seizure management and neuro-rehabilitation (Galeano, 2011; Wada, 2008; Baxendale, 2008).

6. Neuroimaging

Neuroimaging is one of the current mainstays for the study, diagnosis, treatment and follow-up of patients with TLE.

Since Wilhelm Roentgen discovered X-rays in 1895, the most important milestones in the field of neuroimaging are given by the advent of computerized tomography [CT] (Hounsfield - Cormack) in 1971 and magnetic resonance imaging [MRI] (Damadian - Lauterbur - Mansfield) in 1976 (Shorvon, 2009; Canals, 2008). No less important is the development of functional MRI (BOLD) thanks to the work of Ogawa and Kwong in the early 90s (Ogawa, 1992; Kwong, 1992). Magnetic resonance spectroscopy (MRS) was introduced in the field of epilepsy around 1984.

6.1 Radiological anatomy

In the macroscopic examination of the temporal lobe magnetic resonance can recognize two surfaces: lateral, with the superior, middle, inferior and basal temporal gyrus, with fusiform and parahippocampal gyrus. They are delimited by the respective fissures: superior

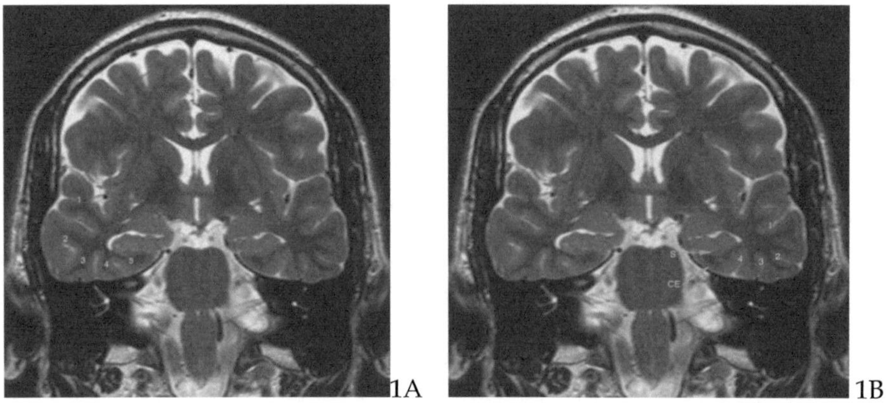

Fig. 1. Normal hippocampus
1A. 1, Superior temporal gyrus. 2, Middle temporal Gyrus. 3, Inferior temporal gyrus. 4, Fusiform gyrus. 5, Parahippocampal gyrus
1B. 1, Superior temporal sulcus. 2, Inferior temporal sulcus. 3, Temporo-occipital sulcus.4, Collateral sulcus. EC, Entorhinal cortex. S, Subiculum

temporal, inferior temporal, temporo-occipital and collateral. The parahippocampal gyrus includes the entorhinal cortex and subiculum (Fig. 1).
Superior to the parahippocampal gyrus is the hippocampal formation (Ammon´s horn and dentate gyrus) which is divided into head (digitations), body and tail (Fig. 2). Anterior, medial and superior to the hippocampal head is the amygdala. Adjacent is the uncus, the medial reference of the temporal lobe.

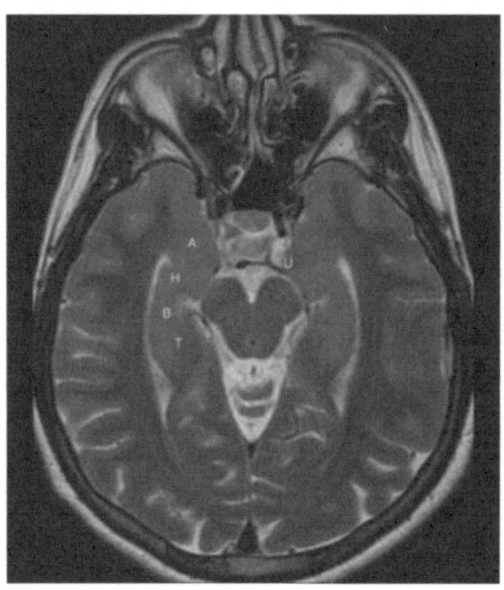

Fig. 2. Normal hippocampus
H=Head, B=Body, T=Tail, A=Amygdala, U=Uncus

Three structures with cerebrospinal fluid (CSF) surround the hippocampus: lateral, temporal horn, medial, the perimesencephalic cistern and superior, the choroid fissure. Hippocampal efferent system is evaluated with the fimbria, the fornix and mamillary body (Fig. 3). It Continues with the mamilothalamic tract that reaches the anterior nuclei of the thalamus and thence to the cingulate gyrus that culminates in the parahippocampal gyrus. It´s the so-called Papez circuit.

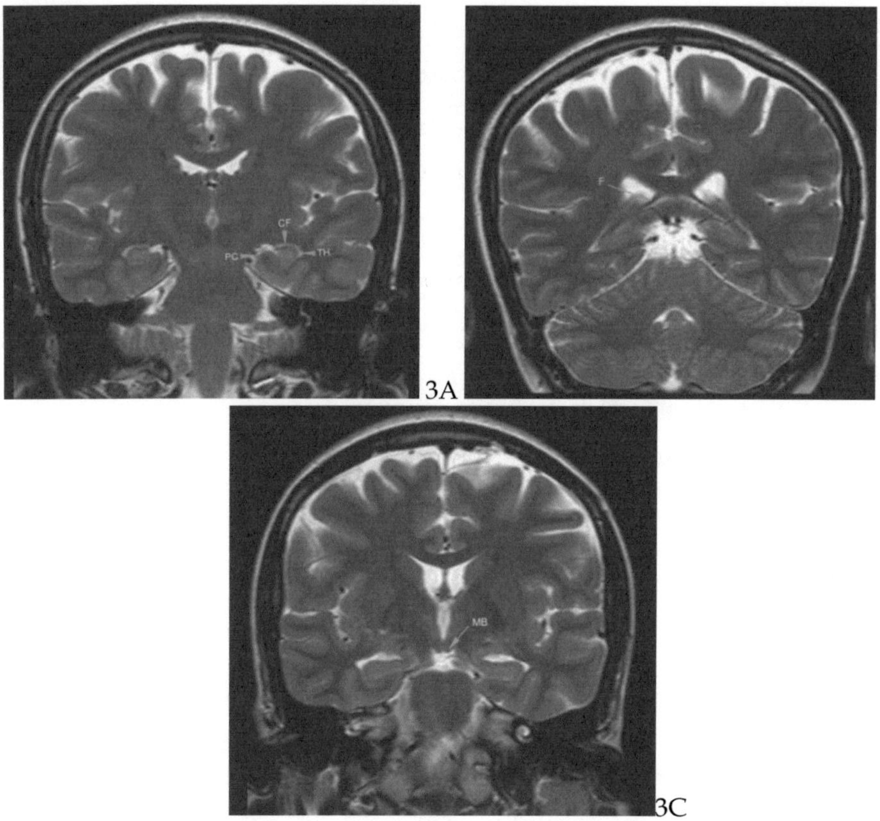

Fig. 3. Normal hippocampus
A. PC = Perimesencephalic cistern, CF = Choroidal fissure, TH = Temporal horn
B. F=Fornix
C. MB= Mamillary body

Keep in mind that irrigation depends mainly on the posterior cerebral artery and in a smaller proportion, to the anterior choroidal artery.

6.2 Anatomical image

It refers to data from CT either sequential, helical or multidetector and magnetic resonance imaging (MRI) of low (<1.5 T), high (1.5-3 T) or ultrahigh field (> 3 T). In the diagnosis of refractory epilepsy we are not going to mention CT because of its poor performance (Bronen, 1996).

The MRI study should be done with high field equipment, with orthogonal planes to the axis of the hippocampal formation with high resolution antenna with the minimum possible slice thickness (Fig. 4). Protocol should include series of T1- weighted volumetric images that allows cuts to resolution of 1 mm (1.5 T) or 0.25 mm (3 T). The routine use of coronal FLAIR is not necessary due to artifacts and can generate false positives when it comes to assessing the hippocampal formation (Vattipally, 2006). Instead, we recommended the STIR sequence that implies the IR series in its acquisition, which is essential to review the cortex in cases of malformation of cortical development.

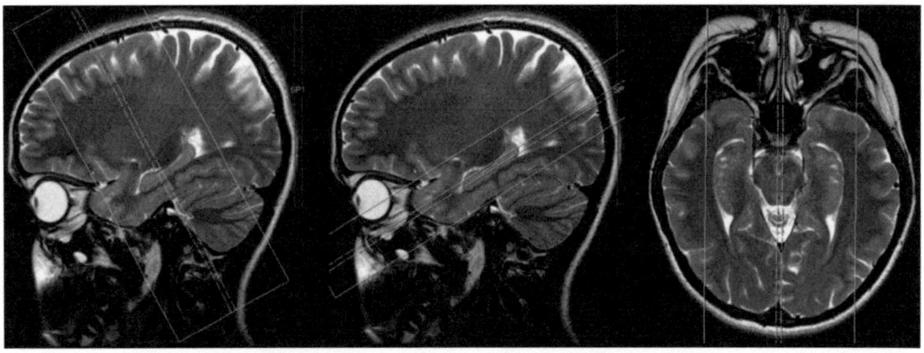

Fig. 4. Cutting planes. The diagram illustrates the orthogonal planes to be acquired in the coronal , axial and sagittal images of the hippocampus.

Due to the detail and the high number of images obtained (about 250) the neuroradiologist should interpret the results on a workstation that allows their proper handling.

Clinicopathological conditions are grouped into the following seven categories for descriptive purposes: variants, hippocampal malrotation, hippocampal sclerosis, malformations of cortical development, tumors, vascular lesions and gliosis.

6.2.1 Variants

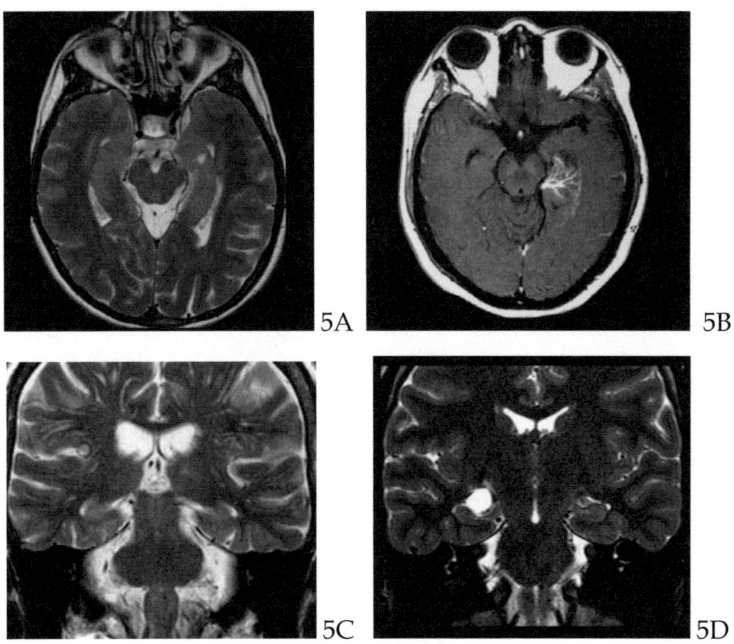

Fig. 5. Variants

A. Cyst of the left hippocampal fissure
B. Anomaly of the venous development of left hippocampus
C. Generalized perivascular spaces
D. Cyst of the right choroidal fissure

About 10-15% of the population may have cystic remnants of the hippocampal fissure, a structure that separates the Ammon´s horn of the dentate gyrus. Is present from week 10 of pregnancy and regularly regresses (Kier, 1997) [Fig 5A]. The medial temporal lobe may be the place of venous developmental abnormalities, disorders have not shown causal effect in terms of epileptogenicity (Topper, 1999) [Fig. 5B]. In the temporal lobe perivascular spaces can be found, defined as round or oval structures in the MRI, sharply defined, isointense to CSF in all sequences, according to the route of the vessel and without mass effect (Ogawa, 1995) [Fig 5C].The presence of a temporal arachnoid cysts or cyst of the choroid fissure are not of great value except if they are of a significant size (Bronen, 1996) [Fig 5D].

6.2.2 Hippocampal malrotation (HIMAL)

Defined in 2000 by Barsi et al. as a group of ten characteristics: incomplete hippocampal investment with rounded shape, unilateral commitment, signal intensity and normal size, internal structure blurred, abnormal angle collateral sulcus, anomalous fornix size and position, temporal lobe size preserved, temporal horn enlargement and normal corpus callosum (Barsi, 2000) [Fig. 6].

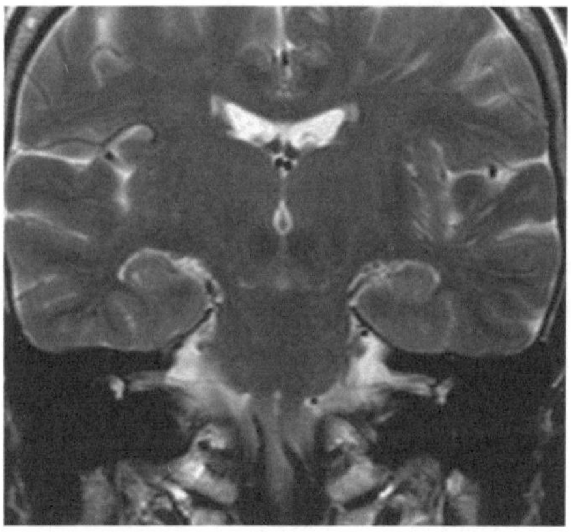

Fig. 6. Left HIMAL

In our experience we found that it can be focal or even bilaterally. This discrepancy can be explained in part by the original study methodology where they used low field resonators (0.5-1 T). Although the original description was present in 6% of 527 epileptic patients examined, it is unclear whether it can have a causal relationship.

6.2.3 Hippocampal sclerosis (HS)

Is the most common pathologic substrate in TLE in most of the series and the MRI is the most sensitive and specific for detection in vivo. Although it may be bilateral or symmetrical, it is more often unilateral or asymmetric (Fig. 7A). Among the characteristic findings are atrophy, loss of internal architecture and the increase in signal intensity on T2 series (Wieser, 2004). It has been proposed, however, that when there is no obvious changes of atrophy and signal alterations, complete loss of hippocampal head fingering has a sensibility of 92% or a specificity of 100% for the diagnosis (Oppenheim, 1998) [Fig. 7B].

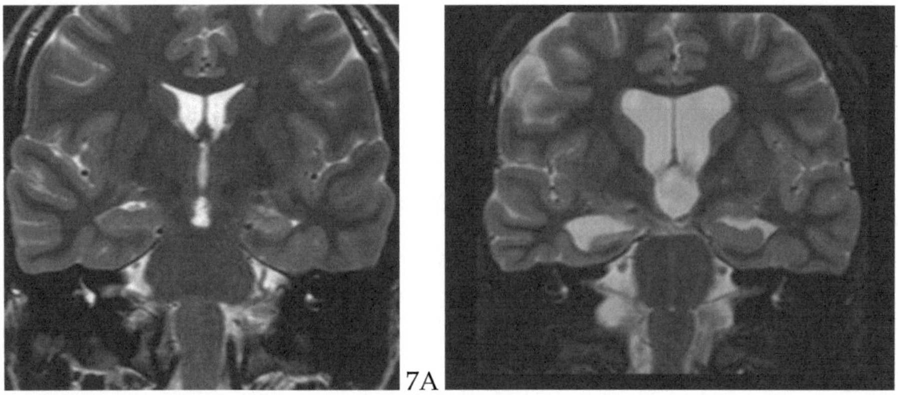

7A 7B

Fig. 7. Hippocampal Sclerosis
A. Atrophy and hyperintensity (T2) of the hippocampal formation
B. Loss of the digitations of right hippocampus head

In many cases ipsilateral extra-hippocampal findings can be observed as:

- Atrophy-signal alterations of the temporal neocortex, temporal white matter, amygdala, fornix, mamillary body, thalamus and basal frontal cortex.
- Atrophy-signal alterations in the contralateral hippocampus
- Dilatation of the ipsilateral and contralateral temporal horn.
- Diffuse ipsilateral hemispheric atrophy (Wieser, 2004; Ng, 1997; Deasy, 2000; Oikawa, 2001)

In approximately 15-20% of cases of HS can be associated with other extra-hippocampal epileptogenic entity, between which are malformations of cortical development (eg. cortical dysplasia) and gliosis in the first instance. It's called dual pathology (Palacios, 2008).

Furthermore, it is important to note that incidental hippocampal sclerosis, an entity recognized in the field of neuroimaging and debated in the epilepsy groups, requires special mention. From the histopathological point of view there are reports of HS in up to 10% of individuals without epilepsy (Menzler, 2010). This incidental MRI finding in patients without epilepsy is rare and requires the strict clinical correlation discarding undocumented seizure syndrome (Kevin, 1999).

6.2.4 Malformations of cortical development

Corresponds to a heterogeneous group of entities characterized by abnormal cerebral cortical structure, usually related to genetic, vascular, infectious and toxic alterations. It may occur during states of proliferation, migration or cellular organization in pre or postnatal stage depending of the case. It should be noted that these processes are synchronous and are continuous from temporal point of view(Abdel, 2009).

Although several classification schemes, the most common and practical approach due to concepts of Barkovich (Barkovich, 1996; Barkovich, 2001; Barkovich, 2005). They can be grouped into three categories according to the original classification based on the alteration in the development process microlisencephaly, hemimegalencephaly and cortical dysplasia (proliferation), complete lissencephaly, congenital muscular dystrophy and heterotopia (migration), polymicrogyria and schizencephaly (organization) [Fig. 8].

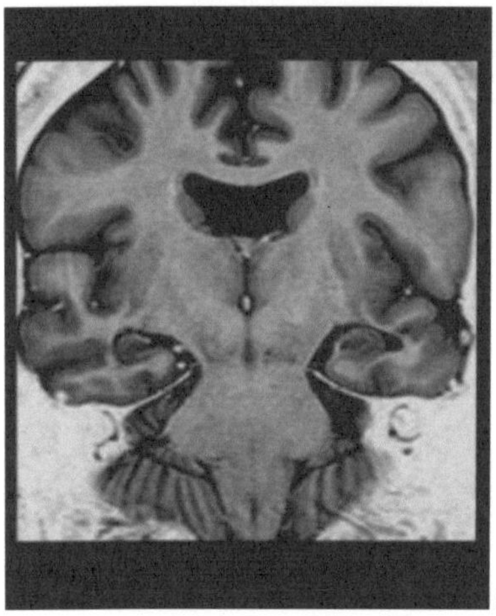
8A

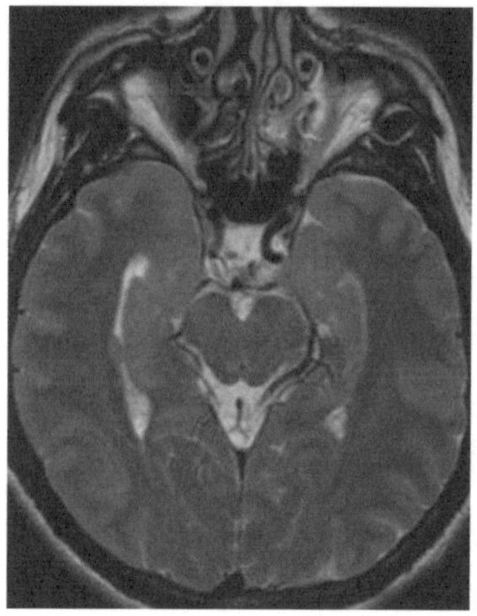
8B

Fig. 8. Malformations of cortical development
A. Polymicrogyria in the right inferior temporal sulcus
B. Subependymal nodular heterotopia of the right temporal horn

Particular interest receives the entity of cortical dysplasia, a source of intense study in recent years. Blümcke recently published an international consensus that modifies the traditional classification of Palmini with the aim of improving the clinical-pathologic characterization of the entity (Blümcke, 2011).
The MRI features include: hyperintensity in T2, FLAIR and STIR (explained by cellularity, gliosis, hypomyelination or ball cells), Giral abnormal pattern, increased cortical thickness, cortical depression and absence of calcification [Fig. 9A] (Widdess, 2006). In the case of transmantle cortical dysplasia it could be found a path that reaches the ventricular surface (Fig. 9B).

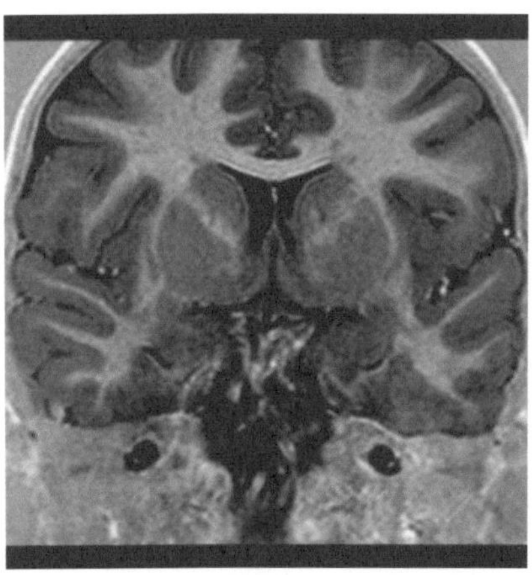
9A

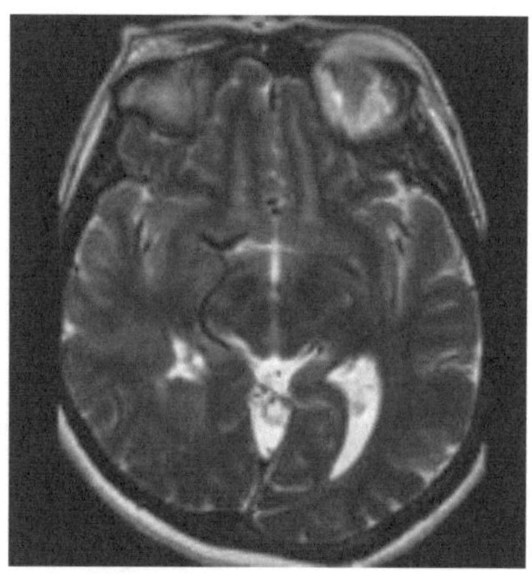
9B

Fig. 9. Cortical dysplasias
A. Dysplasia of the left temporo-occipital and fusiform gyrus
B. Trasmantle right temporal dysplasia

6.2.5 Tumors

Neoplasias are usually of low-grade malignancy predominantly gangliogliomas and dysembryoplastic neuroepithelial tumors (DNET). It is important to remember its close association with malformations of cortical development not only for their coexistence, and similar imaging appearance but by their possible common origin (Urbach, 2004). It´s appearance are small lesions, cortical-subcortical, with varying degrees of calcification, microcystic component and little or no enhancement with gadolinium administration (Fig. 10).

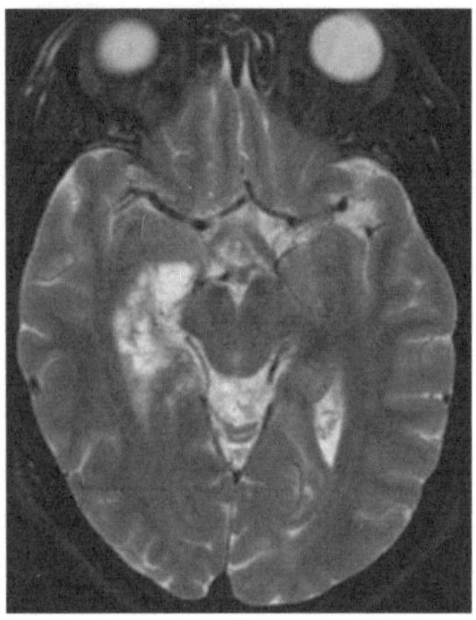
10A

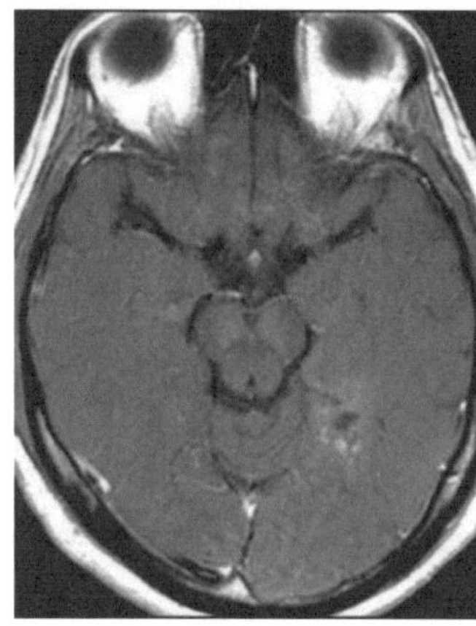
10B

Fig. 10. Tumors
A. DNET of right hippocampus
B. Left temporal medial ganglioglioma

6.2.6 Vascular

Cavernous malformation is the most common vascular disorder, in Lehéricy´s series, these were found in 4.5% of 222 patients with TLE studied with MRI (Lehéricy, 1997). This configuration is called "popcorn" in the T2 series, explained by the presence of central extracellular methemoglobin and peripheral hemosiderin (Fig. 11).

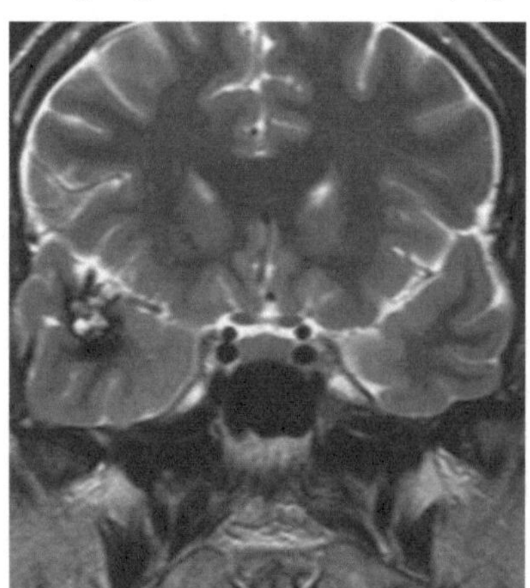

Fig. 11. Cavernous malformation

Image of "popcorn" on the anterior part of the right temporal.

6.2.7 Gliosis

This is the manifestation of a reactive process to different insults. Becomes relevant when talking about post-traumatic, post-infectious and postinfarct epilepsy. However, it is usually an epiphenomenon secondary to trauma in an epileptic patient with ictal onset zone with a different location, and may be indistinguishable from very small cortical dysplasias. Images are observed as hyperintense in FLAIR series (Fig. 12).

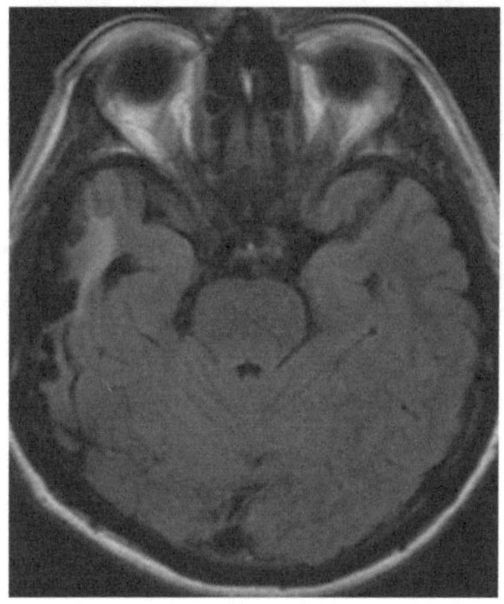

Fig. 12. Gliosis

Traumatic malacia and gliosis in the lateral part of right temporal lobe

6.3 Functional image

It refers to the imaging techniques that allow the assessment of physiological, biophysical and metabolic properties of a tissue. We will talk about images by MRI (MRS, DTI and tractography or BOLD).

The MRS has shown disorders of certain metabolites such as N-acetyl aspartate (NAA), choline (Cho), creatine (Cr), myoinositol (Mio) and lactate (Lac) in TLE. It is well known the decrease in NAA and the indexes of NAA / Cho-Cr in the hippocampus with HS (Wieser, 2004). It has been reported significant hippocampal changes in neocortical TLE (Lee, 2005) and also described a possible relationship with the severity of epilepsy (Hammen, 2007). However, their greatest utility is reserved for patients with normal MRI as a potential lateralizing study. It should be noted that some changes seen in this context may be transient and reversible.

The DTI is based on microstructural tissue organization delimited by the anisotropic diffusion of water in the brain. The approach allows axonal trajectories, that report anomalies in shape, size, number and location of tracts and white matter fibers in addition to their state of myelination. Information closely related to the different cortical abnormalities has been described (Rastogi, 2008). It also has become an element almost for routine surgical planning.

Functional magnetic resonance imaging (fMRI) itself or BOLD (Blood Oxygen Level-Dependent) allows to obtain maps of cortical activity during an specific test (paradigm), based on hemodynamic changes resulting of neuronal activity. With respect to the presurgical evaluation, the most important to consider are language and memory functions (Fig. 13).

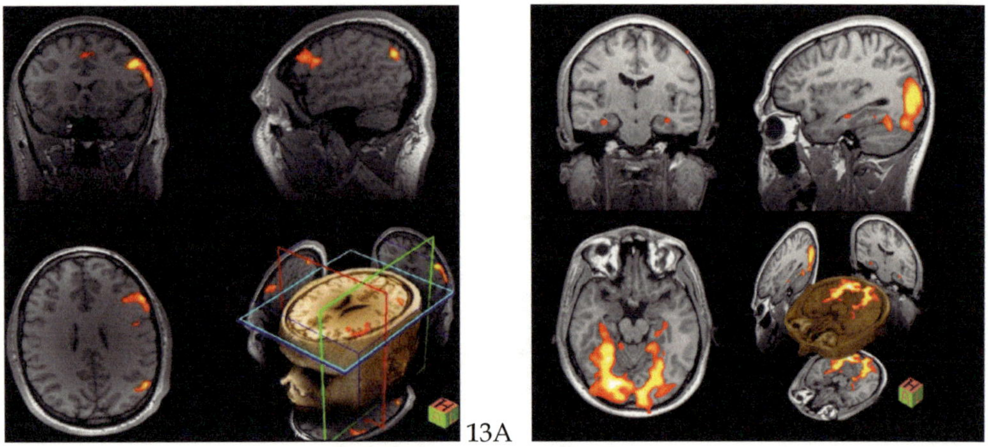

13A 13B

Fig. 13. fMRI
A. Cortical activation of the left inferior frontal and supramarginal gyrus, corresponding to Broca's and Wernicke's areas respectively. Paradigms of Word-generation and comprehension (hear stories).
B. Bilateral medial temporal activation mediated by visual stimuli in a paradigm of memory (complex scenes).

The determination of lateralization of language is critical in TLE since in this population there are higher incidences of atypical dominance. That assessment has been done traditionally with the Intracarotid Amobarbital Procedure (IAP) or Wada test (Wada, 1960). In 1996, Binder made a comparative study in a group of 22 epileptic patients with IAP and a semantic decision paradigm in fMRI. He found a high correlation in terms of laterality indices. Emphasizing the potential of fMRI such as a noninvasive technique, without significant risks, independent of variations in arterial anatomy and easily reproducible (Binder, 1996). Gaillard subsequently studied 30 patients with complex partial epilepsy with a nomination paradigm and identified frontotemporal activation consistent with the IAP and cortical mapping (Gaillard, 2002). An important comparison between the two methods was performed by Woermann in a group of 100 patients, which used the word generation paradigm and showed a concordance of 91% (Woermann, 2003). Despite these good results it shouldn't be forgotten that like any diagnostic test there is always the possibility of false positives and false negatives. For example, Jayakar reported a case of false lateralization of language in a 14-year-old with left-HS who was assessed in the postictal period (Jayakar, 2002). On the other hand, it is necessary to keep in mind the cost of fMRI versus IAP for the assessment of candidates for surgery. A cost analysis study recently showed that the IAT is 3.7 times more expensive than fMRI in the evaluation of language lateralization (Medina, 2004). In contrast to the lateralization, the localization of critical areas for language has been very difficult. It seems that the use of different paradigms (verb generation, nomination, verbal fluency, and reading comprehension) gets more sensitive in the detection of these critical areas (Rutten, 2003).
With respect to the study of memory there are good results in the assessment of episodic memory with paradigms such as encoding of complex scenes, test that have shown good correlation in terms of lateralization with respect to the memory dominance found in IAP (Detre, 2004).

6.4 Future of neuroimaging in temporal lobe epilepsy

Continued progresses in different areas of knowledge converge on technological developments that in the case of magnetic resonance will generate key points in the field of early and accurate diagnosis. In that order of ideas we must note the possibilities that are opened with the use of ultrahigh field in the image not only structural but functional. We should think in the anatomical resolution in microscopic scale which are obtained from images of the hippocampal histologic slices that are now available with equipment of 7 and 9.4 T (Fatterpekar, 2002; Prudent, 2010).

7. Conclusion

The approach and management of patients with refractory epilepsy requires the presence of a multidisciplinary team with different sub-specialties and with the motivations to achieve the best possible outcome. Confirmation of the diagnosis of epilepsy and its medical intractability is the essential prerequisite for epilepsy surgery. The main objective of surgical treatment of epilepsy is seizure control and improvement of quality-of-life of patients with medically intractable epilepsy. The role of the different diagnostic methods with respect to identification of the epileptogenic zone is vital for surgical patient selection and outcome.

Based in our experience with the epilepsy group, and as expressed by many authors, the best results that are obtained when patients are submitted to epilepsy surgery, regarding crisis control, are those in which there is convergence of the different diagnostic methods towards the epileptogenic zone. But in other group of patients, there is no convergence of the diagnostic methods; these do not lateralize or lateralize to the contralateral side of the lesional zone. In this situation, each method takes its own specific weight, and based on the analysis of these results, a surgical decision can be made. Video-EEG is considered for many authors as the "gold standard" in the evaluation of refractory epilepsy and temporal mesial sclerosis. When it does not lateralize, or lateralizes to the contralateral side, other diagnostic methods such as the IAP or MRI take a much more important role, when it comes to decision making. The IAP defines the functional memory reserve, and limits the surgeon when it comes to resecting the affected area, defining if besides the lesion he can proceed with mesial structures, if the contralateral temporal lobe has a normal function. By this, we can avoid an unnecessary invasive intracranial EEG recording in this group of patients. It has been demonstrated that the propagation of ictal activity can be generated in the contralateral side of the lesion and transmitted to other areas using different networks. For example, if the MRI demonstrates a lesion in the contralateral lobe (temporal mesial sclerosis) to the one reported by the video-EEG as the ictal-onset zone, and the IAP reports functional memory reserve contralateral as well, this test would have less importance. In patients with dual pathology, when there is a tumor or a malformation, in addition to the demonstration that the seizure-onset zone is ipsilateral, the IAP has more specific weight. If there is a functional memory reserve contralateral to the lesion, the surgeon can make a wider resection, but if the functional memory reserve is ipsilateral, the surgeon should focus on the specific lesion.

8. References

Abdel, A.A.K., et al. (2009). Disorders of Cortical Formation: MR Imaging Features. *AJNR*, Vol. 30, pp. 4–11.

Abou-Khalil, B. (2007). An update on determination of language dominance in screening for epilepsy surgery: the Wada test and newer noninvasive alternatives. *Epilepsia*, Vol. 48, No. 3, pp. 442-55.

Alssadi, TM., et al. (2001). False lateralization by subdural electrodes in two patients with temporal lobe epilepsy. *Neurology*, Vol. 57, pp. 532-534.

Andrade, R., et al. (2011). Semiología de las crisis en las epilepsias temporales y tipos semiológicos de las epilepsias temporales, In: *Epilepsias del lóbulo temporal*. Cornejo, JW., & Toro, ME., pp. 23-33. ISBN: 978-958-44-8359-1, Medellín.

Andriani Rahal, M., et al. (2006). Somatosensory Aura in Mesial Temporal Lobe Epilepsy: Semiologic Characteristics, MRI Findings and Differential Diagnosis with Parietal Lobe Epilepsy. *J Epilepsy Clin Neurophysiol* , Vol. 12, No. 3, pp. 155-160.

Aoki, C. & Stekevitz, P. (1988). Plasticity in Brain Development. *Scientific American*, Vol. 259, pp. 34-42.

Archarya, V. et al. (1998). Olfactory epileptic auras. *Neurology*, Vol. 51, No. 1, pp. 56-61.

Ardila, A. & Rosselli, M. (1992). *Neuropsicología Clínica*, Manual Moderno, ISBN: 9707292792.

Aull-Watschinger, S., et al. (2008). Sexual auras: Predominance of epileptic activity within the mesial temporal lobe. *Epilepsy & Behavior, Vol.* 12, pp. 124–127.

Barkovich, J., et al. (1996). A classification scheme for malformationsof cortical development. *Neuropediatrics*, Vol. 27, pp. 59–63.

Barkovich, J., et al. (2001). Classification system for malformations of cortical development: update 2001. *Neurology*, Vol. 57, pp. 2168–78.

Barkovich, J., et al. (2005). A developmental and genetic classification for malformations of cortical development. *Neurology* , Vol. 65, pp. 1873–87.

Barsi, P., et al. (2000). Hippocampal malrotation with normal corpus callosum: a new entity?. *Neuroradiology*, Vol. 42, pp. 339-345.

Baxendale, S. (2009). The Wada test. *Curr Opin Neurol*, Vol. 22, No. 2, pp. 185-9.

Baxendale, S., et al. (2008). The role of the Wada test in the surgical treatment of temporal lobe epilepsy: an international survey. *Epilepsia*; Vol. 49, pp. 715–20; discussion 720-7.

Binder, JR., et al. (1996). Determination of language dominance using functional MRI: A comparison with the Wada test. *Neurology*, Vol. 46, No. 4, pp. 978-84.

Biraben, A. et al. (2001). Fear as the main feature of epileptic seizures. *J Neurol Neurosurg Psychiatry*,Vol. 70, No. 2, pp. 186–191.

Blümcke, I., et al. (2011). The clinicopathologic spectrum of focal cortical dysplasias: A consensus classification proposed by an ad hoc Task Force of the ILAE Diagnostic Methods Commission. Epilepsia, Vol. 52, No. 1, pp. 158–174.

Bronen, R., et al. (1996). Refractory Epilepsy: Comparison of MR Imaging, CT, and Histopathologic Findings in 117 Patients. *Radiology*, Vol. 201, pp. 97-105.

Canals, M. (2008). Historia de la resonancia magnética de Fourier a Lauterbur y Mansfield: en ciencias, nadie sabe para quién trabaja. *Rev Chil Radio*, Vol. 14, No. 1, pp. 39-45.

Castilho Garcia, MT. et al. (2010). Auras and clinical features in temporal lobe epilepsy: A new approach on the basis of voxel-based Morphometry. *Epilepsy Research*, Vol. 89, pp. 327—338.

Chelune, GJ. (1995). Hippocampal adequacy versus functional reserve: Predicting memory functions following temporal lobectomy. *Archives of Clinical Neuropsychology*, Vol. 10, pp. 413-432.

Chelune, G., & Najm, IM. (2001). Risk factors associated with postsurgical decrements in memory. In: *Epilepsy Surgery.* Lüders, H., & Comair, Y., editors. pp. 497-504, Lippincott Williams & Wilkins, Philadelphia.

Chiosa, V., et al. (2010). Temporal Lobe Epilepsy: From Electro-Clinical Semiology to Surgical Outcome. *Epileptologie,* Vol. 27, pp. 94 - 100.

Chiosa, V., M.S., S. Vulliémoz. (2010). Temporal Lobe Epilepsy: From Electro-Clinical Semiology to Surgical Outcome.*Epileptologie,* Vol. 27, pp. 94 - 100.

Dantas, FG., et al. (1998). Clinical and EEG analysis of mesial and lateral temporal lobe seizures. *Arq Neuropsiquiatr.,* Vol. 56(3A), pp. 341-9.

Deasy, N., et al. (2000). Thalamic changes with mesial temporal sclerosis: MRI. *Neuroradiology,* Vol. 42, pp. 346-351.

Dericioglu, N., & Saygi, S. (2008). Ictal scalp EEG findings in patients with mesial temporal lobe epilepsy. *Clin EEG Neurosci.,* Vol. 39, No. (1), pp. 20-7.

Detre J. (2004). fMRI: Applications in Epilepsy. *Epilepsia,* Vol. 45 (Suppl. 4), pp. 26–31.

Devinsky, O., et al. (1995). Ictus emeticus; further evidence of non-dominant temporal involvement. *Neurology,* Vol. 45, pp. 1158-1160.

Di Gennaro, G., et al. (2004). Ictal heart rate increase precedes EEG discharge in drug-resistant mesial temporal lobe seizures. *Clin Neurophysiol.,* Vol. 115, pp. 1169-77.

Drake, M., et al. (2002). Evaluación neuropsicológica y test de Wada en el pronóstico de la lobectomía temporal en pacientes con epilepsia del lóbulo temporal mesial. *Rev. Neur Argentina,* Vol. 27, pp. 254-260.

Dubeau, F., & McLachlan, RS. (2000). Invasive electrographic recording techniques in temporal lobe epilepsy. *Can J Neurol Sci.,* Vol. 27, No. 1, pp. 29-34.

Dupont, S., et al. (2010). Functional MR imaging or Wada test: which is the better predictor of individual postoperative memory outcome?. *Radiology,* Vol. 255, No. 1, pp. 128-34.

Ebersole, JS., & Pacia, SV. (1996). Localization of temporal lobe foci by ictal EEG patterns. *Epilepsia,* Vol. 37, No. 4, pp. 386-99.

Ebner, A., et al. (1995). Automatisms with preserved responsiveness: a lateralizing sign in psychomotor seizures. *Neurology,* Vol. 45, pp. 61-64.

Eisenschenk, S., et al. (2001). Lateralization of temporal lobe foci: depth versus subdural electrodes. *J Clin Neurophysiol,* Vol. 112, pp. 836-844.

Engel, Jr J., & Ojemann, GA. (1993). *Surgical treatment of the epilepsies.* [ed.] Jr J Engel. Raven Press, pp. 319-329, New York.

Fatterpekar, G., et al. (2002). Cytoarchitecture of the Human Cerebral Cortex: MR Microscopy of Excised Specimens at 9.4 Tesla. *AJNR,* Vol. 23, pp. 1313–21.

Fernádez-Torre JL. (2002). Auras epilépticas: clasificación, fisiopatología, utilidad práctica, diagnóstico diferencial y controversias. *Rev Neurol,* Vol. 34, No. 10, pp. 977-983.

French, JA., et al. (1993). Characteristics of medial temporal lobe epilepsy. I. Results of history and physical examination. *Ann Neurol,* Vol. 34, pp. 774–80.

Fried, I. et al. (1995). The anatomy of epileptic auras: focal pathology and surgical outcome. *J Neurosurg,* Vol. 83, No. 1, pp. 60-66.

Gaillard, WD., et al. (2002). Language dominance in partial epilepsy patients identified with an fMRI reading task. *Neurology,* Vol. 59, pp. 256-65.

Galeano, LM., et al. (2011). Importancia del procedimiento con amobarbital intracarotideo en la evaluación prequirurgica del paciente con epilepsia del lóbulo temporal, In:

Epilepsias del lóbulo temporal. Cornejo, JW., & Toro, ME., pp. 181-193. ISBN: 978-958-44-8359-1, Medellín.

Gates, JR., & Cruz-Rodriguez, R. (1990). Mesial temporal sclerosis: pathogenesis, diagnosis and management. *Epilepsia*, Vol. 32, pp. 55-65.

Geyer, JD., et al. (1999). Significance of interictal temporal lobe delta activity for localization of the primary epileptogenic region. *Neurology*, Vol. 52, pp. 202-5.

Gil-Nagel, A., & Risinger MW. (1997). Ictal semiology in hippocampal versus extrahippocampal temporal lobe epilepsy. *Brain*, Vol. 120, pp. 183-92.

Gloor, P. (1990). Experiential phenomena of temporal lobe epilepsy. Facts and hypotheses. *Brain*; Vol. 113 (Pt 6), pp. 1673–94.

Hammen, T. et al. (2007). H-MR Spectroscopy Indicates Severity Markers in Temporal Lobe Epilepsy: Correlations between Metabolic Alterations, Seizures, and Epileptic Discharges in EEG. *Epilepsia*, Vol. 48, No. 2, pp. 263–269.

Hausser-Hauw, C. et al. (1987). Gustatory hallucinations in epileptic seizures. Electrophysiological, clinical and anatomical correlates. *Brain*, Vol. 110, No. 2, pp. 339–359.

Henkel, A., et al. (2002). The localizing value of the abdominal aura and its evolution: a study in focal epilepsies. *Neurology*, Vol. 58, No. 2, pp. 271-276.

Immonen, A., et al. (2010). Long-term epilepsy surgery outcomes in patients with MRI-negative temporal lobe epilepsy. *Epilepsia*, Vol. 51, pp. 2260-2269.

Jasper, H. (1958). The ten-twenty electrode system of the International Federation. *Electroencephalogr Clin Neurophysiol*, Vol. 10, pp. 371-5.

Jayakar, P., et al. (2002) False lateralization of language cortex on functional MRI after a cluster of focal seizures. *Neurology*, Vol. 58, pp. 490-2.

Jones-Gotman, M., et al. (2000). Neurosychological assessment for temporal lobe epilepsy surgery. *Can J Neurol Sci*, Vol. 27 (Suppl. 1), pp. S42-S46.

Kaplan, PW., et al. (1999). Ictus expectoratus: a sign of complex parcial seizures usually of non dominant temporal lobe origin. *Seizure*, Vol. 8, pp. 480-484.

Kasper, BS., et al. (2010). Phenomenology of hallucinations, illusions, a delusions as part of seizure semiology. *Epilepsy Behav*,Vol. 18, No. 1-2, pp. 13-23.

Kesavadas, C., & Thomas, B. (2008). Clinical applications of functional MRI in epilepsy. *Indian J Radiol Imaging*, Vol. 18, No. 3, pp. 210-7.

Kevin, R., et al. (1999). Incidental Detection of Hippocampal Sclerosis on MR Images: Is It Significant?. *AJNR*, Vol. 20, pp. 1609–1612.

Kier, E., et al. (1997). Embryology of the Human Fetal Hippocampus: MR Imaging, Anatomy, and Histology. *AJNR*, Vol. 18, pp. 525–532.

Kotagal, P., et al. (1995). Psychomotor seizures of temporal lobe onset: analysis of symptom clusters and sequences. *Epilepsy Res*, Vol. 20, pp. 49-67, 1995.

Koutroumanidis, M., et al. (2004). Interictal temporal delta activity in temporal lobe epilepsy: correlations with pathology and outcome. *Epilepsia*, Vol. 45, No. 11, pp. 11351-67.

Kuba, R., et al. (2010). Peri-ictal yawning lateralizes the seizure onset zone to the nondominant hemisphere in patients with temporal lobe epilepsy. *Epilepsy Behav.*, Vol. 19, No. 3, pp. 311-4

Kwong, KK., et al. (1992). Dynamic magnetic resonance imaging of human brain activity during primary sensory stimulation. *Proc Natl Acad Sci USA*, Vol. 89, pp. 5675-9.

Lee, S., et al. (2005). Effect of seizure on hippocampus in mesial temporal lobe epilepsy and neocortical epilepsy: an MRS study. *Neuroradiology,* Vol. 47, pp. 916–23.

Lehéricy, S., et al. (1997). Temporal lobe epilepsy with varying severity: MRI study of 222 patients. *Neuroradiology,* Vol. 39, pp. 788-96.

Lin, K., et al. (2009). Sign of the Cross (Signum Crucis): Observation of an uncommon ictal manifestation of mesial temporal lobe epilepsy. *Epilepsy & Behavior, Vol.* 14, pp. 400–403.

Loddenkemper, T., & Kotagal, P. (2005). Lateralizing signs during seizures in focal epilepsy. *Epilepsy Behav,* Vol. 7, pp. 1-17.

Loring, D., & Meador, K. (2001). Wada testing to define Hippocampal Function. In: *Epilepsy Surgery.* Lüders, H., & Comair, Y., editors. pp. 531-536. Lippincott Williams & Wilkins, Philadelphia.

Lüders, HO. (2008). *Textbook of Epilepsy Surgery,* Informa Healthcare UK Ltd., ISBN-10: 1841845760, London.

Lüders, HO. (1999). Chapter 16 Mesial Temporal Sclerosis, In: *The Epilepsies: Etiologies and Prevention.* Kotagal, P., & Lüders, HO. Academic Press, San Diego.

Maestú, F., et al. (2000). Evaluation of epilepsy surgery. *Rev Neurol,* Vol. 15, No. 5, pp. 477-82.

Maestú, F., et al. (1999). Neuropsicología y deterioro cognitivo en epilepsia. *Rev Neurol,* Vol. 28, pp. 793-798.

Manford, M. et al. (1996). An analysis of clinical seizure patterns and their localizing value in frontal and temporal lobe epilepsies. *Brain,* Vol. 119, pp. 17–40.

McIntyre, DC., & Gilby K. (2008). Mapping seizure pathways in the temporal lobe., *Epilepsia,* Vol. 49, pp. 23-30.

Medina, LS., et al. (2004). Functional MR Imaging versus Wada Test for Evaluation of Language Lateralization: Cost Analysis. *Radiology,* Vol. 230, pp. 49-54.

Meletti, S., et al. (2003). The expression of interictal, pericital, y postictal facial-wiping behavior in temporal lobe epilepsy: a neuro-ethological analysis and interpretation. *Epilepsy & Behavior,* Vol. 4, pp. 635-643.

Menzler, K., et al. (2010). Evaluation of MRI criteria (1.5T) for the diagnosis of hippocampal sclerosis in healthy subjects. *Epilepsy Research,* Vol. 89, No. 2, pp. 349-354.

Milner, B. (1966). Amnesia following operation on the temporal lobes. In: Amnesia. Whitty,CWM. & Zangwill, OL., editors. pp. 109–33. Butterworths, London.

Mintzer, S., Lopez, F. (2002). Comorbidity of ictal fear and panic disorder. *Epilepsy and Behavior,* Vol. 3, No. 4, pp. 330–337.

Mohammed, M., et al. (2010). Electroencephalographic Features of Temporal Lobe Epilepsy. *Can. J. Neurol. Sci.,* Vol. 37, pp. 439-448.

Morris, HH., et al. (1987). Value of closely spaced electrodes in the localization of epileptiform foci: a study of 26 patients with complex partial seizures. *Electroencephalogr Clin Neurophysiol,* Vol. 63, pp. 107-11.

Napolitano, CE., & Orriols, MA. (2010). Graduated and sequential propagation in mesial temporal epilepsy: analysis with scalp ictal EEG. *J Clin Neurophysiol,* Vol. 27, No. 4, pp. 285-291.

Napolitano, CE., & Orriols, M. (2008). Two types of remote propagation in mesial temporal epilepsy: analysis with scalp ictal EEG. *J Clin Neurophysiol,* Vol. 25, pp. 69-76.

Ng, S., et al. (1997). MRI of the fornix and mamillary body in temporal lobe epilepsy. *Neuroradiology*, Vol. 39, pp. 551–5.

Noachtar, S., & Rémi, J. (2009). The role of EEG in epilepsy: a critical review. *Epilepsy Behav.*, Vol. 15, No. 1, pp. 22-33.

Oddo S., et al. (2000). Protocolo de evaluación neuropsicológica para pacientes candidatos a cirugía de la epilepsia. *Rev Neurol. Arg.*, Vol. 25 (S2), pp. 68.

Ogawa, S., et al. (1992). Intrinsic signal changes stimulation: functional brain mapping with magnetic resonance imaging. *Proc Natl Acad Sci USA*, Vol. 89, pp. 5951-5.

Ogawa, T., et al. (1995). Unusual Widening of Virchow-Robin Spaces: MR Appearance. *AJNR*, Vol. 16, pp. 1238–1242.

Oikawa, H., et al. (2001). The circuit of Papez in mesial temporal sclerosis: MRI. *Neuroradiology*, Vol. 43, pp. 205-210.

Oppenheim, C., et al. (1998). Loss of Digitations of the Hippocampal Head on High-Resolution Fast Spin-Echo MR: A Sign of Mesial Temporal Sclerosis. *AJNR*, Vol. 19, pp. 457–463.

Orozco-Giménez, C., et al. (2002). Neuropsicología Clínica en la Cirugía de Epilepsia del lóbulo Temporal. *Rev Neurol*, Vol. 35, No. 12, pp. 1116-1135.

Ostrowsky, K., et al. (2000). Functional mapping of the insular cortex: clinical implication in temporal lobe epilepsy. *Epilepsia*; Vol. 41, pp. 681-686.

Palacios, R., et al. (2008). Hippocampal Sclerosis: Histopathology Substrate and Magnetic Resonance Imaging. *Semin Ultrasound CT MRI*, Vol. 29, pp. 2-14.

Paolicchi, JM. (2008). Is the Wada test still relevant? Yes. *Arch Neurol*, Vol. 65, No. 6, pp. 838-40.

Parra, J., & Iriarte, J. (1999). Valor del registro ictal con vídeo-EEG en la evaluación prequirúrgica de pacientes con epilepsia del lóbulo temporal. Semiología y patrones electroencefalográficos. *Rev Neurol*, Vol. 28, No. 9, pp. 898-908.

Placantonakis, DG., et al. (2010). Bilateral intracranial electrodes for lateralizing intractable epilepsy: efficacy, risk, and outcome. *Neurosurgery*, Vol. 66, pp. 274-283.

Prudent, V., et al. (2010). Human Hippocampal Subfields in Young Adults at 7.0 T: Feasibility of Imaging. *Radiology*, Vol. 254, No. 3, pp. 900-6.

Rastogi, S., et al. (2008). Neuroimaging in Pediatric Epilepsy: A Multimodality Approach. *RadioGraphics*, Vol. 28, pp. 1079–95.

Ray, A., & Kotagal, P. (2005). Temporal lobe epilepsy in children: overview of clinical semiology. *Epileptic Disord*, Vol. 7, No.4, pp. 299-307.

Rausch, R. (2001). Psychological evaluation. In: *Surgical treatment of epilepsies*. Raven Press, New York.

Rodriguez, AJ., et al. (2007). Temporal lobe seizure semiology during wakefulness and sleep. *Epilepsy Research*, Vol. 74, No. 2-3, pp. 211—214.

Rutten, GJ., et al. (2003). Toward functional neuronavigation: implementation of functional magnetic resonance imaging data in a surgical guidance system for intraoperative identification of motor and language cortices. *Neurosurgical Focus* , Vol. 15, No. 1, pp. 1-6.

Saygi, S., et al. (1994). Differentiation of temporal lobe ictal behavior associated with hippocampal sclerosis and tumors of temporal lobe. *Epilepsia*, Vol. 35, pp. 737-42.

Sammaritano, M., et al. (1987). False lateralization by surface EEG of seizure onset in patients with temporal lobe epilepsy and gross focal cerebral lesions. *Ann Neurol*, Vol. 21, pp. 361-369.

Sakai, Y., et al. (2002). Localization of epileptogenic zone in temporal lobe epilepsy by ictal scalp EEG. *Seizure*, Vol. 11, pp. 163–168.

Serrano-Castro, PJ., et al. (1998). Mesial temporal sclerosis (II); Clinical features and complementary studies. *Rev Neurol*, Vol. 26, No. 152, pp. 592-597.

Sharan, A., et al. (2010). Intracarotid amobarbital procedure for epilepsy surgery. *Epilepsy Behav*. 2010 Dec 27. [Epub ahead of print]

Shorvon, SD. (2009). History of epilepsy 1909–2009: The ILAE century. *Epilepsia*, Vol. 50 (Suppl. 3), pp. 39–49.

Silverman, D. (1960). The anterior temporal electrode and the ten-twenty system. *Electroencephalogr Clin Neurophysiol*, Vol. 12, pp. 735-7.

Spencer, DC., et al. (2000). The role of the intracarotid amobarbital procedure in evaluation of patients for epilepsy surgery. *Epilepsia*, Vol. 41, No. 3, pp. 320-5.

Topper, R., et al. (1999). Clinical significance of intracranial developmental venous anomalies. *J Neurol Neurosurg Psychiatry*, Vol. 67, pp. 234–8.

Trenerry, M., & Loring, D. (2006). The intracarotid Amobarbital Procedure. In: The *Treatment of Epilepsy: Principles and Practice.* Wyllie, Elaine, Editor. pp. 1043-1052. Lippincott Williams & Wilkins, Philadelphia.

Urbach, H., et al. (2004). MR Imaging in the Presurgical Workup of Patients with Drug-Resistant Epilepsy. *AJNR*, Vol. 25, pp. 919-26.

Vattipally, V., & Bronen, R. (2006). MR Imaging of Epilepsy: Strategies for Successful Interpretation. *Radiol Clin N Am*, Vol. 44, pp. 111–133.

Van Buren, JM. (1963). The abdominal aura: a study of abdominal sensations occurring in epilepsy and produced by depth stimulation. *Electroenceph Clin Neurophysiol*,Vol. 15, pp. 1–19.

Vossler, DG., et al. (1998). Temporal ictal electroencephalographic frequency correlates with hippocampal atrophy and sclerosis. *Ann Neurol.*, Vol. 43, pp. 756-62.

Wada JA. (2008). A fateful encounter: sixty years later - reflections on the Wada test. *Epilepsia*, Vol. 49, pp. 726–727.

Wada, J., & Rasmussen, T. (1960). Intracarotid injection of sodium amytal for the lateralization of cerebral speech dominance. *J Neurosurg*, Vol. 17, pp. 266-82.

Widdess-Walsh, P., et al. (2006). Neuroimaging of Focal Cortical Dysplasia. J *Neuroimaging*, Vol. 16, pp. 185-96.

Walczak, T., et al. (1992). Accuracy and interobserver reliability of scalp ictal EEG. *Neurology*, Vol. 42, pp. 2279-85.

Wieser, HG. (1983). Electroclinical Features of the Psychomotor Seizure: A Stereoelectroencephalographic Study of Ictal Symptoms and Chronotopographical Seizure Patterns Including Clinical Effects of Intracerebral Stimulation. London: Butterworths.

Wieser, H.G. (2004). ILAE Comisión Report. Mesial Lobe Temporal Epilepsy with Hippocampal Sclerosis. *Epilepsia*, Vol. 45, No. 6, pp. 695-714.

Woermann, FG., et al. (2003). Language lateralization by Wada Test and fMRI in 100 patients with epilepsy. *Neurology*, Vol. 61, pp. 699-701.

Yu, HY., et al. (2010). The Wada memory test and prediction of outcome after anterior temporal lobectomy. *J Clin Neurosci.*, Vol. 17, No. 7, pp. 857-61. Epub 2010 May 14.

Zapata, JF., et al. (2010). Ictal electrocorticographic dissemination pattern in mesial temporal epilepsy with epileptogenic zone discordance. Proceedings of 6th Latin American Congress on Epilepsy (LACE), Cartagena, August 2010.

15

Clinical Development of Corpus Callosotomy in Treating Refractory Seizure

Jiwen Xu[1], Ping Zheng[2] and Hongyu Zhou[1]
[1]*Shanghai Renji Hospital,*
[2]*Shanghai Pudong New area People's Hospital,*
China

1. Introduction

For those patients with refractory seizures who are not candidates for focal respective surgery, corpus callosotomy can decrease the severity and attacking rate, but its outcome, complications and indications are still worrying the clinical doctors. In this text, we review the history, development and recent progress of corpus callosotomy in treating the refractory seizure.

The corpus callosum serves to integrate the activity of the two hemispheres and permits them to communicate with each other. The primary purpose of the corpus callosum may be to equalize the activity of both hemispheres to permit optimal integration of cortical responses. The purpose of this article is to provide a comprehensive review of clinical and practical aspects of callosotomy including rations, beneficial effects, adverse effects and prognostic factors for surgery success.

2. Anatomy and physiology of corpus callosum

The corpus callosum is a large bundle of mostly myelinated and some nonmyelinated fibers, the great white commissure, that cross the longitudinal cerebral fissure and interconnect the hemispheres. The body of the corpus callosum is arched; its anterior curved portion, the genu, continues anteroventrally as the rostrum. The thick posterior portion terminates in the curved splenium, which lies over the midbrain (Waxman, 2003).

The corpus callosum is topographically organized with anterior fibers connecting frontal regions of the two hemispheres and posterior fibers connecting posterior cortical structures. This anterior-to-posterior organization results in modality-specific regions of the corpus callosum. For example, the rostrum transfers higher cognitive information; the anterior midbody transfers motoric information by connecting fibers from the premotor, motor, anterior insular, and anterior cingulate cortical areas; the posterior midbody transfers somatosensory information; the isthmus transfers auditory signals; and the splenium transfers visual information (Wong et al., 2006; Funnell et al., 2000). Thus, the fiber tract in the anterior half of the corpus callosum is essential for the generalization of tonic and tonic-clonic convulsions, as well as atonic seizures (Wong et al., 2006). The corpus callosum is the major anatomical substratum for seizure bilateralization and bisynchronization (Reeves & Roberts, 1995).

3. Surgery rationale of corpus callosotomy

There are six midline commissural structures connecting the cerebral hemispheres, including the corpus callosum, anterior commissure, posterior commissure, hippocampal commissures, massa intermedia, and fornix. Of these, the most significant is the corpus callosum, which covers the most part of cortex (Wyllie, 1993). Curtis found that cortical stimulation of one hemisphere evoked potential on the opposite hemisphere (Curtis, 1940). Crowell and Ajmone reported that experimentally induced cortical epileptic activities of one hemisphere were also found in the homotonic area of the opposite hemisphere. Therefore, they suggested that a cortical epileptic discharge in one hemisphere is transferred to the other to induce epileptic synchronization (Crowell & Ajmone, 1972). Erickson's experimental report revealed that the corpus callosum was a major pathway for interhemispheric generalization of seizures in monkeys (Erickson, 1940). The rationale underlying the amelioration of seizures by corpus callosotomy is based on the hypothesis that the corpus callosum is the most important pathway for interhemispheric spread of epileptic activity (Reeves & Roberts, 1995).

4. Application of corpus callosotomy in refractory seizure

4.1 History

The history of corpus callosotomy began with a publication by Dandy (Dandy, 1936) in 1936 of patients who had partial callosal resection during surgeries of pineal tumors. Dandy reported that there were no resultant gross neurologic deficits in his patients. Corpus callosotomy as a treatment of epilepsy was first described in a series of 10 patients by Van Wagenen and Herren (Van & Herren, 1940) in 1940. The authors had observed that patients with tumors of the corpus callosum initially presented with generalized seizures. As the tumors grew and destroyed more of the corpus callosum, the seizures became less frequent and were more often unilateral. Their results at the time were variable and the follow-up period was brief. Interest in callosotomy remained stagnant until the 1960s when Bogen and Vogel (Bogen & Vogel, 1963) published their articles on the clinical and neuropsychological outcome of the surgery. Luessenhop (Luessen et al., 1970) reported the corpus callosotomy could replace the hemispherectomy. Adding with the report from Wilson (Wilson & Reevesm, 1978), the corpus callosotomy has earned widespread consideration.

4.2 Evolution of corpus callosotomy

Since the 1960s numerous studies regarding the indication and outcomes of corpus callosotomies have been published (Bogen & Vogel, 1963; Luessen et al., 1970; Wilson & Reevesm, 1978). The goal of a callosotomy procedure is to reduce the frequency and severity of seizures by interrupting common seizure spread pathways. Traditionally anterior two-third corpus callosotomy has been performed with great success. Different series have reported 50% or more reduction in seizure frequency in 55–100% of patients following this procedure (Wong et al., 2006; Maehara & Shimizu, 2001).

As a result of these data, corpus callosotomy has been increasingly utilized to control intractable generalized epilepsy. However, no standardized guidelines have been universally accepted for the selection of callosotomy patients for anterior two-third versus total callosotomy. In the past it had been thought that anterior two-third callosotomy would prevent postoperative neurologic deficits such as the disconnection syndrome marked by mutism, hemiataxia, and/or alexia (Harbaugh et al., 1983). Thus many neurosurgeons preferentially performed anterior two-third callosotomy initially with completion of the callosotomy during a second procedure if seizures were not properly controlled. Results of a second procedure for completion of the callosotomy were not impressive along with the associated increased morbidity with a second craniotomy procedure (Wyllie, 1993). Maxwell reported a modified surgical approach, using a more anterior interhemispheric approach, which decreased the surgical complications (Engel, 1993). Wyler suggested sectioning the corpus callosum between the bilateral pericallosal arteries (Wyllie, 1993).

4.3 Contemporary concept of corpus callosotomy

With the evolution of the operation technique and concept of corpus callosotomy, this procedure has been used more frequently and for a wider range of epilepsy disorders. It can be considered that decreasing the surgical complications and the seizure incidence rate, improving the cognitive and psychology function is much important to younger patients.

4.3.1 Surgical complications

Permanent serious complications are rare after callosotomy; most adverse effects are temporary. These include acute epidural hematoma, hydrocephalus, subdural cerebrospinal fluid accumulation, and infections (e.g., meningitis, osteomyelitis) (Wong et al., 2006; Maehara & Shimizu, 2001; Nei et al., 2006), possibly because of brain retraction and trans-ventricular approach. Disconnection syndrome is more common with total section than anterior callosotomy (Maehara & Shimizu, 2001; Kim et al., 2004; Rossi et al., 1996). Objects presented solely to the hemisphere that is not dominant for language may not be verbally reported by the patient. For example, rapid presentation of visual stimuli in the non-dominant visual field is not reported by the patient, as the language-dominant hemisphere has no access to the information. The nondominant hand no longer responds reliably to verbal commands, because the dominant hemisphere may not readily transfer information to the nondominant motor cortex (Kim et al., 2004; Reeves & Roberts, 1995). Most patients are unaware of the deficit (Kim et al., 2004). Transient postoperative apathy is sometimes observed and is probably related to mesial and convexity frontal lobe disconnections. The symptoms usually diminish with time, but are permanent to some extent and may fluctuate over the years. There remains debate over the extent of callosal damage necessary to produce disconnection syndrome (Geschwind, 1995). It typically appears in the setting of a complete disconnection (callosotomy), but we have rarely observed it after an anterior callosal section as well. It is quite unlikely to occur in patients with significant unilateral cerebral injury, for example, porencephaly, prior to surgery.

4.3.2 Overall daily function and behavioral consequences

In recent years, the implications of corpus callosotomy on the cognitive status of epilepsy patients have been emphasized. In one study, overall daily function, as assessed by families, improved in 62% of patients. Changes included improvement in hyperactivity (93%), emotional well-being (42%), social contacts (36%), speech function (21%), and memory function (17%) (Maehara & Shimizu, 2001). In another study, nearly three-fourths of the parents appreciated improvements in behavior and attentiveness of their children (Turanli et al., 2006). Activities of daily living including level of self-care, family life, and even school attendance may improve significantly (Turanli et al., 2006). Intelligence quotient scores do not usually change significantly after callosotomy. However, in some patients with marked impairment of cognitive and language functions in whom a favorable seizure outcome has been achieved, an improvement in overall intelligence and language abilities has been observed (Maehara & Shimizu, 2001; Turanli et al., 2006; Rathore et al., 2007). This improvement is probably due to the decrease in seizure frequency or consequent decrease in antiepileptic drug load, or both. In one study, a close relationship was observed between improvement in quality of life and seizure relief regardless of the age and operation and psychological status (Rougier et al., 1997). Improvement in quality of life is more common in children (>70%) than in adults (>45%). One possible explanation for the better functional outcome in children is that a child's brain is more flexible and has better compensatory mechanisms to make up for the disconnected corpus callosum (Maehara & Shimizu, 2001). No association has been found between the extent of callosotomy and changes in Intelligence Quotient score or neuropsychological outcome in one study (Mamelak et al., 1993).

4.3.3 Patient selection

Corpus callosotomy is a palliative procedure for patients with medically un- controllable seizures not amenable to focal resection. Clinically, ictal EEG with bilateral synchronization has been associated with good outcome in some studies. In one study, ictal EEG was important as a predictive factor for outcome after callosotomy. The patterns with generalized slow spike-wave, electrodecrement, or nonevolving low-amplitude fast activity were associated with absence seizures, tonic and atonic seizures, or axial spasms, all of which can cause drop attacks. Patients with these patterns demonstrated a marked reduction in seizure frequency, and 10 of 11 (91%) demonstrated a 90% or greater decrease in their seizure frequency. The ictal EEG can efficiently identify patients with drop attacks who have a likelihood of good outcome after callosotomy (Hanson et al., 2002).

Most epilepsy patients, especially in children, have light or seriously lower Intelligence Quotient score. Although this is not the surgery contraindication, it exerts important implication on the outcome of patients. Rathore (Rathore et al., 2007) reported that those who with serious lower Intelligence Quotient score had a significant improve in cognitive function and social psychological status, in spite of not good control of seizure as expected. Therefore, it is thought that to improve the quality of life of patients after surgery is more important and meaningful, compared to sheer control of seizure attack.

5. Conclusion

Corpus callosotomy is a reasonably safe and effective palliative surgical procedure for some patients with intractable seizures who are not amenable to focal resection. This is a feasible and cost-effective treatment for some patients, even those in developing countries and with limited resources (Asadi-Pooya & Sperling, 2008). New imaging techniques may serve to further understanding of the role of callosal connections in generating and propagating seizures. Other areas for research include development of a reliable prognostic and outcome scoring system, development and evaluation of new techniques for surgery (e.g., gamma knife or endoscopic surgery), better characterization of specific deficits after surgery, and implementation of surgical and medical preventive measures to prevent postoperative complications.

In conclusion, the corpus callosotomy can be viewed as a feasible alternative to the standard surgical procedure in patients with refractory seizures. When physicians, patients, and their families choose a treatment for seizure control, several factors should be considered, including the control of seizure frequency and severity, patient expectations, and relative risk of the procedure.

6. References

Asadi-Pooya AA, Sperling MR. (2008) Strategies for surgical treatment of epilepsies in developing countries. *Epilepsia*, Vol. 49, pp. (381–385).

Bogen JE, Vogel PJ. (1963) Treatment of generalized seizures by cerebral commissar- otomy. *Surg Forum.* Vol. 14, pp. (431–435).

Crowell RM, Ajmone-Marsan C. (1972) Topographical distribution and patterns of unit activity during electrically induced after-discharge. *Electroencephalogr Clin Neurophysio,l* Vol. Suppl 31, pp. (59-73).

Curtis HJ. (1940) Intercortical connections of corpus callosum as indicated by evoked potentials. *J Neurophysio,l* Vol. 3, pp. (407-413).

Dandy WE. (1936) Operative experiences in cases of pineal tumors. *Arch Surg* Vol.33, pp. (19–46).

Engel, JJ. (Ed). (1993). *Surgical treatment of the epilepsies* (2ed). Lippincott Williams & Wilkins, 088167988, Newyork

Erickson TC. (1940) Spread of the epileptic discharge. An experimental study of the after ischarge induced by electrical stimulation of the cerebral cortex. *Arch Neurol Psych,* Vol. 43, pp. (429-452).

Funnell MG, Corballis PM, & Gazzaniga MS. (2000) Cortical and subcortical inter-hemispheric interactions following partial and complete callosotomy. *Arch Neurol* Vol. 57, pp. (185–189).

Geschwind DH, Iacoboni M, Mega MS, et al. (1995) Alien hand syndrome: interhemispheric motor disconnection due to a lesion in the midbody of the corpus callosum. *Neurology,* Vol. 45, pp. (802–808).

Hanson RR, Risinger M, Maxwell R. (2002) The ictal EEG as a predictive factor for outcome following corpus callosum section in adults. *Epilepsy Res,* Vol. 49, pp. (89–97).

Harbaugh RE, Wilson DH, Reeves AG, et al. (1983) Forebrain commissurotomy for epilepsy. Review of 20 consecutive cases. *Acta Neurochir,* Vol. 68, pp. (263–275).

Kim DS, Yang KH, Kim TG, et al. (2004) The surgical effect of callosotomy in the treatment of intractable seizure. *Yonsei Med J,* Vol. 45, pp. (233–240).

Luessen AJ, Dela Cruz TC, Fenichel GM. (1970) Surgical disconnection of the cerebral hemispheres for intractable seizures. Results in infancy and childhood. *JAMA*, Vol. 213, pp. (1630-1636).

Maehara T, Shimizu H. (2001) Surgical outcome of corpus callosotomy in patients with drop attacks. *Epilepsia,* Vol. 42, pp. (67-71).

Mamelak AN, Barbaro NM, Walker JA, et al. (1993) Corpus callosotomy: a quantitative study of the extent of resection, seizure control, and neuropsychological outcome. *J Neurosurg,* Vol. 79, pp. (688–695).

Nei M, O'Connor M, Liporace J, et al. (2006) Refractory generalized seizures: response to corpus callosotomy and vagal nerve stimulation. *Epilepsia,* Vol.47, pp. (115–122).

Rathore C, Abraham M, Rao RM, et al. (2007) Outcome after corpus callosotomy in children with injurious drop attacks and severe mental retardation. *Brain Dev,* Vol.29, pp. (577–585).

Reeves AG, Roberts DW, editors. (1995). *Epilepsy and the corpus callosum 2,* Plenum, 978-0-306-45134-8, New York.

Rossi GF, Colicchio G, Marchese E, et al. (1996) Callosotomy for severe epilepsies with generalized seizures: outcome and prognostic factors. *Acta Neurochir (Wien),* Vol.138, 221–227.

Rougier A, Claverie B, Pedespan JM, et al. (1997) Callosotomy for intractable epilepsy: overall outcome. *J Neurosurg Sci* , Vol. 41, pp. (51–57).

Turanli G, Yalnizoglu D, Genc-Acikgoz D, et al. (2006) Outcome and long term follow-up after corpus callosotomy in childhood onset intractable epilepsy. *Childs Nerv Syst,* Vol. 22, pp. (1322–1327).

Van WP, Herren RY. (1940) Surgical division of commissural pathways in the corpus callosum. Relation to spread of an epileptic attack. *Arch Neurol Psychiatry* Vol.44, pp. (740–759).

Waxman, SG. (2003). *Clinical neuroanatomy* (25th ed), McGraw-Hill, 0071212264, New York.

Wilson DH, Reevesm GM. (1978) Division of the corpus callosum for uncontrollable epilepsy. Neurology, Vol. 28, pp. (649-653).

Wong TT, Kwan SY, & Chang KP, et al. (2006) Corpus callosotomy in children. *Childs Nerv Syst* Vol. 22, pp. (999–1011).

Wyllie, E. (1993). The treatment of epilepsy: principle and practices(2ed), Lea & Febiger, 0-8121-1504-X, Philadelphia.

16

Neuromodulatory Treatment of Medically Refractory Epilepsy

Mark Witcher and Thomas L. Ellis
Wake Forest University School of Medicine, Department of Neurosurgery, Medical Center Blvd., Winston-Salem, USA

1. Introduction

Epilepsy is a common chronic neurologic disorder affecting 0.5 to 1 percent of the population. (Hauser, 1993 4131) More than one-third of all epilepsy patients have incompletely controlled seizures or debilitating medication side effects in spite of optimal medical management. (Kwan et al. 2000; Sillanpaa et al. 2006; Sander et al. 1993) Medically refractory epilepsy is associated with excess injury and mortality, psychosocial dysfunction, and significant cognitive impairment. (Brodie et al. 1996) Treatment options for these patients include new anti-epileptic drugs (AEDs), which may lead to seizure freedom in 7 percent of patients (Fisher et al. 1993) and resective surgery which is associated with long-term seizure freedom in 60-80% of patients.(Engel et al. 2003 ;Lee et al. 2005) Surgery for patients whose epilepsy has proven refractory to AEDs provides a high likelihood of reduction in seizure frequency, is generally safe, and is recommended for selected patients with refractory partial seizures. In spite of improvements in surgical technique, approximately 4 percent of patients will suffer death or permanent neurologic disability (A global survey on epilepsy surgery, 1980-1990: a report by the Commission on Neurosurgery of Epilepsy, the International League Against Epilepsy 1997). Moreover, more than one-third of patients will not be candidates for surgical resection (Kwan et al. 2000). For patients who are not candidates for resective surgery, there are limited options. Neuromodulatory treatment, which consists of administering electrical pulses to neural tissue to modulate its activity leading to a beneficial effect, may be an option for these patients. The interest in neuromodulation for neurological disorders is driven by a desire to discover less invasive surgical treatments, as well as new treatments for patients whose medical conditions remain refractory to existing modalities. Vagal nerve stimulation (VNS) is one example of neuromodulation that was developed in the 1980s, and which is now routinely available. (Ben-Menachem et al. 2002) VNS, as an adjunct to medical management, may yield up to a 50 percent reduction in seizure frequency (A randomized controlled trial of chronic vagus nerve stimulation for treatment of medically intractable seizures. The Vagus Nerve Stimulation Study Group. 1995) although most of these patients will not be seizure-free. Deep brain stimulation (DBS) is another example of neuromodulation. Given the significant experience and success of DBS for movement disorders (Krack et al. 2003) combined with its reversibility, programmability, and low risk of morbidity, there has been a resurgence of interest in using DBS devices for treating medically refractory epilepsy. Responsive neurostimulation is a technology that detects seizure activity at a previously defined focus and applies an electrical stimulus to the site of seizure onset to terminate the seizure. Transcranial magnetic stimulation (TMS) is a nearly 25-year-old technology initially introduced as a means to noninvasively investigate corticospinal circuits. Currently, TMS is used primarily in clinical neurophysiology. Importantly, TMS can be used to evaluate and manipulate excitatory and inhibitory intracortical circuits with post-stimulatory effect, allowing for a developing use in epileptic neuromodulation.

In summary, resective epilepsy surgery is not an ideal option for all patients with medically refractory epilepsy. It is an invasive, irreversible procedure which will not lead to a cure in all patients. It is associated with only modest success in patients with a normal MRI or a diffuse ictal onset zone. It has a significant risk of neurological or neuropsychological decline postoperatively. These factors in combination drive the search for alternative treatment options such as neuromodulation.

2. Vagal nerve stimulation

The vagal nerve has a complex anatomical arrangement which projects to the autonomic and reticular structures and well as limbic and thalamic neurons. Stimulation of the vagus nerve and its bilateral multisynaptic targets has become a common technology for the treatment of epilepsy. To date, over 50,000 patients have been treated with the technology, and current reports indicate an approximate 50% efficacy in seizure reduction, rivaling the efficacy of antiepileptic treatment, and often decreasing dependence on them (Labar et al. 2002). Efficacy has also been shown to increase over time (Vonck et al. 1999). The low side effect profile of vagal nerve stimulation (VNS) has also proven to be advantageous for users. Reported side effects mainly include hoarseness, paresthesias, shortness of breath, headache, and coughing (Morris et al. 1999) . These effects are typically stimulation-related and resolve over time. (Boon et al. 1999) The mechanism of efficacy remains unknown, though certain structures within the brain appear to be affected by VNS. As evidenced by studies using positron-emission technology (PET), the thalamus is consistently affected by VNS stimulation, and bloodflow to the cerebellum and cerebral structures is consistently altered (Ko et al. 1996; Henry et al. 1999; Henry et al. 1998; Ben-Menachem et al. 2002). Thalamic involvement has also been supported through SPECT (Van et al. 2000; Vonck et al. 2000) and functional MRI.(Liu et al. 2003; Narayanan et al. 2002) analysis.

2.1 Animal studies

Studies of VNS have been reported from multiple vertebrate models including rodents (McLachlan et al. 1993), canines(Zabara et al. 1992) and lower primates. (Lockard et al. 1990) In the rodent penicillin/pentylenetetrazol model, interictal spike frequency was reduced by 33%(McLachlan et al. 1993) the effect of which was later found to be greatest in continuous stimulation and reduced in a time-dependent fashion after stimulation. (Takaya et al. 1996) Later tests have shown that cortical excitability in rats can be modulated through VNS.(De et al. 2010) Canine strychnine and pentylenetetrazol models show similar efficacy with lasting reduction in motor seizures and tremors. (Zabara et al. 1992) In the aluminagel monkey model, seizures were eliminated in half of test animals during stimulation periods with some persistence into post-stimulation periods. (Lockard et al. 1990)

2.2 Clinical studies

Clinical trials began in 1988 with the first open trial; preliminary results showed that such a therapy was potentially efficacious and safe with only transient side effects.(Penry et al. 1990) This was followed by a series of clinical trials from 1988 through 1995 which included two double-blind, randomized, controlled studies.(Handforth et al. 1998) Results indicated seizure reduction at both low and high stimulation paradigms, with significantly greater reduction in the high-stimulation group(Handforth et al. 1998) and overall efficacy showed a mean seizure reduction of approximately 35-45%.(Morris et al. 1999) Safety of the therapy was also established in this series of trials, with few patients discontinued secondary to adverse events.(Handforth et al. 1998) Vagal innervation of the larynx produced typical side effects including cough, dyspnea, and local paresthesia, though distal effects on the vagus were not appreciated. (Handforth, et al. 1998) The findings of these trials led to the widespread use of VNS therapy for complex partial and secondary generalized seizures in patients over 12 years of age.(Saillet et al. 2009) Since that time, data from pediatric studies have shown similar outcomes in younger patients.(Wheless et al. 2002)

In 2005, PuLsE: an open, prospective, randomized, parallel group study directly comparing best medical practice with and without adjunctive VNS Therapy was initiated (http://clinicaltrials.gov/ct2/show/NCT01281280). Long-term data were collected on both health outcomes and seizure frequency to determine if a possible significant clinical benefit in health outcomes over time of best medical practice with or without adjunctive VNS Therapy in patients with drug-resistant epilepsy with partial-onset seizures. Due to lower than anticipated enrollment, this study was discontinued in July 2008. The study was inconclusive due to inability to meet the primary objective with appropriate statistical power. However, due to a relatively large number of participants (n=121) randomized in the original PuLsE study, industry decided to implement an observational long-term follow-up of the participants enrolled in the original PuLsE study. This post-market study is designed to identify clinically and statistically significant predictors of response in patients with drug-resistant epilepsy with partial-onset seizures treated with best medical practice with or without adjunctive VNS Therapy. This is a 5-year study set to open in 2011 (http://clinicaltrials.gov/ct2/show/NCT01281280).

3. Transcranial magnetic stimulation

Transcranial magnetic stimulation (TMS) of cortical tissues was initially reported by Barker and colleagues and quickly found acceptance as a research vehicle for neurophysiologists.(Barker et al. 1985) TMS was first applied to the study of the motor system(Barker et al. 1985) and this use has since expanded to include investigations in psychiatric conditions(Pascual-Leone et al. 1996), migraine headache(Lipton et al. 2010) and other neurologic conditions. Importantly, it has also become a viable option for the treatment of drug resistant epilepsy. TMS exerts its effects through repetitive noninvasive stimulation in which a pulsed magnetic field creates current flow in the brain which can temporarily excite or inhibit target areas.(Hallett et al. 2000)

3.1 Animal studies

The basis of TMS as a therapeutic intervention in epilepsy is derived from the lasting effects that from the application of a train of transcranial stimuli. Theoretically, the lasting effects of

TMS can be used to modulate activity in focal areas of cortex.(Fregni et al. 2007) The TMS-induced effect depends on the nature of the stimulation; that is, the frequency, the timing, the focus, and the intensity of the repetitive stimulation. (Kimiskidis et al. 2010) While some paradigms have been studied using animal models, the numbers of basic studies particular to epilepsy are somewhat limited.

Early study within the mouse hippocampal-entorhinal cortex slice model indicated that repetitive direct (i.e., non-transcranial) stimulation at 1 Hz can depress the generation of ictal activity in a 4-aminopyridine model(Barbarosie et al. 1997), which later was shown to have a frequency-dependent effect.(D'Arcangelo, et al. 2005) This frequency dependence has been replicated in TMS. Low-frequency TMS stimulation shows the tendency to lower seizure activity. One study found that in rats, 1000 pulses of low-frequency TMS (0.5 Hz) reduced susceptibility to the induction of status epilepticus and also to increase the latency to onset of pentylenetetrazol-induced seizures.(Akamatsu et al. 2005) A later study indicated that in rats genetically modified as models of absence seizures, TMS could be used at 0.5 Hz to reduce spike wave discharge for a short, albeit statistically insignificant manner with maximal effect at 30 minutes.(Godlevsky et al. 2006) A more recent study suggests that TMS can suppress kainate-induced seizures in rats at frequencies of 0.5 and 0.75Hz though not at 0.25 Hz, demonstrating a frequency dependence on seizure control.(Rotenberg et al. 2008)

On the other hand, higher frequency stimulation has been shown to have confounding effects. Using male Wistar rats, it was shown that in the pentylenetrazole model of clonic seizures, chronic high-frequency stimulation (50Hz) may induce kindling of seizure activity, though this effect was not appreciated with acute-only stimulation.(Jennum et al. 1996) Later work indicated that an acute high-frequency (20 Hz) TMS train significantly increased the threshold for induction of epileptic after-discharges in amygdala-kindled rats, with effects lasting at least 2 weeks, though it was not directly compared with chronic stimulation.(Ebert et al. 1999) High frequency stimulation has been shown therefore to potentially have both protective and inductive effects dependent on the chronicity of treatment and potentially other, unexplored, factors.

3.2 Clinical studies

Similar results have been identified in human studies. High frequency TMS (>5 Hz) has been shown to enhance cortical excitability at high intensities.(Berardelli et al. 1998) Alternatively, low-frequency TMS (i.e. ≤1 Hz), has been shown to reduce cortical excitability, potentially secondary to an increase in the refractory neuronal period(Cincotta et al. 2003) as well as decreased strength of neuronal signaling.(Muellbacher et al. 2000)

As detailed by Kimiskidis (Kimiskidis 2010), the clinical effects are theoretically similar to long term potentiation (LTP) and long-term depression (LTD) elicited by high- and low-frequency electrical stimulation, respectively. It is therefore possible that TMS at lower frequencies may exert its effect through the initiation of LTD, while at higher frequencies, the proconvulsant effect may be initiated through the induction of an LTP-type effect.(Ziemann U. et al. 2005)

Multiple investigations into the effect of low-frequency TMS on multiple seizure types have been reported utilizing variable targeting, frequency, intensities, and train parameters. One of the first open-label pilot trials of this technology demonstrated at least a six-week reduction in the frequency of epileptic events using a frequency of 0.33 Hz (Tergau et al.

1999) Theodore et al. reported a statistically insignificant and short-lived trend towards seizure reduction in a randomized trial of 12 focal epilepsy patients at a frequency of 1 Hz.(Theodore et al. 2002) A later trial involving 17 patients utilizing both frequencies demonstrated seizure reduction at the lower frequency of 0.33 Hz only.(Tergau et al. 2003) TMS applied at a frequency of 0.5 Hz in a single session was associated with an approximate 42% reduction of epileptiform discharges lasting at least 30 days in a population of cortical dysplasia patients in an open-label study.(Fregni et al. 2005) A larger, randomized follow-up trial using a frequency of 1 Hz showed a reduction of seizure activity when compared with the sham group, with effects lasting at least 60 days.(Fregni et al. 2006) In another extratemporal focal epilepsy series, TMS applied at a frequency of 0.9 Hz, demonstrated a favorable though statistically insignificant trend towards seizure reduction.(Kinoshita et al. 2005) Larger randomized trials have indicated encouraging though statistically insignificant decreases in epileptic activity. In a series of 35 patients with focal, nonfocal and multifocal epilepsy, stimulation at vertex and temporal targets at a frequency of 0.5 Hz reduced interictal spikes by greater than 50%, though seizure reduction was non-significant. It should be noted that the trend was toward reduction, and target of TMS was non-influential on the outcome.(Joo et al. 2007) Cantello et al.(Cantello et al. 2007) similarly found an appreciable decrease in interictal epileptiform abnormalities in approximately one-third of a series of 43 patients with mostly focal epilepsy in a randomized double-blind study, though the clinical antiepileptic activity was insignificant

As can be appreciated from these findings, the antiepileptic effects of TMS show somewhat ambiguous results even when accounting for different stimulation paradigms and locations. The efficacy of this technology will therefore need careful scrutiny from the perspective of larger randomized trials and carefully conducted meta-analyses accounting for differences in localization of epilepsy, stimulation paradigms, frequency, target and repetition and potential placebo effects.(Bae et al. 2011) The safety of this therapy may also be of concern, as there have been reports of seizures related to therapy.(Tergau et al. 1999; Bae et al. 2007; Rotenberg et al. 2009) Generally, however, the therapy is considered safe, with common adverse effects including headache (<10%) and mild discomfort.(Bae et al. 2007)

4. Deep brain stimulation (open-loop)

DBS lead implantation within the anterior nucleus of the thalamus (ANT), as well as other central nervous system (CNS) targets - including the caudate nucleus, centromedian nucleus of the thalamus, cerebellum, hippocampus, and subthalamic nucleus - results in seizure reduction in selected patients.(Vercueil et al. 1998; Shandra et al. 1990; Mirski et al. 1986; Bragin et al. 2002) In all of these studies, the stimulation was delivered in an open-loop fashion, that is, in a pre-defined manner, independent of the momentary physiological activity of the brain. The exact mechanism of action of DBS in reducing seizure activity is unknown. It is known that stereotactic lesions of the ANT in humans can result in reduction in seizure frequency. (Mullan et al. 1967) Some evidence suggests that DBS may interfere with synchronized oscillations by neurotransmitter release.(Lee et al. 2005) Other evidence suggests that the most likely mechanism may involve stimulation-induced modulation of pathologic neural networks.(McIntyre et al. 2004) High-frequency DBS appears to reproduce the clinical effect of ablative procedures.(Benabid et al. 1987) Moreover, at high frequencies, DBS may abolish cortical epileptiform activity.(Lado et al. 2003) A microthalamotomy effect has been postulated based on the observation that some patients obtain reduction in seizure frequency prior to activation of the pulse generator.(Lim et al. 2007 ; Andrade et al. 2006)

Although the precise mechanism by which DBS reduces seizure activity is unclear, inhibition of neurons immediately adjacent to the area of applied current is likely involved. A "reversible functional lesion" may be generated in structures integral to initiating or sustaining epileptic activity.(Boon et al. 2007) The applied current may inhibit neurons with a pathologically lowered threshold of activation. Alternatively, DBS may act on neuronal network projections to nearby or remote CNS structures originating from the area of stimulation. This might take place through either activation of inhibitory projections or through the inhibition of excitatory projections.

DBS for movement disorders has met with widespread success (Nguyen et al. 2000; Pollak et al. 2002; Volkmann et al. 2004) and is increasingly being investigated for new indications such as chronic pain, obsessive-compulsive disorders, and even headache. (Gybels et al. 1993; Leone et al. 2005; Leone et al. 2003) While DBS of targets such as the thalamus, cerebellum, and locus ceruleus was performed in the past in patients with psychiatric disorders or spasticity who also had seizures, technical limitations prevented it from becoming an appropriate treatment option for patients with epilepsy alone. (Cooper et al. 1976; Wright et al. 1984; Upton et al. 1985; Feinstein et al. 1989) A renewed interest in DBS for epilepsy has arisen from success with the technique in movement disorders, along with technological improvements in the equipment. Multiple epilepsy centers throughout the world have performed trials over the years using DBS for epilepsy, targeting a variety of CNS structures. (Fisher et al. 1992; Velasco et al. 1995; Chkhenkeli et al. 1997; Chabardes et al. 2002; Hodaie et al. 2002; Velasco et al. 2005) These trials can be summarized based on two different strategies.

One strategy is to target CNS structures believed to have a "gating" role in the epileptogenic network, such as the subthalamic nucleus or thalamus.(Iadarola et al. 1982) The other strategy is to target the ictal onset zone with the theory that stimulation may lead to interference with seizure initiation. The latter strategy might ideally be used in patients with mesial temporal lobe (MTL) epilepsy given the success in reducing seizures in patients after anterior temporal lobectomy. (Engel et al. 2003) MTL epilepsy is the most common form of medically refractory partial epilepsy. These patients have a long-term freedom from seizure rate of 60 to 75 percent after undergoing temporal lobectomy. In spite of undergoing satisfactory preoperative Wada testing, however, many of these patients will demonstrate a verbal memory deficit on postoperative neuropsychological evaluation. (Helmstaedter et al. 2003; Gleissner et al. 2004) Given that some of these patients must undergo implantation of electrodes prior to considering resection, they may be ideal candidates for using DBS with the same electrodes used for diagnostic purposes.

4.1 Animal studies at various anatomic sites

Numerous animal models have been used to elucidate DBS mechanism of action and its potential usefulness in the treatment of epilepsy.(Ziai et al. 2005; Wyckhuys et al. 2007; Usui et al. 2005; Shi et al. 2006; Nishida et al. 2007; Lian et al. 2003; Jensen et al. 2007) Animal epilepsy models have utilized pentylenetetrazol (PTZ), kainic acid (KA), bicuculline (BIC), picrotoxin, and kindling to induce seizures.(Ziai et al. 2005; Usui et al. 2005; Shi et al. 2006; Nishida et al. 2007; Lian et al. 2003; Jensen et al. 2007; Mirski et al. 1986) Sinusoidal alternating current (AC) versus direct current (DC) stimulation protocols, synaptic versus non-synaptic inhibition, regional alterations in neurochemistry, and differing anatomic targets are among many variables investigated in these models.(Ziai et al. 2005; Nishida et al. 2007; Lian et al. 2003; Jensen et al. 2007)

4.1.1 Cerebellum

Cooke and Snider(Cooke et al. 1955) demonstrated that cerebellar stimulation (CS) can modify or abruptly terminate seizure activity in various cerebral areas. Iwata and Snider (IWATA et al. 1959) observed that CS could terminate hippocampal seizures and prolonged afterdischarges (AD) that had been induced by electrical stimulation. In 1962, Dow et al.(Dow et al. 1962) showed that CS could alter electroencephalogram (EEG) activity and reduce frontal lobe seizures in a model of chronic epilepsy in awake unanesthetized rats. Fanardjian and Donhoffer (Fanardjian & Donhoffer 1964) found CS induced slow waves in the normal hippocampus while activation-like patterns appeared simultaneously in the cerebrum. In 1980, Laxer et al.(Laxer et al. 1980) found inconsistent results when reviewing studies from 22 groups using CS with a wide range of stimulation parameters. They were nonetheless able to draw two conclusions: (a) stimulation of the vermis and superomedial surface is more effective than stimulation of the lateral hemisphere, and (b) CS is most effective in epilepsy of the limbic system, and least effective in models of focal epilepsy of the sensorimotor cortex.

4.1.2 Hippocampus

Lian et al. (Lian et al. 2003) tested the effects of DC stimulation and low-duty cycle AC stimulation (which more closely approximates that used clinically) in a hippocampal slice epilepsy model. They demonstrated that continuous sinusoidal, 50% duty-cycle sinusoidal, and 1.68% duty-cycle pulsed stimulation (120μsec, 140Hz) all suppressed low-Ca^{2+} epileptiform activity. Continuous sinusoidal stimulation was also found to completely suppress picrotoxin-induced epileptiform activity. AC stimulation resulted in an increase in extracellular potassium concentration and neuronal depolarization blockade, and was not found to be slice orientation-selective. DC stimulation by contrast, suppressed epileptiform activity only in the region surrounding the electrode, and did so by membrane hyperpolarization.

Jensen and Durand (Jensen & Durand 2007) recently demonstrated that in vitro sinusoidal high frequency stimulation of rat hippocampal slices suppresses axonal conduction. Stimulation was found to suppress the alvear compound action potential as well as the antidromic evoked potential. The stimulation frequency at which maximal suppression occurred was between 50 and 200 Hz, similar to that observed in most clinical DBS studies. The degree of suppression of axonal conduction correlated with a rise in extracellular potassium demonstrating that stimulation may block axonal activity through non-synaptic mechanisms.

4.1.3 STN and SNr

DBS of the substantia nigra pars reticulata (SNr) completely blocked amygdala-kindled seizures in 10 of 23 (43.5%) rats studied by Shi (Shi 2006). Microwire electrodes were implanted into the SNr and amygdala of adult male rats. Seizures were produced by daily amygdala kindling, and DBS was delivered to the SNr bilaterally 1 sec after kindling stopped. When the same amygdala kindling procedure was performed 24h later without

DBS, the kindling failed to elicit any seizures in 6 of the 10 rats. In 3 animals, only mild seizures appeared following amygdala kindling. Only 1 of the 10 responders exhibited stage 5-kindled seizures 24h after DBS was discontinued. In 9 of the 10 responders, the period of seizure suppression or reduction lasted for up to 4 days. The authors concluded that highly plastic neural networks may be involved in amygdala-kindled seizures and that DBS may exert long lasting effects on these networks.
In contrast, when Usui et al. (Usui et al. 2005) tested SNr DBS in rats with KA induced seizures they found no treatment effect. They compared one group of rats with a unilateral SNr electrode to a second group with a unilateral subthalamic nucleus (STN) electrode. A control group received no electrodes. KA was systemically administered to all three groups to induce limbic seizures, and DBS of the STN or SNr was begun immediately afterward. EEG changes and the magnitude of clinical seizures were then evaluated. They demonstrated that unilateral STN stimulation significantly reduced the duration of generalized seizures on EEG. Interestingly, the duration of focal seizures on EEG was prolonged by STN DBS, a result felt possibly due to the suppression of secondary generalization. In addition, STN DBS reduced the severity of clinical seizures. The group receiving SNr DBS demonstrated no significant effect when compared to the controls. They concluded that unilateral STN DBS suppresses secondary generalization of limbic seizures. The failure of SNr DBS to reduce secondary generalization was felt to imply that, while nigral influence on seizure propagation may be important, other antiepileptic mechanisms such as antidromic stimulation of the corticosubthalamic pathway may also be involved.

4.1.4 Anterior nucleus of the thalamus

The hypothesis that the ANT participates in the propagation of some forms of seizures is supported by experimental animal studies. Low frequency (8Hz) stimulation of the ANT has been found to be epileptogenic (Lado et al. 2003). Seizures can be induced in guinea pigs by microinjection of KA, BIC, or PTZ into the ANT. (Mirski et al. 1986) Hamani et al.(Hamani et al. 2004) discovered that bilateral, high frequency ANT DBS delays the onset of status epilepticus (SE) after exposure to pilocarpine. In their study, adult Wistar rats underwent unilateral or bilateral ANT lesioning, or unilateral or bilateral ANT DBS electrode placement. The control group received bilateral ANT electrodes but no stimulation. Seven days later, the animals were given pilocarpine, after which EEG recordings and ictal behavior were evaluated. In the control group, 67% of the animals developed SE with a latency of 15.3 +/- 8.8 minutes after pilocarpine administration. Neither unilateral ANT lesions nor unilateral ANT DBS significantly reduced the likelihood or latency of SE. Bilateral ANT DBS did not prevent SE (observed in 56% of the animals), but did significantly prolong the latency to 48.4 +/- 17.7 min ($p = 0.02$). Interestingly, no animals with bilateral ANT lesions developed SE with pilocarpine.

4.2 DBS clinical studies at various anatomic sites

4.2.1 Cerebellum

Cooper et al. (Cooper et al. 1976) were the first to report on CS for epilepsy, and observed that 10 of the 15 patients in the trial experienced a reduction in seizure frequency of ≥50% when followed up to 3 years. Stimulation of the anterior lobe appeared to be more effective than that of the posterior lobe. Cerebellar biopsies, obtained in five patients at the time of lead placement, revealed a reduction in the molecular layer, decreased or absent Purkinje cells, and decreased stellate cells. One patient, who failed to respond to stimulation, died as a result of a seizure 17 months after implantation. Davis and Emmonds(Davis, 1992 4120) subsequently discovered that 23 of 27 evaluable patients who underwent long-term (average follow-up 14.3 years) CS had an overall reduction in seizure frequency. Interestingly, 12 of the patients had a non-functioning stimulator at the time of the report and yet 5 were found to be seizure-free, while 7 had experienced a reduction in seizure frequency.

Wright et al. (Wright et al. 1984) examined twelve patients with severe, intractable epilepsy who underwent CS under double-blind conditions for six months. The trial was divided into three phases, each lasting two months. Patients received two months of continuous stimulation (alternating from one cerebellar hemisphere to the other every minute), two months of contingent stimulation (during which both hemispheres were stimulated only while a button was depressed by the patient or family member), and two months of no stimulation. The sequence of phases was randomly assigned and the patients, family members, and evaluators were blinded to each epoch. No reduction in seizure frequency occurred that could be attributed to stimulation. However, most patients reported a reduction in the duration and severity of seizures although these were not measured during the study. Eleven of the patients considered that the trial had helped them and wished to continue "stimulation" at the conclusion of the trial.

Velasco et al. (Velasco et al. 2005), in a more recent double-blind trial with two years of follow-up in five patients undergoing CS, demonstrated improvement in seizure control. Beginning one month after implantation and for a period of 3 months, 3 patients were assigned randomly to receive stimulation while 2 others had their stimulators left OFF. After the fourth month, all patients were then ON stimulation for the next 6 months. During the 3-month double-blind phase, the two patients with stimulation OFF demonstrated no difference in mean seizure rate compared to baseline. During the same phase, the 3 patients with stimulation ON demonstrated a reduction in seizure rate to 33% of baseline. At the end of the subsequent 6 months, all five patients had a mean seizure rate of 41%(range 14-75%) of baseline. The improvement in generalized tonic-clonic seizures occurred earlier and to a greater degree than that for tonic seizures.

It is likely that CS results in the activation of Purkinje cells which exert inhibitory output on the deep cerebellar nuclei. CS likely reduces excitatory cerebellar output from these nuclei to the thalamus, leading to a reduction in output from excitatory thalamocortical projections, and thus inhibition of cortical activity. (Molnar et al. 2004)

4.2.2 Hippocampus

Evidence strongly suggests that the hippocampus is involved in the initiation and propagation of temporal lobe seizures. (Swanson et al. 1995; Sperling et al. 1992) Velasco et al. (Velasco et al. 2000) demonstrated that hippocampal stimulation using electrode grids or depth electrodes significantly reduced interictal spikes and abolished complex partial and secondarily generalized tonic-clonic seizures in 7 of 10 patients with intractable temporal lobe epilepsy. The same group, in a subsequent study, observed that chronic hippocampal stimulation in three patients reduced seizure activity without affecting short-term memory. (Velasco et al. 2001)

Vonck et al. (Vonck et al. 2002) conducted an open label trial involving three patients with complex partial seizures who underwent DBS of the amygdalohippocampal region. Two DBS electrodes were implanted in each hemisphere through two occipital burr holes. This procedure was performed on the same day as placement of subdural grids and strips. The most anterior electrode on each side was placed in the amygdala. The second electrode was placed more posteriorly in the anterior part of the hippocampus on each side. AEDs were gradually tapered until seizures were observed. During a trial phase, stimulation was applied to both the amygdalar and hippocampal electrodes. The frequency was set to 130Hz and pulse width to 450μsec. Seizure frequency during the chronic stimulation condition was then compared with the mean monthly seizure frequency recorded 6 months before DBS placement. At a mean follow-up of 5 months (range, 3-6 months), all three patients had a greater than 50% reduction in seizure frequency. In two of the patients, AEDs were tapered. No side effects of stimulation were noted by the patients.

4.2.3 Centromedian nucleus of the thalamus (CMT)

The CMT arises from the diencephalon and brain stem, projecting diffusely to the cerebral cortex as part of the ascending subcortical system. The CMT may play a role in the pathophysiology and propagation of seizures. (Velasco et al. 2000) DBS of the CMT may result in hyperpolarization and desynchronization of the ascending reticular and cortical neurons. (Velasco et al. 2000)

Fisher et al. (Fisher et al. 1992) implanted programmable stimulators into CMT bilaterally in 7 patients with intractable epilepsy to test feasibility and safety. Stimulation was ON or OFF in 3-month blocks, with a 3-month washout period in a double-blind, cross-over protocol. The stimulation was delivered as 90 μsec pulses at 65 pulses/sec, 1 min. of each 5 min. for 2 hours/day. They noted a mean reduction of tonic-clonic seizure frequency of 30% with respect to baseline when the stimulator was ON compared to a decrease of 8% when the stimulator was OFF. Stimulation at low intensity produced no changes in the EEG, but high-intensity stimulation induced slow waves or 2-3 Hz spike-waves with ipsilateral frontal maximum. When the stimulator trains were continued for 24 hours/day, 3 of 6 patients reported at least a 50% decrease in seizure frequency. There were no side effects reported.

A recent trial of CMT DBS in 13 patients with Lennox-Gastaut Syndrome (LGS) revealed an overall seizure reduction rate of 80 percent, and significant gains in quality of life. (Velasco et al. 2006) LGS is one of the most severe forms of childhood epilepsy characterized by drug-resistant generalized seizures in conjunction with mental deterioration. The overall prognosis is very poor with 90% of patients being mentally retarded and 80% continuing seizures into adulthood. The 13 patients implanted in this study tolerated the procedure well, although two had to be explanted due to multiple repeated erosions through the skin. Three patients experienced no improvement in their ability scale score due to persistent seizures. Two patients became seizure-free during the 18 month follow-up, while 8 experienced progressive improvement (5 of the 8 became completely independent).

4.2.4 Subthalamic nucleus

The abundant experience of STN DBS for treating patients with Parkinson's disease makes STN a familiar and attractive target (Halpern et al. 2007). The substantia nigra pars reticulata (SNr) appears to be involved in propagation of seizures through GABAergic projections to the superior colliculus (Gale et al. 1986). It is recognized that STN outputs produce excitatory influence over the SNr system, and that electrical or pharmacologic inhibition of the STN in rats can result in seizure suppression. (Vercueil et al. 1998)

High frequency bilateral STN DBS in a child with cortical dysplasia and inoperable epilepsy resulted in an 83 percent improvement in seizure frequency at 30 months, reduction in seizure severity, and a recovery of motor function. (Benabid et al. 2001) In the same report, Benabid noted a 50% reduction in seizures in one patient with severe myoclonic epilepsy undergoing bilateral STN DBS.

Loddenkemper et al. (Loddenkemper et al. 2001) reported on five patients undergoing STN DBS implantation for pharmacologically intractable seizures. The patients underwent constant stimulation at a frequency of 100Hz, and stimulus duration of 60 μsec. In 2 of the 5 patients, an 80% reduction of seizures was noted after 10 months and 60% reduction at 16 months. They hypothesized that the dorsal midbrain anticonvulsant zone in the superior colliculus is under inhibitory control of efferents from the SNr. In this model, inhibition of the STN is believed to reduce the inhibitory effect of the SNr on the dorsal midbrain anticonvulsant zone, thereby raising the seizure threshold.

Chabardes et al. (Chabardes et al. 2002), in an open label study of STN DBS, implanted 5 patients with medically intractable seizures who were considered unsuitable for resective surgery. A 67-80% reduction in seizure frequency was noted in 3 of the 5 patients. A fourth patient with severe myclonic epilepsy (Dravet syndrome) had a less impressive reduction. The fifth patient, who showed no improvement with the treatment, suffered from an autosomal dominant form of frontal lobe epilepsy.

More recently, Handforth et al. (Handforth et al. 2006) reported their results in two patients with refractory partial onset seizures who were treated with bilateral STN DBS. In one patient, seizure frequency was reduced by one-third, and the patient's quality of life was improved as a result of milder, less harmful seizures. The other patient continued to have seizure-related injuries in spite of a 50% reduction in seizure frequency. To better understand the potential of STN DBS as a treatment for medically refractory epilepsy, more trials will be necessary.

4.2.5 Caudate nucleus

The caudate loop is a functional unit made up of the neocortex, thalamus, and head of the caudate nucleus (HCN) (Heuser et al. 1961). Chkhenkeli et al. (Chkhenkeli et al 2004) examined 57 patients with test stimulation of the HCN, 17 of whom went on to have implantation of a neurostimulator for therapeutic purposes. They discovered that short duration, high frequency (2-5s, 30-100Hz) stimulation of the dorsal and ventral HCN produced enhancement of epilieptiform spike and/or sharp wave activity. By contrast, low frequency (4 to 8Hz) stimulation of similar duration reduced the frequency of sharp transients in the interictal epileptic activity and truncated epileptic discharges from the temporal neocortex. Overall, 14 of 17 patients experienced a reduction in seizure frequency. They postulated that activation of the head of the CN results in hyperpolarization of cortical neurons, and that stimulation-induced inhibition can theoretically suppress seizure activity.

4.2.6 Anterior nucleus of the thalamus (ANT)

Low frequency (8Hz) stimulation of the ANT has been found to be epileptogenic.(Lado et al. 2003) Seizures can be induced in guinea pigs by microinjection of the excitatory agents KA, BIC, or PTZ into the ANT. (Mirski et al. 1986) Placement of DBS electrodes bilaterally into ANT delays the onset of status epilepticus after exposure to pilocarpine. (Hamani et al. 2004) Given the absence of anticonvulsant effect noted in numerous studies, as well as the proconvulsant effects noted in others, the efficacy of chronic ANT DBS for epilepsy in animal studies remains incompletely defined. (Hamani et al. 2004; Lado et al. 2006)

Upton et al. (Upton et al. 1987) treated six patients (five male, one female, mean age 23.7 years) with debilitating, medically refractory seizures by pulsed electrical stimulation of the ANT. In four of the six patients, statistically significant reduction in seizure frequency was obtained. In two of the six patients, they observed changes in regional cerebral glucose metabolism, serum levels of AEDs, and serum cortisol levels ON and OFF stimulation. They concluded that stimulation of the ANT produces not only clinical and electroencephalographic changes, but also changes in cerebral metabolic, endocrinologic and pharmacokinetic responses.

Recently, Osorio et al. (Osorio et al. 2007) reported on the safety and efficacy of high frequency ANT stimulation in patients with inoperable MTL epilepsy. Four patients underwent bilateral implantation of DBS leads in the ANT, followed six weeks later by generator implantation. The mean stimulation parameters were: 175 Hz, 4.1V, pulse width of 90*μsec*. The stimulation was intermittent with one minute ON and five minutes OFF. The efficacy of stimulation was evaluated by comparing seizure frequency during a 36-month treatment period to a 6-month baseline obtained prior to implantation. They noted a mean reduction in seizure frequency of 75.6% (range 53-92%). Quality of life indices improved in all four subjects, and there were no serious adverse events reported. They concluded that high frequency intermittent thalamic stimulation is safe and efficacious for inoperable MTL.

Lee et al. (Lee et al. 2006) reported on six patients with medically refractory, surgically inoperable epilepsy who were implanted with DBS electrodes (three in ATN, three in STN). Seizure frequency and severity were observed and compared to baseline. The stimulators were turned ON one week after insertion of the electrodes. The patients undergoing implantation within ANT experienced a 75.4% reduction in seizure frequency, while those with STN electrodes had their seizure frequency reduced by 49.1%.

Long-term follow-up was reported by Lim et al. (Lim et al. 2007) in four patients who underwent bilateral DBS implantation within the ANT. Initial stimulation parameters were 90-110Hz, 4-5V, and 60-90μsec. For each patient, seizure frequency at baseline and after implantation was analyzed. An average reduction in seizure frequency of 67% (range 44-94%), was noted during the sham interval. Once the stimulators were turned ON, a 49% (range 35-76%) reduction in seizure frequency was noted over the subsequent follow-up period (mean 43.8 months, range 33-48 months). One patient inadvertently had the stimulator turned OFF from months 7-12, during which the seizure frequency increased compared to baseline. No significant difference in seizure frequency was noted between the cycling and continuous stimulation intervals. One patient was seizure-free on medication for 15 months after implantation. No permanent neurological morbidity was observed. While a reduction in seizure frequency was noted during this study, the authors could not demonstrate whether a lesioning effect, subsequent stimulation, or changes in AEDs had the greatest impact.

Hodaie et al. (Hodaie et al. 2002) implanted bilateral DBS electrodes in the ANT of five patients with medically refractory epilepsy who were not eligible for resective surgery. The stimulators were then turned ON 4 weeks after implantation. Stimulation parameters were: 100Hz, 10V, 90μsec pulse width, cycling one minute ON and five minutes OFF, alternating left and right sides. AEDs were unchanged for the duration of the study. For each of the patients, pre- and post-operative seizure rates were evaluated using a one-way analysis of variance (ANOVA; F test). The average follow-up time was 14.9 months (range 10.6-20.7

months). The seizure reduction rate ranged between 24 and 89% (mean 53.8%, $p<0.05$). Two of the patients had >75% reduction in seizure frequency. They noted that merely inserting the electrodes resulted in reduced seizure frequency, and that turning the stimulator ON at 4 weeks yielded no additional reduction. After an interval of continuous stimulation ranging from 7-17 months, each of the patients had their stimulators turned OFF in a blinded fashion for 2 months. Seizure rates were then compared between these ON and OFF intervals. No significant difference in the rate of seizure reduction was observed between the two intervals. The only adverse surgical event was erosion of the skin over the DBS site, requiring wound revision in one patient.

Kerrigan et al. (Kerrigan et al. 2004) conducted an open-label pilot study in 5 patients to investigate the safety and tolerability of bilateral stimulation of the ANT and to investigate the range of appropriate stimulation parameters. Patients enrolled in the study had medically intractable partial seizures and were not candidates for surgical resection. Four of the five patients also had secondarily generalized seizures. After completing implantation, long-term ANT stimulation was then performed intermittently, with the stimulator on each side programmed to produce 1 min of stimulation every 10 min. Stimulation on each side was offset by 5 min. Stimulation parameters were: frequency of 100 Hz, pulse width of 90μsec and intensity of 1-10V. The voltage was incrementally increased over a period of 12-30 weeks, depending on the clinical response of each patient. Seizure counts were monitored through the use of daily diaries and were compared to baseline. AEDs were unchanged during the first 3 months of stimulation, but were adjusted thereafter. The baseline average monthly seizure frequency across all five patients was 46.8 +/- 26.4 (mean +/- SD). During the 12-month treatment period of high-frequency stimulation, the average monthly seizure frequency for the group dropped to 25.0 +/- 11.5 (mean +/- SD), although this was not a statistically significant difference. Only one subject had a statistically significant ($p < 0.05$) reduction in overall seizure frequency. However, 4 of the 5 patients demonstrated reduction in the incidence of injurious seizures to <50% of their baseline incidence.

Andrade et al. (Andrade et al. 2006) reported the long-term follow-up of 6 patients who underwent bilateral ANT DBS for epilepsy. Three patients had generalized epilepsy with tonic-clonic seizures while the other three had multi-focal/partial epilepsy with secondarily generalized seizures. Programming was initiated 1 month after insertion of electrodes. AEDs were not changed for the two years of follow-up. Stimulation parameters were: frequency of 100-185Hz, intensity of 1-10V, and pulse duration of 90-120μsec. The first five patients implanted underwent a 2-month, single-blind period of sham stimulation, during which the generator was OFF. Implantation of the DBS electrodes resulted in statistically significant reduction in seizure frequency in all six patients. Five of the patients had a 50% or greater reduction, although two of the patients received no benefit until years 5 and 6, and only after changes in AEDs. Changes made to stimulation parameters could not be correlated with success in seizure control. Moreover, during the single-blind, 2-month period of stimulation OFF, there was no difference in seizure rates. The only adverse event was a 4-day period of lethargy in one of the patients. Otherwise, even at maximum voltage, the patients were not able to tell if their stimulators were ON or OFF.

5. Responsive neurostimulation (closed-loop)

In contrast to open-loop stimulation, contingent or closed-loop stimulation is designed to suppress epileptiform activity by stimulating a target directly in response to abnormal EEG activity. This form of closed-loop, responsive brain stimulation, is currently available in a clinical setting in the form of the RNS system by Neuropace (Mountain View, CA). It is currently being evaluated in a multi-center, double-blinded, randomized trial to assess the safety and efficacy.

5.1 Animal studies

In 1983, Psatta first examined the effects of low-frequency (5 hz) feedback caudate nucleus stimulation on the interictal spiking activity of epileptic foci detected in adult cats.(Psatta et al. 1983) Spike depression was found to occur immediately after the onset of feedback stimulation and became stable after 3-4 days. Similar effects were not observed when the caudate nucleus was stimulated randomly, nor as a result of contingent stimulation of other subcortical structures. He hypothesized the existence of a recurrent inhibitor caudate-cortical loop as the anatomic mechanism for the normalization of cortical excitability.

In 1991 Nakagawa and Durand presented the effects of applied current on spontaneous epileptiform activity in the CA1 region of the rat hippocampus.(Nakagawa & Durand 1991) A computer-controlled system was used to detect spontaneous, abnormal EEG activity in a slice model using elevated potassium artificial CSF. The system, in response to the abnormal EEG activity, delivered electrical currents (average 12.5 microA) to the stratum pyramidale which suppressed interictal bursts in 90% of the slices. Using intracellular recordings, they determined that the currents induced hyperpolarization of the somatic membrane, thereby inhibiting neuronal firing.

In 1998, Kayyali and Durand reported their results from recordings of the CA1 region in a rat hippocampal slice model in which low-Ca2+ artificial CSF was used to induce spontaneous epileptiform events.(Kayyali, & Durand 1991) Activity was recorded with a glass pipette electrode and voltage threshold detector, after which current (average 3.8 microA) was injected in the stratum pyramidale via a tungsten electrode placed 150 microns from the recording site. They observed a complete suppression of epileptiform events by subthreshold anodic current pulses that in some cases were shorter in duration than the event itself.

5.2 Clinical studies

The first clinical experiments demonstrating the application of responsive stimulation were trials conducted on patients undergoing invasive monitoring and stimulation mapping to localize seizure onset prior to a planned epilepsy surgery. In stimulation mapping, electrical pulses are applied at increasing amplitudes until a clinical alteration or after-discharge is evoked. Lesser et al. reported that short duration (0.3-2 s) pulses were more effective than longer duration (4-5 s for typical stimulation mapping) pulses in reducing after-discharges.(Lesser et al. 1999) Specifically, they noted that for a every 1-s increase in stimulation duration, there was a 40% reduction in eliminating after-discharges. In a related report, Motamedi et al. (Motamedi et al. 2002) demonstrated that stimulation pulses were more effective in eliminating after-discharges if applied early.

Although after-discharges are similar in morphology to spontaneous discharges and can evolve into seizures, they are not the same as spontaneous epileptiform activity. Delivering a stimulation in response to spontaneous epileptiform activity requires an integrated system that analyzes the EEG in real-time and automatically produces pulses in response to a detected event. Peters et al. described such a system in 2001 consisting of a combination of custom-written software and commercially available hardware and software.(Peters et al. 2001) The custom-written software included a unique detection algorithm to detect events early and nearly in real time.(Osorio et al. 1998) Using this system, the authors were able to detect electrographic seizure onset with a latency of approximately 4-12 seconds, noting that in most of their patients the clinical onset was multiple tens of seconds later. (Osorio et al. 2002; Osorio et al. 2005) This system was evaluated in a trial of eight patients. In four of these patients, the stimulation was automatically delivered to the ANT, while the other four had responsive stimulation administered into the epileptogenic zone. The authors observed three of four responders (>50% seizure reduction) in the group with direct stimulation of the epileptogenic zone, and two of four responders in the patients receiving stimulation to the ANT.

Kossoff et al. reported on four patients treated with responsive stimulation while implanted with electrodes for purposes of localization.(Kossoff et al. 2004) This open trial evaluated clinical and EEG responses to stimulation from an external device that detected electrographic seizures and delivered preprogrammed stimulation. In all four patients responsive stimulation appeared to be safe and well tolerated, although two patients experienced sensations in the face and tongue. While the study was designed to evaluate efficacy, stimulation appeared to reduce the number of clinical and electrographic seizures.

5.3 The neuropace RNS system

Success with external responsive neurostimulators in the prior animal and clinical studies led to the development of the first implantable system for epilepsy, the RNS system by Neuropace. This device is capable of performing real-time seizure detection and applying responsive electrical stimulation to abort seizures. The device is made up of intracranial depth and strip leads and an implanted neurostimulator. The system is controlled by a microprocessor, powered by a battery, and continuously monitors electrographic activity from the leads, applying preprogrammed stimulation in response to detected events. Because the system has two leads (each with four electrode contacts) , it can monitor and deliver responsive neurostimulation to two different epileptogenic regions simultaneously.

In addition to the implantable hardware, the system includes a patient data transmitter, a physician programming device, and a telemetry wand. The transmitter allows the patient to upload data between visits to allow remote monitoring. The programmer is utilized by the physician to retrieve stored information from the neurostimulator, and to program detection and stimulation settings. The telemetry wand provides wireless communication between the neurostimulator and the programmer. The system and patient data can be uploaded to a central patient data management system via the web allowing the physician to monitor the patient remotely.

The stimulator delivers constant-current, biphasic, charge-balanced pulses upon detection of an seizure. The detection tools can be adjusted by the physician to optimize the trade-off between sensitivity and specificity for a given patient. Two detectors can be independently programmed for either of the two sensing channels. The device can be programmed by the physician to deliver stimulation frequencies ranging from 1-333 Hz, pulse widths from 40 to 1000 mic sec, and current amplitudes from 1-12 mA. Stimulation can be configured to apply current between any combination of electrodes and the device case. Parameters for stimulation are empirically determined, although the system is designed to limit current density to less than 25 micC/cm^2 per phase. In addition, programming options include bipolar stimulation across electrode pairs or stimulating across all eight electrodes to the case.

Experience with the RNS system includes a feasibility study of 65 patients which revealed excellent safety and tolerability and preliminary evidence of efficacy.(Sun et al. 2008) An interim analysis of 39 of the subjects revealed no serious device-related unanticipated adverse events. In the first 24 patients who had complete data, the responder rate (>50% reduction in seizures) was 43% for complex partial seizures and 35% for simple partial, complex partial or secondarily generalized tonic-clonic seizures. At the time of this writing, a double-blinded, randomized, multicenter clinical trial is underway to determine whether the RNS System is safe and effective as an adjunctive treatment for medically refractory partial-onset seizures.

6. Conclusion

In spite of optimal medical management, many patients with epilepsy remain medically refractory and suffer from debilitating seizures. Many of the medically refractory patients are not candidates for surgery because of the inability to localize a resectable focus. Some of these patients may benefit from neuromodulatory treatment. A variety of targets may be suitable for implantation and no current studies exist to favor one target over another, or even one modality over another. Additional studies are needed to identify the appropriate patient population for neuromodulation, the optimal target, the best stimulation modality, and the best stimulation parameters within that modality. It may be that a complex pathologic entity as heterogeneous as epilepsy cannot be addressed via a single target or even technology. Differences in stimulation parameters within the same anatomic target make it difficult to compare the available animal and clinical studies, perhaps raising more questions than have been answered. Is unilateral DBS sufficient or is bilateral stimulation necessary to prevent seizures? What is the ideal voltage, current, and frequency of stimulation that results in suppression of seizures while minimizing damage to the underlying tissue? What is the ideal waveform? Is the most effective stimulation paradigm continuous or intermittent? If intermittent, should the stimulus be at regular intervals or closed-loop, contingent upon detection of a seizure? If the stimulus needs to be bilateral and intermittent at regular intervals, should it alternate from side to side? If so, how often? Further studies are needed to determine whether open-loop or closed loop stimulation paradigms are more effective. Ultimately, the two methods may be found to be complementary and used in differing populations of patients. It is conceivable that they may even be combined within the same patient: open-loop stimulation for seizure prophylaxis and closed-loop stimulation for acute seizure interruption. The appearance of a lesioning effect arising in some studies but not others is problematic, making it difficult to compare ON and OFF intervals. This must be resolved before DBS can be embraced as a treatment option for epilepsy.

Advanced diagnostics, including magnetoencephalography and modern functional imaging, are likely to play an increasing role in determining appropriate treatment targets. Although it has already met with some success in the clinical arena, the successful future of DBS for the treatment of refractory epilepsy is contingent on the continued collaboration of clinician and scientist. Our technical capabilities have grown at a rate that may well have surpassed our understanding of the complex neurobiology that we aim to modulate. A greater knowledge of what local electrical and neurochemical alterations have led to success in current stimulation models will help ensure reproducibility in those to come. Understanding these relationships may enable future technologies, perhaps even nanotechnologies, to flourish in the developing field of therapeutic neuromodulation.

7. References

A randomized controlled trial of chronic vagus nerve stimulation for treatment of medically intractable seizures. The Vagus Nerve Stimulation Study Group. *Neurology 45*:224-230, 1995

A global survey on epilepsy surgery, 1980-1990: a report by the Commission on Neurosurgery of Epilepsy, the International League Against Epilepsy. *Epilepsia 38*:249-255, 1997

kamatsu N: [Newer treatment of epilepsy--brain pacemakers and transcranial magnetic stimulation]. *Rinsho Shinkeigaku 45*:928-930, 2005

Andrade DM, Zumsteg D, Hamani C, et al: Long-term follow-up of patients with thalamic deep brain stimulation for epilepsy. *Neurology 66*:1571-1573, 2006

Bae EH, Schrader LM, Machii K, et al: Safety and tolerability of repetitive transcranial magnetic stimulation in patients with epilepsy: a review of the literature. *Epilepsy Behav 10*:521-528, 2007

Bae EH, Theodore WH, Fregni F, et al: An estimate of placebo effect of repetitive transcranial magnetic stimulation in epilepsy. *Epilepsy Behav 20*:355-359, 2011

Barbarosie M, Avoli M: CA3-driven hippocampal-entorhinal loop controls rather than sustains in vitro limbic seizures. *J Neurosci 17*:9308-9314, 1997

Barker AT, Jalinous R, Freeston IL: Non-invasive magnetic stimulation of human motor cortex. *Lancet 1*:1106-1107, 1985

Ben-Menachem E: Vagus-nerve stimulation for the treatment of epilepsy. *Lancet Neurol 1*:477-482, 2002

Benabid AL, Koudsie A, Benazzouz A, et al: Deep brain stimulation of the corpus luysi (subthalamic nucleus) and other targets in Parkinson's disease. Extension to new indications such as dystonia and epilepsy. *J Neurol 248 Suppl 3*:III37-III47, 2001

Benabid AL, Pollak P, Louveau A, et al: Combined (thalamotomy and stimulation) stereotactic surgery of the VIM thalamic nucleus for bilateral Parkinson disease. *Appl Neurophysiol 50*:344-346, 1987

Berardelli A, Inghilleri M, Rothwell JC, et al: Facilitation of muscle evoked responses after repetitive cortical stimulation in man. *Exp Brain Res 122*:79-84, 1998

Boon P, Vonck K, D'Have M, et al: Cost-benefit of vagus nerve stimulation for refractory epilepsy. *Acta Neurol Belg 99*:275-280, 1999

Boon P, Vonck K, De H, V, et al: Deep brain stimulation in patients with refractory temporal lobe epilepsy. *Epilepsia 48*:1551-1560, 2007

Bragin A, Wilson CL, Engel J, Jr.: Rate of interictal events and spontaneous seizures in epileptic rats after electrical stimulation of hippocampus and its afferents. *Epilepsia 43 Suppl 5*:81-85, 2002

Brodie MJ, Dichter MA: Antiepileptic drugs. *N Engl J Med 334*:168-175, 1996

Cantello R, Rossi S, Varrasi C, et al: Slow repetitive TMS for drug-resistant epilepsy: clinical and EEG findings of a placebo-controlled trial. *Epilepsia 48*:366-374, 2007

Chabardes S, Kahane P, Minotti L, et al: Deep brain stimulation in epilepsy with particular reference to the subthalamic nucleus. *Epileptic Disord 4 Suppl 3*:S83-S93, 2002

Chkhenkeli SA, Chkhenkeli IS: Effects of therapeutic stimulation of nucleus caudatus on epileptic electrical activity of brain in patients with intractable epilepsy. *Stereotact Funct Neurosurg 69*:221-224, 1997

Chkhenkeli SA, Sramka M, Lortkipanidze GS, et al: Electrophysiological effects and clinical results of direct brain stimulation for intractable epilepsy. *Clin Neurol Neurosurg 106*:318-329, 2004

Cincotta M, Borgheresi A, Gambetti C, et al: Suprathreshold 0.3 Hz repetitive TMS prolongs the cortical silent period: potential implications for therapeutic trials in epilepsy. *Clin Neurophysiol 114*:1827-1833, 2003

Cooke PM, Snider RS: Some cerebellar influences on electrically-induced cerebral seizures. *Epilepsia 4*:19-28, 1955

Cooper IS, Amin I, Riklan M, et al: Chronic cerebellar stimulation in epilepsy. Clinical and anatomical studies. *Arch Neurol 33*:559-570, 1976

D'Arcangelo G, Panuccio G, Tancredi V, et al: Repetitive low-frequency stimulation reduces epileptiform synchronization in limbic neuronal networks. *Neurobiol Dis 19*:119-128, 2005

Davis R, Emmonds SE: Cerebellar stimulation for seizure control: 17-year study. *Stereotact Funct Neurosurg 58*:200-208, 1992

De H, V, De WJ, Raedt R, et al: Modulation of seizure threshold by vagus nerve stimulation in an animal model for motor seizures. *Acta Neurol Scand 121*:271-276, 2010

Dow RS, FERNANDEZ-GUARDIOLA A, Manni E: The influence of the cerebellum on experimental epilepsy. *Electroencephalogr Clin Neurophysiol 14*:383-398, 1962

Ebert U, Ziemann U: Altered seizure susceptibility after high-frequency transcranial magnetic stimulation in rats. *Neurosci Lett 273*:155-158, 1999

Engel J, Jr., Wiebe S, French J, et al: Practice parameter: temporal lobe and localized neocortical resections for epilepsy. *Epilepsia 44*:741-751, 2003

Fanardjian VV, DONHOFFER H: AN ELECTROPHYSIOLOGICAL STUDY OF CEREBELLOHIPPOCAMPAL RELATIONSHIPS IN THE UNRESTRAINED CAT. *Acta Physiol Acad Sci Hung 24*:321-333, 1964

Feinstein B, Gleason CA, Libet B: Stimulation of locus coeruleus in man. Preliminary trials for spasticity and epilepsy. *Stereotact Funct Neurosurg 52*:26-41, 1989

Fisher RS: Emerging antiepileptic drugs. *Neurology 43*:S12-S20, 1993

Fisher RS, Uematsu S, Krauss GL, et al: Placebo-controlled pilot study of centromedian thalamic stimulation in treatment of intractable seizures. *Epilepsia 33*:841-851, 1992

Fregni F, Otachi PT, Do VA, et al: A randomized clinical trial of repetitive transcranial magnetic stimulation in patients with refractory epilepsy. *Ann Neurol 60*:447-455, 2006

Fregni F, Pascual-Leone A: Technology insight: noninvasive brain stimulation in neurology-perspectives on the therapeutic potential of rTMS and tDCS. *Nat Clin Pract Neurol 3*:383-393, 2007

Fregni F, Thome-Souza S, Bermpohl F, et al: Antiepileptic effects of repetitive transcranial magnetic stimulation in patients with cortical malformations: an EEG and clinical study. *Stereotact Funct Neurosurg 83*:57-62, 2005

Gale K: Role of the substantia nigra in GABA-mediated anticonvulsant actions. *Adv Neurol 44*:343-364, 1986

Gleissner U, Helmstaedter C, Schramm J, et al: Memory outcome after selective amygdalohippocampectomy in patients with temporal lobe epilepsy: one-year follow-up. *Epilepsia 45*:960-962, 2004

Godlevsky LS, Kobolev EV, van Luijtelaar EL, et al: Influence of transcranial magnetic stimulation on spike-wave discharges in a genetic model of absence epilepsy. *Indian J Exp Biol 44*:949-954, 2006

Gybels J, Kupers R, Nuttin B: Therapeutic stereotactic procedures on the thalamus for pain. *Acta Neurochir (Wien) 124*:19-22, 1993

Hallett M: Transcranial magnetic stimulation and the human brain. *Nature 406*:147-150, 2000

Halpern C, Hurtig H, Jaggi J, et al: Deep brain stimulation in neurologic disorders. *Parkinsonism Relat Disord 13*:1-16, 2007

Hamani C, Ewerton FI, Bonilha SM, et al: Bilateral anterior thalamic nucleus lesions and high-frequency stimulation are protective against pilocarpine-induced seizures and status epilepticus. *Neurosurgery 54*:191-195, 2004

Handforth A, DeGiorgio CM, Schachter SC, et al: Vagus nerve stimulation therapy for partial-onset seizures: a randomized active-control trial. *Neurology 51*:48-55, 1998

Handforth A, DeSalles AA, Krahl SE: Deep brain stimulation of the subthalamic nucleus as adjunct treatment for refractory epilepsy. *Epilepsia 47*:1239-1241, 2006

Hauser WA, Annegers JF, Kurland LT: Incidence of epilepsy and unprovoked seizures in Rochester, Minnesota: 1935-1984. *Epilepsia 34*:453-468, 1993

Helmstaedter C, Kurthen M, Lux S, et al: Chronic epilepsy and cognition: a longitudinal study in temporal lobe epilepsy. *Ann Neurol 54*:425-432, 2003

Henry TR, Bakay RA, Votaw JR, et al: Brain blood flow alterations induced by therapeutic vagus nerve stimulation in partial epilepsy: I. Acute effects at high and low levels of stimulation. *Epilepsia 39*:983-990, 1998

Henry TR, Votaw JR, Pennell PB, et al: Acute blood flow changes and efficacy of vagus nerve stimulation in partial epilepsy. *Neurology 52*:1166-1173, 1999

HEUSER G, Buchwald NA, WYERS EJ: The "caudatespindle". II. Facilitatory and inhibitory caudate-cortical pathways. *Electroencephalogr Clin Neurophysiol 13*:519-524, 1961

Hodaie M, Wennberg RA, Dostrovsky JO, et al: Chronic anterior thalamus stimulation for intractable epilepsy. *Epilepsia 43*:603-608, 2002

Iadarola MJ, Gale K: Substantia nigra: site of anticonvulsant activity mediated by gamma-aminobutyric acid. *Science 218*:1237-1240, 1982

IWATA K, SNIDER RS: Cerebello-hippocampal influences on the electroencephalogram. *Electroencephalogr Clin Neurophysiol 11*:439-446, 1959

Jennum P, Klitgaard H: Repetitive transcranial magnetic stimulations of the rat. Effect of acute and chronic stimulations on pentylenetetrazole-induced clonic seizures. *Epilepsy Res 23*:115-122, 1996

Jensen AL, Durand DM: Suppression of axonal conduction by sinusoidal stimulation in rat hippocampus in vitro. *J Neural Eng 4*:1-16, 2007

Joo EY, Han SJ, Chung SH, et al: Antiepileptic effects of low-frequency repetitive transcranial magnetic stimulation by different stimulation durations and locations. *Clin Neurophysiol 118*:702-708, 2007

Kayyali H, Durand D: Effects of applied currents on epileptiform bursts in vitro. *Exp Neurol 113*:249-254, 1991

Kerrigan JF, Litt B, Fisher RS, et al: Electrical stimulation of the anterior nucleus of the thalamus for the treatment of intractable epilepsy. *Epilepsia 45*:346-354, 2004

Kimiskidis VK: Transcranial magnetic stimulation for drug-resistant epilepsies: rationale and clinical experience. *Eur Neurol 63*:205-210, 2010

Kinoshita M, Ikeda A, Begum T, et al: Low-frequency repetitive transcranial magnetic stimulation for seizure suppression in patients with extratemporal lobe epilepsy-a pilot study. *Seizure 14*:387-392, 2005

Ko D, Heck C, Grafton S, et al: Vagus nerve stimulation activates central nervous system structures in epileptic patients during PET H2(15)O blood flow imaging. *Neurosurgery 39*:426-430, 1996

Kossoff EH, Ritzl EK, Politsky JM, et al: Effect of an external responsive neurostimulator on seizures and electrographic discharges during subdural electrode monitoring. *Epilepsia 45*:1560-1567, 2004

Krack P, Batir A, Van BN, et al: Five-year follow-up of bilateral stimulation of the subthalamic nucleus in advanced Parkinson's disease. *N Engl J Med 349*:1925-1934, 2003

Kwan P, Brodie MJ: Early identification of refractory epilepsy. *N Engl J Med 342*:314-319, 2000

Labar DR: Antiepileptic drug use during the first 12 months of vagus nerve stimulation therapy: a registry study. *Neurology 59*:S38-S43, 2002

Lado FA: Chronic bilateral stimulation of the anterior thalamus of kainate-treated rats increases seizure frequency. *Epilepsia 47*:27-32, 2006

Lado FA, Velisek L, Moshe SL: The effect of electrical stimulation of the subthalamic nucleus on seizures is frequency dependent. *Epilepsia 44*:157-164, 2003

Laxer KD, Robertson LT, Julien RM, et al: Phenytoin: relationship between cerebellar function and epileptic discharges. *Adv Neurol 27*:415-427, 1980

Lee KH, Hitti FL, Shalinsky MH, et al: Abolition of spindle oscillations and 3-Hz absence seizurelike activity in the thalamus by using high-frequency stimulation: potential mechanism of action. *J Neurosurg 103*:538-545, 2005

Lee KJ, Jang KS, Shon YM: Chronic deep brain stimulation of subthalamic and anterior thalamic nuclei for controlling refractory partial epilepsy. *Acta Neurochir Suppl 99*:87-91, 2006

Lee SK, Lee SY, Kim KK, et al: Surgical outcome and prognostic factors of cryptogenic neocortical epilepsy. *Ann Neurol 58*:525-532, 2005

Leone M, Franzini A, Broggi G, et al: Hypothalamic deep brain stimulation for intractable chronic cluster headache: a 3-year follow-up. *Neurol Sci 24 Suppl 2*:S143-S145, 2003

Leone M, Franzini A, D'Andrea G, et al: Deep brain stimulation to relieve drug-resistant SUNCT. *Ann Neurol 57*:924-927, 2005

Lesser RP, Kim SH, Beyderman L, et al: Brief bursts of pulse stimulation terminate afterdischarges caused by cortical stimulation. *Neurology 53*:2073-2081, 1999

Lian J, Bikson M, Sciortino C, et al: Local suppression of epileptiform activity by electrical stimulation in rat hippocampus in vitro. *J Physiol 547*:427-434, 2003

Lian J, Bikson M, Sciortino C, et al: Local suppression of epileptiform activity by electrical stimulation in rat hippocampus in vitro. *J Physiol 547*:427-434, 2003

Lim SN, Lee ST, Tsai YT, et al: Electrical stimulation of the anterior nucleus of the thalamus for intractable epilepsy: a long-term follow-up study. *Epilepsia 48*:342-347, 2007

Lipton RB, Pearlman SH: Transcranial magnetic simulation in the treatment of migraine. *Neurotherapeutics* 7:204-212, 2010

Liu WC, Mosier K, Kalnin AJ, et al: BOLD fMRI activation induced by vagus nerve stimulation in seizure patients. *J Neurol Neurosurg Psychiatry* 74:811-813, 2003

Lockard JS, Congdon WC, DuCharme LL: Feasibility and safety of vagal stimulation in monkey model. *Epilepsia 31 Suppl 2*:S20-S26, 1990

Loddenkemper T, Pan A, Neme S, et al: Deep brain stimulation in epilepsy. *J Clin Neurophysiol 18*:514-532, 2001

McIntyre CC, Savasta M, Kerkerian-Le GL, et al: Uncovering the mechanism(s) of action of deep brain stimulation: activation, inhibition, or both. *Clin Neurophysiol 115*:1239-1248, 2004

McLachlan RS: Suppression of interictal spikes and seizures by stimulation of the vagus nerve. *Epilepsia 34*:918-923, 1993

Mirski MA, Ferrendelli JA: Anterior thalamic mediation of generalized pentylenetetrazol seizures. *Brain Res 399*:212-223, 1986

Mirski MA, McKeon AC, Ferrendelli JA: Anterior thalamus and substantia nigra: two distinct structures mediating experimental generalized seizures. *Brain Res 397*:377-380, 1986

Molnar GF, Sailer A, Gunraj CA, et al: Thalamic deep brain stimulation activates the cerebellothalamocortical pathway. *Neurology 63*:907-909, 2004

Morris GL, III, Mueller WM: Long-term treatment with vagus nerve stimulation in patients with refractory epilepsy. The Vagus Nerve Stimulation Study Group E01-E05. *Neurology 53*:1731-1735, 1999

Motamedi GK, Lesser RP, Miglioretti DL, et al: Optimizing parameters for terminating cortical afterdischarges with pulse stimulation. *Epilepsia 43*:836-846, 2002

Muellbacher W, Ziemann U, Boroojerdi B, et al: Effects of low-frequency transcranial magnetic stimulation on motor excitability and basic motor behavior. *Clin Neurophysiol 111*:1002-1007, 2000

Mullan S, Vailati G, Karasick J, et al: Thalamic lesions for the control of epilepsy. A study of nine cases. *Arch Neurol 16*:277-285, 1967

Nakagawa M, Durand D: Suppression of spontaneous epileptiform activity with applied currents. *Brain Res 567*:241-247, 1991

Narayanan JT, Watts R, Haddad N, et al: Cerebral activation during vagus nerve stimulation: a functional MR study. *Epilepsia 43*:1509-1514, 2002

Nguyen JP, Lefaucher JP, Le GC, et al: Motor cortex stimulation in the treatment of central and neuropathic pain. *Arch Med Res 31*:263-265, 2000

Nishida N, Huang ZL, Mikuni N, et al: Deep brain stimulation of the posterior hypothalamus activates the histaminergic system to exert antiepileptic effect in rat pentylenetetrazol model. *Exp Neurol 205*:132-144, 2007

Osorio I, Frei MG, Giftakis J, et al: Performance reassessment of a real-time seizure-detection algorithm on long ECoG series. *Epilepsia 43*:1522-1535, 2002

Osorio I, Frei MG, Sunderam S, et al: Automated seizure abatement in humans using electrical stimulation. *Ann Neurol 57*:258-268, 2005

Osorio I, Frei MG, Wilkinson SB: Real-time automated detection and quantitative analysis of seizures and short-term prediction of clinical onset. *Epilepsia 39*:615-627, 1998

Osorio I, Overman J, Giftakis J, et al: High frequency thalamic stimulation for inoperable mesial temporal epilepsy. *Epilepsia 48*:1561-1571, 2007

Pascual-Leone A, Rubio B, Pallardo F, et al: Rapid-rate transcranial magnetic stimulation of left dorsolateral prefrontal cortex in drug-resistant depression. *Lancet 348*:233-237, 1996

Penry JK, Dean JC: Prevention of intractable partial seizures by intermittent vagal stimulation in humans: preliminary results. *Epilepsia 31 Suppl 2*:S40-S43, 1990

Peters TE, Bhavaraju NC, Frei MG, et al: Network system for automated seizure detection and contingent delivery of therapy. *J Clin Neurophysiol 18*:545-549, 2001

Pollak P, Fraix V, Krack P, et al: Treatment results: Parkinson's disease. *Mov Disord 17 Suppl 3*:S75-S83, 2002

Psatta DM: Control of chronic experimental focal epilepsy by feedback caudatum stimulations. *Epilepsia 24*:444-454, 1983

Rotenberg A, Bae EH, Muller PA, et al: In-session seizures during low-frequency repetitive transcranial magnetic stimulation in patients with epilepsy. *Epilepsy Behav 16*:353-355, 2009

Rotenberg A, Muller P, Birnbaum D, et al: Seizure suppression by EEG-guided repetitive transcranial magnetic stimulation in the rat. *Clin Neurophysiol 119*:2697-2702, 2008

Saillet S, Langlois M, Feddersen B, et al: Manipulating the epileptic brain using stimulation: a review of experimental and clinical studies. *Epileptic Disord 11*:100-112, 2009

Sander JW: Some aspects of prognosis in the epilepsies: a review. *Epilepsia 34*:1007-1016, 1993

Shandra AA, Godlevsky LS: Antiepileptic effects of cerebellar nucleus dentatus electrical stimulation under different conditions of brain epileptisation. *Indian J Exp Biol 28*:158-161, 1990

Shi LH, Luo F, Woodward D, et al: Deep brain stimulation of the substantia nigra pars reticulata exerts long lasting suppression of amygdala-kindled seizures. *Brain Res 1090*:202-207, 2006

Sillanpaa M, Schmidt D: Natural history of treated childhood-onset epilepsy: prospective, long-term population-based study. *Brain 129*:617-624, 2006

Sperling MR, O'Connor MJ, Saykin AJ, et al: A noninvasive protocol for anterior temporal lobectomy. *Neurology 42*:416-422, 1992

Sun FT, Morrell MJ, Wharen RE, Jr.: Responsive cortical stimulation for the treatment of epilepsy. *Neurotherapeutics 5*:68-74, 2008

Swanson TH: The pathophysiology of human mesial temporal lobe epilepsy. *J Clin Neurophysiol 12*:2-22, 1995

Takaya M, Terry WJ, Naritoku DK: Vagus nerve stimulation induces a sustained anticonvulsant effect. *Epilepsia 37*:1111-1116, 1996

Tergau F, Naumann U, Paulus W, et al: Low-frequency repetitive transcranial magnetic stimulation improves intractable epilepsy. *Lancet 353*:2209, 1999

Tergau F, Neumann D, Rosenow F, et al: Can epilepsies be improved by repetitive transcranial magnetic stimulation?--interim analysis of a controlled study. *Suppl Clin Neurophysiol 56*:400-405, 2003

Theodore WH, Hunter K, Chen R, et al: Transcranial magnetic stimulation for the treatment of seizures: a controlled study. *Neurology 59*:560-562, 2002

Upton AR, Amin I, Garnett S, et al: Evoked metabolic responses in the limbic-striate system produced by stimulation of anterior thalamic nucleus in man. *Pacing Clin Electrophysiol 10*:217-225, 1987

Upton AR, Cooper IS, Springman M, et al: Suppression of seizures and psychosis of limbic system origin by chronic stimulation of anterior nucleus of the thalamus. *Int J Neurol 19-20*:223-230, 1985

Usui N, Maesawa S, Kajita Y, et al: Suppression of secondary generalization of limbic seizures by stimulation of subthalamic nucleus in rats. *J Neurosurg 102*:1122-1129, 2005

Van LK, Vonck K, Boon P, et al: Vagus nerve stimulation in refractory epilepsy: SPECT activation study. *J Nucl Med 41*:1145-1154, 2000

Velasco AL, Velasco F, Jimenez F, et al: Neuromodulation of the centromedian thalamic nuclei in the treatment of generalized seizures and the improvement of the quality of life in patients with Lennox-Gastaut syndrome. *Epilepsia 47*:1203-1212, 2006

Velasco AL, Velasco M, Velasco F, et al: Subacute and chronic electrical stimulation of the hippocampus on intractable temporal lobe seizures: preliminary report. *Arch Med Res 31*:316-328, 2000

Velasco F, Carrillo-Ruiz JD, Brito F, et al: Double-blind, randomized controlled pilot study of bilateral cerebellar stimulation for treatment of intractable motor seizures. *Epilepsia 46*:1071-1081, 2005

Velasco F, Velasco M, Velasco AL, et al: Electrical stimulation of the centromedian thalamic nucleus in control of seizures: long-term studies. *Epilepsia 36*:63-71, 1995

Velasco F, Velasco M, Velasco AL, et al: Electrical stimulation for epilepsy: stimulation of hippocampal foci. *Stereotact Funct Neurosurg 77*:223-227, 2001

Velasco M, Velasco F, Velasco AL, et al: Acute and chronic electrical stimulation of the centromedian thalamic nucleus: modulation of reticulo-cortical systems and predictor factors for generalized seizure control. *Arch Med Res 31*:304-315, 2000

Vercueil L, Benazzouz A, Deransart C, et al: High-frequency stimulation of the subthalamic nucleus suppresses absence seizures in the rat: comparison with neurotoxic lesions. *Epilepsy Res 31*:39-46, 1998

Volkmann J, Allert N, Voges J, et al: Long-term results of bilateral pallidal stimulation in Parkinson's disease. *Ann Neurol 55*:871-875, 2004

Vonck K, Boon P, Achten E, et al: Long-term amygdalohippocampal stimulation for refractory temporal lobe epilepsy. *Ann Neurol 52*:556-565, 2002

Vonck K, Boon P, D'Have M, et al: Long-term results of vagus nerve stimulation in refractory epilepsy. *Seizure 8*:328-334, 1999

Vonck K, Boon P, Van LK, et al: Acute single photon emission computed tomographic study of vagus nerve stimulation in refractory epilepsy. *Epilepsia 41*:601-609, 2000

Wheless JW, Maggio V: Vagus nerve stimulation therapy in patients younger than 18 years. *Neurology 59*:S21-S25, 2002

Wright GD, McLellan DL, Brice JG: A double-blind trial of chronic cerebellar stimulation in twelve patients with severe epilepsy. *J Neurol Neurosurg Psychiatry 47*:769-774, 1984

Wyckhuys T, De ST, Claeys P, et al: High frequency deep brain stimulation in the hippocampus modifies seizure characteristics in kindled rats. *Epilepsia 48*:1543-1550, 2007

Zabara J: Inhibition of experimental seizures in canines by repetitive vagal stimulation. *Epilepsia 33*:1005-1012, 1992

Ziai WC, Sherman DL, Bhardwaj A, et al: Target-specific catecholamine elevation induced by anticonvulsant thalamic deep brain stimulation. *Epilepsia 46*:878-888, 2005

Ziemann U.: Evaluation of epilepsy and anticonvulsants, in Hallett M, Chokroverty A. (eds): *Magnetic Stimulation in Clinical Neurophysiology*. Elsevier, 2005, pp 253-270

17

Surgical Treatment of Intractable Epilepsy Associated with Focal Cortical Dysplasia

Zhao Jizong[1], Fei Zhou[2] and Bai Hongmin[3]
[1]*Department of neurosurgery, Tiantan hospital,*
[2]*Neurosurgical department of Xijing hospital, The Forth Military Medical University,*
[3]*Neurosurgical department of Liuhuaqiao hospital,*
[1,2,3]*China*

1. Introduction

Focal cortical dysplasias (FCDs), initially thought to be rare, are a common cause of drug-refractory epilepsy in both children and adults. Successful resection and subsequent characterization of FCDs was first described by Taylor et al. in 1971 from pathological specimens obtained in patients treated for intractable temporal lobe epilepsy (Tassi, et al.,2001; Becker, et al.,2002; Tassi, et al.,2002; Urbach, et al.,2002; Nobili, et al.,2009). The dysplasias include abnormalities of cellular proliferation, migration, and differentiation. From recent published reports, patients with cortical dysplasia constitute approximately 14% of all patients undergoing epilepsy neurosurgery. Cortical dysplasia is the most common etiology in younger surgical patients. Using the UCLA cohort as an example, cortical dysplasia was the histopathologic substrate identified in 75% of infants and children operated in the first 2 years of life. By comparison, cortical dysplasia was found in less than 10% in those having surgery who were older than age 21 years (Diaz, et al., 2008).
Surgical evaluation and treatment of FCDs requires an understanding of pathological, presurgical imaging, EEG findings and intraoperative mapping of epileptogenic zone and functional areas (Sisodiya,2011).

2. Histopathological characteristics of FCD

The establishment of a uniform terminology and classification of histopathological findings associated with FCDs has recently been proposed by a consensus panel of neuropathologists, neuroepileptologists, and neuroradiologists.
The Palmini classification has been adopted most widely to categorize these heterogeneous lesions. Palmini et al. determined that several distinct histopathological features of the cortex must be present for a lesion to be considered a true FCD. These include architectural abnormalities, either dyslamination or columnar disorganization with or without dysmorphic neurons, giant cells, or balloon cells. Palmini et al. described 2 major types and 4 subtypes of FCD: Type 1 dysplasia refers to the most subtle alterations in cortical lamination and ectopic neurons in the white matter or immediately adjacent to layer 1. 1a with isolated architectural abnormalities alone; Type 1b, including giant neurons; Whereas type 2 dysplasia refers to areas of more extensive dyslamination outside of layer 1 with the

absence (type 2a) or presence (type 2b) of cytomegalic or balloon cells (Crino,2009; Gumbinger, et al.,2009; Nobili, et al.,2009; Wong,2009; Kim, et al.,2010; Krsek, et al.,2010). (Table 1)

Type	Subtype	Pathology features
FCD type 1	1a	Architectural cortical abnormalities ±feature of mild MCD
	1b	Architectural abnormalities and giant or immature neurons
FCD type 1	2a	Architectural abnormalities with dysmorphic neurons but no balloon cells
	2b	Architectural abnormalities with dysmorphic neurons and balloon cells

Table 1. Pathological features of FCD subtypes as outlined in the system by Palmini et al.(2004)

Macroscopic abnormalities may be present in surgical resections from FCD cases. There may be apparent thickening of the cortical gray matter, blurring of the gray-white border and the tissue may appear firmer (Figure 1). The overall lesion size varies and can be up to several centimetres broad, involving both sulci and gyri. On histological examination, abnormalities of cortical laminar architecture (also called 'dyslamination') are common to all types of FCD with loss of distinction between cortical layers, more easily visualized with Nissl stain or NeuN immunohistochemistry(Crino,2009; Gumbinger, et al.,2009; Nobili, et al.,2009; Wong,2009; Krsek, et al.,2010; Wong,2010).

Patients with mild Palmini type 1 CD represent about 50% of the surgical cases, and these lesions tend to occur most often in the temporal lobe, often associated with hippocampal sclerosis. By comparison, patients with severe type 2 CD present at younger ages, often with multilobar extratemporal lesions, and more aggressive seizures(Morales, et al.,2009; Blumcke, et al.,2011; Palmini,2011).

Although strictly a pathological classification, an expected correlation with neuroimaging results was summarized within the classification system. Mild MCDs and Type 1a and 1b FCDs were not considered likely to have correlating characteristics on MR images, unlike Type II which would probably exhibit changes including increased cortical thickness, blurring of grey-white junction, and extension of cortical tissue toward the ventricle.

The etiology of these lesions is poorly understood, and has been postulated to be due to possible in utero focal insults to cortex or to genetic mutations responsible for disordered cell proliferation or differentiation. Tuberous sclerosis complex (TSC) represents a more specific form of type 2b FCD, with the presence of areas of dysplasia containing giant cytomegalic cells as well as dysplastic neurons and astrocytes, termed "tubers." TSC1 and TSC2 are the genes that are found to be mutated in TSC, and encode for hamartin and tuberin, respectively(Lugnier, et al.,2009; Wong,2010). Hamartin and tuberin cooperatively inhibit excessive protein translation by acting to down-regulate the mammalian target of rapamycin (mTOR). The mTOR pathway has been shown to be upregulated in TSC, and some of its components are also overactive in non-TSC FCDs, suggesting that this pathway may be common to a wide range of cortical dysplasias(Crino,2009; Gumbinger, et al.,2009; Nobili, et al.,2009; Wong,2009; Krsek, et al.,2010; Wong,2010; Blumcke, et al.,2011; Palmini,2011).

The epileptogenicity of FCDs is hypothesized to be caused by abnormal synaptogenesis and dysregulated gaminobutyric acid-mediated inhibitory signalling. Enhanced neuronal hyperexcitability may also play a role in the abnormal synchronization of neuronal populations, leading to prolonged trains of epileptic activity (Sisodiya, et al.,2009).

3. Preoperative evaluation

The presurgical evaluation for pharmacoresistant patients with cortical dysplasia is often challenging. There is no particular seizure semiology that characterizes patients with cortical dysplasia from other epilepsy surgery patients with lesions in different locations within the brain. Furthermore, there are no distinctive interictal or ictal scalp EEG "signatures" that are exclusively associated with cortical dysplasia in patients with refractory epilepsy. No one single test of the presurgical evaluation in CD patients is 100% accurate. Based on retrospective cohort studies, the accuracy of investigations are: interictal scalp EEG, 50%; ictal scalp EEG, 65%; MR), 66%; FDG-PET, 81%; and ictal SPECT, 57%. Combined evaluation of detailed history and physical examination, EEG, MRI and other functional Neuroimaging plays a vital role in presurgical planning in patients with intractable epilepsy (Duchowny,2009; Gumbinger, et al.,2009; Roper,2009; Sisodiya, et al.,2009).

3.1 Clinical findings

The preoperative evaluation in a patient with medically refractory seizure starts with a detailed history and physical examination. Seizure type may provide information about the location of the epileptogenic zone, and can contribute to the prognosis of seizure control after resection. Neurological deficits identified on physical examination may point to the area of cortex most affected and provide clues as to the focal, multifocal, or diffuse nature of the underlying pathological entity (Goldring,1987; Crino,2009; Nobili, et al.,2009; Sisodiya, et al.,2009; Tassi, et al.,2009; Kim, et al.,2010).

3.2 EEG

Patients with medically intractable seizures should undergo preoperative evaluation with video-assisted scalp EEG to correlate ictal EEG graphic events with the seizure semiology. The ictal onset zone is defined as the region showing focal rhythmic activity, bursts of high-frequency discharges, repetitive spiking, or electrodecremental patterns(Jiang, et al.,2010). The disadvantage of scalp EEG is that in patients with FCDs there is a high incidence of widespread interictal spiking, which may obscure identification of the epileptogenic zone. Interictal and ictal EEG findings often poorly localize to the MRI-identified lesion in patients with cortical dysplasia. Interictal findings localize on scalp EEG to the eventual area of resection in 48%, and ictal findings localize to one area in 68% of epilepsy surgery patients with cortical dysplasia (Francione, et al.,2003; Aubert, et al.,2009; LeVan, et al.,2010).

3.3 MRI

Identifying a focal lesion on MRI in patients with medically refractory epilepsy remains one of the most important factors in determining surgical outcomes. Therefore, there has been ongoing interest in utilizing new technologies to improve the rate of detection and thereby improve surgical outcomes. Although a number of lesions can result in epilepsy, FCDs remain the most difficult to detect. With new high-field and multichannel technology, the maximum gains in signal to noise are at the cortical surface, making patients with focal-onset refractory epilepsy the most likely to benefit from these technical advances (Bernasconi, et al.,2011; Kim, et al.,2011).

Patients with medically intractable epilepsy should undergo MR imaging in 3 planes for best characterization of the potential underlying FCD. If a temporal lobe lesion is suspected, preoperative MR imaging should include T1-weighted sagittal studies, coronal MPRAGE, coronal FLAIR, and fast T2-weighted coronal sequences. Preoperative MR images obtained in patients with a suspected extratemporal lesion consists of axial fast FLAIR, fastT2-weighted axial, T1-weighted sagittal, and coronal MPRAGE MR imaging sequences.

Imaging findings of CDs include thickening of the cortex, blurring of the gray–white matter junction, abnormal cortical signal and increased T2/FLAIR (fluid-attenuated inversion recovery) and/or T1 hypointense signal extending from the ependymal surface to the cortical surface. Additional imaging features that have been described include focal hypoplasia, a deep sulcus with malformations at the depths of the sulci, broadening of the gyri, and white matter atrophy. Many of these features can be seen on both T1- and T2-weighted images, although the CD for a given patient maybe more apparent on any one of these imaging sequences. FLAIR, especially volumetric FLAIR at 3T, is very sensitive for identifying white matter involvement (Figure 1). There has been ongoing interest in utilizing new advanced MRI techniques to improve the ability to identify, diagnose, characterize, and delineate cortical dysplasias. Technologic gains such as multichannel coils(32 phased array and beyond) and higher field strengths (3T, 7T, and greater) coupled with newer imaging sequences such as arterial spin labeling (ASL), susceptibility weighted imaging(SWI) and diffusion tensor/spectrum imaging(DTI/DSI) are likely to increase yield(Diehl, et al.,2010).

To improve diagnostic accuracy, automated techniques are being developed that identify areas for closer scrutiny by an experienced neuroradiologist. One method for automated lesion detection is voxel-based morphometry. This technique employs the statistical parametric mapping techniques developed for functional MRI to allow voxel-based comparisons between patients and a cohort of control subjects with the goal of identifying areas of the brain that may be different in volume, signal intensity, texture, or sharpness of boundaries. However, in voxel-based morphometry it is difficult to interpret positive results, as differences in image intensity can occur due to differences in gyral folding, differences in relative cortical gray-to-white matter volume, incorrect segmentation, or other factors. Similarly, false-negative findings can be caused by the blurring of gray-white matter boundaries, which results when control groups are averaged (Chiang, et al.,2009; Rajan, et al.,2009).

3.4 MEG

In patients with seizures, MEG is usually most useful in patients with interictal activity, as ictal events are often associated with motion artifact. MEG and EEG appear to have similar sensitivity to record interictal events, with MEG and EEG often providing complementary data. In up to one-third of EEG-negative patients, MEG can be expected to detect interictal epileptiform activity and is particularly effective in neocortical epilepsy and FCDs (Andrade,2009; Beleza,2009; Fauser, et al.,2009) .

3.5 Other functional imaging

With patients presenting with nonlocalized scalp EEG and subtle or normal MRI scans, many centers incorporated additional functional and neuroimaging studies into the multimodality presurgical evaluation to increase the detection of patients with cortical dysplasia. Of these tools, FDG-PET has been shown to be one of the more sensitive techniques in identifying areas of cortical dysplasia. Contemporary studies indicate that FDG-PET detects interictal hypometabolism that localized to areas of cortical dysplasia in approximately 81% of patients. By comparison, 57% of cortical dysplasia patients have localized ictal SPECT scans. For both FDG-PET and ictal SPECT, some patients with normal MRI show positive scans. Hence, adjunctive neuroimaging methods, such as FDG-PET, ictal SPECT, and MEG, have an important role in the presurgical evaluation of patients with cortical dysplasia (Fedi, et al.,2003; Chassoux, et al.,2010; Phi, et al.,2010).

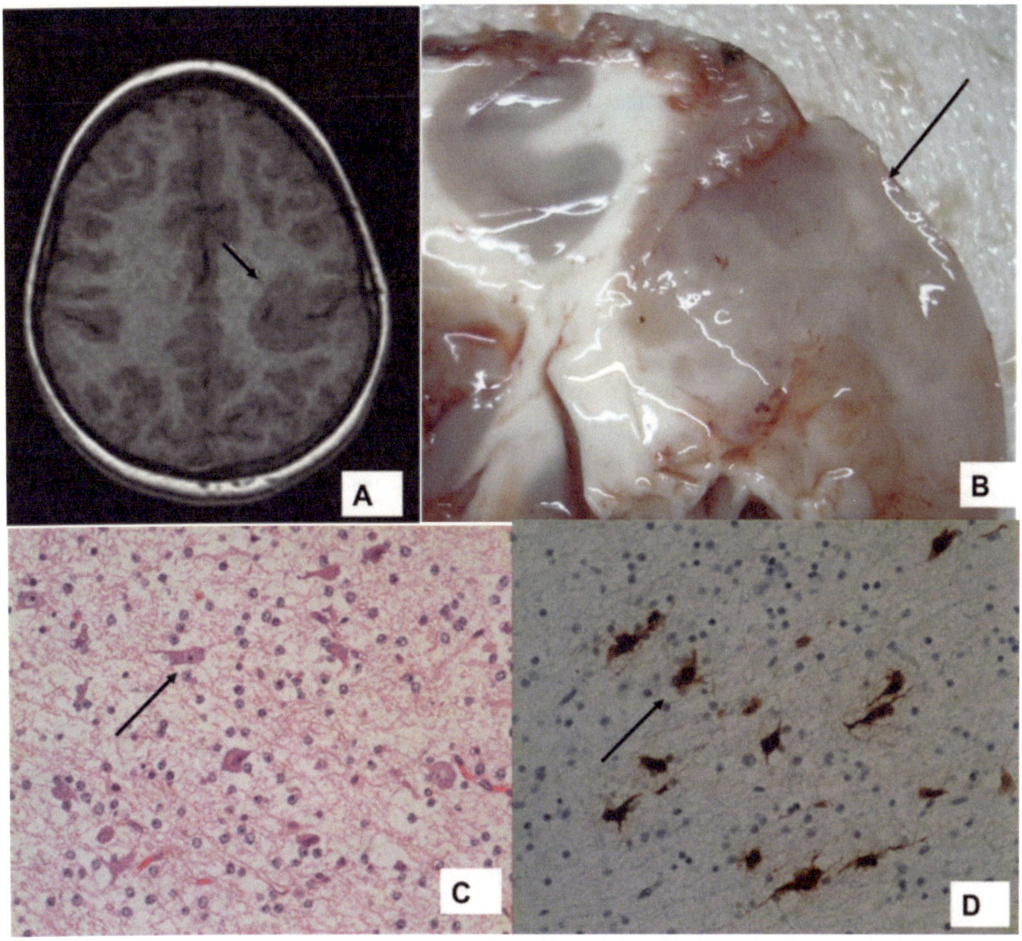

Fig. 1. The T1 weighted MRI(A), macroscopic findings(B) and microscopic findings with H & E stain (C) and in-situ immunohistochemistry with NeuN

4. Surgical considerations

The goal of clinical, EEG, and neuroimaging preoperative assessment is to identify the cortical area producing seizures and generating discharges and its anatomical and functional relationships. Concordance amongst the different modalities used to identify the lesion producing seizures is critical for surgical planning. Preoperative understanding of the epileptogenic zone, surrounding, or encompassing functional cortex, and the characteristic vascularization of the area in individual patients provides a map for planning the surgical approach, the limits of excision, and determining the potential risk to function(Diaz, et al.,2008).

The purpose of surgical intervention in the management intractable epilepsy with underlying histological evidence of cortical dysplasia is to improve seizure control and maximize the potential for normal neuropsychological development. The surgical approach to FCD is dependent on the presence of a lesion visible on MR imaging, its location to eloquent cortex, and the concordance of presurgical EEG and functional neuroimaging with identifiable lesions. If a well-defined lesion is visible on MR imaging that correlates with EEG localization of the epileptogenic focus, resection may be performed in a single-stage procedure with intraoperative electrocorticography as a guide. If no lesion is visible on MR images or if it is localized within eloquent cortex based on the results of noninvasive preoperative studies, a 2-stage procedure with invasive EEG monitoring should be considered for the purpose of locaizing the primary and secondary ictal epileptogenic zones, irritative zones, and cortical mapping of eloquent cortex to guide the focal cortical resection.

Once the epileptogenic zone is identified, different surgical strategies can be used: lesionectomy, focal cortical resections, or regional or hemispheric surgical disconnection. En-bloc resection between cortical vessels, sparing as many vessels as possible to avoid local arterial or venous infarction is essential. An important reason for incomplete resection is the intentional avoidance of the eloquent cortex. Intraoperative corticography or invasive EEG monitoring prior to extension of resection may be considered if the lesion is not well defined on preoperative neuroimaging or noninvasive EEG studies. The extent of further surgery after a first procedure is often limited by the proximity of the remnant epileptogenic zone to the functional cortex. Subsequently, there is a greater risk of neurological impairments such as paresis or visual field deficits after repeated surgery, depending on the location of the surgical target. Mapping studies of epilepsy surgical patients reveals a close association between dysplastic tissue, the epileptogenic zone, and eloquent cortical function. Seizure onset commonly occurs within or near cortical areas for language, motor function, or vision. Structural and functional overlap is frequent in FCD(Goldring,1987; Diaz, et al.,2008; Crino,2009; Duchowny,2009; Roper,2009; Kim, et al.,2010).

Invasive video-EEG monitoring with subdural grids or depth electrodes may be indicated to aid in localization of the epileptogenic zone particularly in patients with cryptogenic lesions on MR imaging, lesions located in or near eloquent cortex, or evidence of bilateral or multifocal seizure onset as determined by scalp video-EEG. Subdural electrodes allow extraoperative mapping of the eloquent cortex including critical somatosensory, motor, and language areas. These techniques can be used on any patient, but may be more important in children in whom intraoperative cortical mapping is impossible. This technique provides important information about the function and spatial relationship of the epileptogenic zone to functional cortex (Goldring,1987; Crino,2009; Duchowny,2009; Roper,2009; Kim, et al.,2010).

5. Seizure outcome after surgery

Contemporary series report that 62% of patients with CD are seizure free after resective neurosurgery, with higher rates for complete (77%) compared with incomplete (20%) removal of the lesion. Temporal location of FCDs lesions is associated with an 87% rate of freedom from seizures. Negative prognostic factors include long duration of epilepsy before surgery, older age at surgery, multiple seizure types, the occurrence of secondary generalized seizures after surgery, the need for invasive EEG recording, and incomplete resection of the epileptogenic area. In a series of patients who underwent frontal lobectomy for frontal lobe epilepsy, independent predictors of seizure recurrence were no MCD/FCD found on MRI, extrafrontal MR imaging abnormalities, generalized ictal EEG patterns, acute postoperative seizures, and incomplete resection. When no lesion was visible on pre-operative MR images, only 37% of adults and children were seizure-free 1 year postoperatively. Positive prognostic factors for good seizure control include the presence of local epileptogenic discharges, a well-defined lesion on preoperative MR images, and coincidence of ictal SPECT findings with the resection site. The completeness of resection appears to have the most predictive power for long-term seizure-free outcome.Surgical failure, defined as the presence of persistent or recurrent seizure activity, is highly dependent on the completeness of resection of the epileptogenic cortex. Intra-operative challenges to complete resection include poorly defined epileptogenic zone margins on neuroimaging or EEG, the presence of important vascular structures in the epileptogenic zone, proximity of the epileptogenic zone to eloquent cortex, or an epileptogenic zone that has important cortical function. It is important to understand that epileptic foci and underlying cortical dysplasia may occur outside of the clearly delineated areas of abnormality demonstrated on MR imaging (Diaz, et al.,2008).

Morbidity (<3%) and mortality (0.2%) are low for patients with CD undergoing epilepsy neurosurgery. The rate of transient postoperative complications after cortical resection, lobectomy, or hemispherectomy for cortical dysplasia has been reported as 10.9%. Significant permanent neurological deficits are rare, but initial neurological deterioration (for example hemiparesis, dysphasia, dysnomia, and/or memory disturbance) is very common in a high proportion of cases(Krsek, et al.,2010; Phi, et al.,2010; Tassi, et al.,2010).

6. Challenges and future directions

Future challenges include the noninvasive identification of patients with CD with 100% accuracy, evaluation of long-term out comes in surgical patients, and devising new treatments based on a better understanding of the neurobiology leading to seizures in CD tissue.

6.1 Identify refractory epilepsy patients with cortical dysplasia with 100% accuracy

A substantial proportion of epilepsy surgery patients with cortical dysplasia have non localizing foci using scalp EEG and "normal" MRI scans. Many of these are patients have mild cortical dysplasia. Thus how many patients with cortical dysplasia are we missing using current presurgical protocols that rely on structural MRI scans? We need more precise presurgical protocols and technologies that can screen patients with refractory epilepsy noninvasively for the presence of subtle cortical dysplasia (Bernasconi, et al., 2011; Kim, et al., 2011).

6.2 Determine the long-term outcomes for epilepsy surgery patients with mild and severe cortical dysplasia

At present, there appear to be minimal differences for patients with type 1 and type 2 cortical dysplasia in the percentage of patient's seizure free 1–2 years after surgery, if the lesion is completely removed. However, it is unclear if patients remain seizure free many years after surgery. In addition, we do not know if patients have long-term improvements in assessments of quality of life and psychosocial outcomes. Hence, long-term outcome studies are needed to determine if there are differences in the percentage of patients who are seizure free along with developmental and psychosocial results, for patients with mild and severe cortical dysplasia (Diaz, et al.,2008).

6.3 Devise new and improved treatments for drug-refractory epilepsy patients with cortical dysplasia

A proportion of medically refractory patients with cortical dysplasia are poor surgical candidates because the lesion cannot be completely removed if it involves areas of important functional cortex. A future challenge will be to develop new therapies that control seizures so that more patients with cortical dysplasia can be treated successfully without increasing the risk of new neurologic deficits. This may involve remedies based on mechanisms learned from the basic science laboratory involving abnormal cells and circuits in cortical dysplasia tissue. These therapies will also need to include emerging knowledge of the genetic abnormalities that may be different in patients with mild and severe cortical dysplasia. Hence, there is a need for more research to understand mechanisms of epileptogenesis and pathogenesis along with genetics in patients with cortical dysplasia, and whether these mechanisms are different in those with mild and severe disease. The use of human tissue may be an important research opportunity for patients with cortical dysplasia, as it offers the opportunity to try new pharmacologic treatments on this disease. In the future, we hope to understand more about the clinical characteristics and mechanisms of epileptogenesis in patients with mild and severe cortical dysplasia that can be translated into novel therapies(Beleza,2009; Crino,2009; Duchowny,2009; Roper,2009).

7. Acknowledgements

We thank professor Wang Weimin and doctor Wang Wei at the Neurosurgical Department of Liuhuaqiao Hospital for providing clinical data.

8. References

Andrade, D.M. (2009). Genetic basis in epilepsies caused by malformations of cortical development and in those with structurally normal brain. *Hum Genet*, 126,173-93.

Aubert, S., Wendling, F., Regis, J., et al. (2009). Local and remote epileptogenicity in focal cortical dysplasias and neurodevelopmental tumours. *Brain*, 132,3072-86.

Becker, A.J., Urbach, H., Scheffler, B., et al. (2002). Focal cortical dysplasia of Taylor's balloon cell type: mutational analysis of the TSC1 gene indicates a pathogenic relationship to tuberous sclerosis. *Ann Neurol*, 52,29-37.

Beleza, P. (2009). Refractory epilepsy: a clinically oriented review. *Eur Neurol*, 62,65-71.

Bernasconi, A., Bernasconi, N., Bernhardt, B.C., Schrader, D. (2011). Advances in MRI for 'cryptogenic' epilepsies. *Nat Rev Neurol*, 7,99-108.

Blumcke, I., Thom, M., Aronica, E., et al. (2011). The clinicopathologic spectrum of focal cortical dysplasias: a consensus classification proposed by an ad hoc Task Force of the ILAE Diagnostic Methods Commission. *Epilepsia*, 52,158-74.

Chassoux, F., Rodrigo, S., Semah, F., et al. (2010). FDG-PET improves surgical outcome in negative MRI Taylor-type focal cortical dysplasias. *Neurology*, 75,2168-75.

Chiang, K.L., Wong, T.T., Kwan, S.Y., Hsu, T.R., Wang, C.H., Chang, K.P. (2009). Finding on brain MRI mimicking focal cortical dysplasia in early Rasmussen's encephalitis: a case report and review. *Childs Nerv Syst*, 25,1501-6.

Crino, P.B. (2009). Focal brain malformations: seizures, signaling, sequencing. *Epilepsia*, 50 Suppl 9,3-8.

Diaz, R.J., Sherman, E.M., Hader, W.J. (2008). Surgical treatment of intractable epilepsy associated with focal cortical dysplasia. *Neurosurg Focus*, 25,E6.

Diehl, B., Tkach, J., Piao, Z., et al. (2010). Diffusion tensor imaging in patients with focal epilepsy due to cortical dysplasia in the temporo-occipital region: electro-clinico-pathological correlations. *Epilepsy Res*, 90,178-87.

Duchowny, M. (2009). Clinical, functional, and neurophysiologic assessment of dysplastic cortical networks: Implications for cortical functioning and surgical management. *Epilepsia*, 50 Suppl 9,19-27.

Fauser, S., Sisodiya, S.M., Martinian, L., et al. (2009). Multi-focal occurrence of cortical dysplasia in epilepsy patients. *Brain*, 132,2079-90.

Fedi, M., Reutens, D.C., Andermann, F., et al. (2003). alpha-[11C]-Methyl-L-tryptophan PET identifies the epileptogenic tuber and correlates with interictal spike frequency. *Epilepsy Res*, 52,203-13.

Francione, S., Nobili, L., Cardinale, F., Citterio, A., Galli, C., Tassi, L. (2003). Intra-lesional stereo-EEG activity in Taylor 's focal cortical dysplasia. *Epileptic Disord*, 5 Suppl 2,S105-14.

Goldring, S. (1987). Pediatric epilepsy surgery. *Epilepsia*, 28 Suppl 1,S82-102.

Guerrini, R., Barba, C. (2010). Malformations of cortical development and aberrant cortical networks: epileptogenesis and functional organization. *J Clin Neurophysiol*, 27,372-9.

Gumbinger, C., Rohsbach, C.B., Schulze-Bonhage, A., et al. (2009). Focal cortical dysplasia: a genotype-phenotype analysis of polymorphisms and mutations in the TSC genes. *Epilepsia*, 50,1396-408.

Jiang, Y.J., Ang, L.C., Blume, W.T. (2010). Extent of EEG epileptiform pattern distribution in "focal" cortical dysplasia. *J Clin Neurophysiol*, 27,309-11.

Kim, D.W., Lee, S.K., Nam, H., et al. (2010). Epilepsy with dual pathology: surgical treatment of cortical dysplasia accompanied by hippocampal sclerosis. *Epilepsia*, 51,1429-35.

Kim, Y.H., Kang, H.C., Kim, D.S., et al. (2011). Neuroimaging in identifying focal cortical dysplasia and prognostic factors in pediatric and adolescent epilepsy surgery. *Epilepsia*, 52,722-7.

Krsek, P., Jahodova, A., Maton, B., et al. (2010). Low-grade focal cortical dysplasia is associated with prenatal and perinatal brain injury. *Epilepsia*, 51,2440-8.

LeVan, P., Tyvaert, L., Moeller, F., Gotman, J. (2010). Independent component analysis reveals dynamic ictal BOLD responses in EEG-fMRI data from focal epilepsy patients. *Neuroimage*, 49,366-78.

Lugnier, C., Majores, M., Fassunke, J., et al. (2009). Hamartin variants that are frequent in focal dysplasias and cortical tubers have reduced tuberin binding and aberrant subcellular distribution in vitro. *J Neuropathol Exp Neurol*, 68,1136-46.

Morales, C.L., Estupinan, B., Lorigados, P.L., et al. (2009). Microscopic mild focal cortical dysplasia in temporal lobe dual pathology: an electrocorticography study. *Seizure*, 18,593-600.

Nobili, L., Cardinale, F., Magliola, U., et al. (2009). Taylor's focal cortical dysplasia increases the risk of sleep-related epilepsy. *Epilepsia*, 50,2599-604.

Palmini, A. (2011). Revising the classification of focal cortical dysplasias. *Epilepsia*, 52,188-90.

Phi, J.H., Cho, B.K., Wang, K.C., et al. (2010). Longitudinal analyses of the surgical outcomes of pediatric epilepsy patients with focal cortical dysplasia. *J Neurosurg Pediatr*, 6,49-56.

Phi, J.H., Paeng, J.C., Lee, H.S., et al. (2010). Evaluation of focal cortical dysplasia and mixed neuronal and glial tumors in pediatric epilepsy patients using 18F-FDG and 11C-methionine pet. *J Nucl Med*, 51,728-34.

Rajan, J., Kannan, K., Kesavadas, C., Thomas, B. (2009). Focal Cortical Dysplasia (FCD) lesion analysis with complex diffusion approach. *Comput Med Imaging Graph*, 33,553-8.

Roper, S.N. (2009). Surgical treatment of the extratemporal epilepsies. *Epilepsia*, 50 Suppl 8,69-74.

Sisodiya, S. (2011). Epilepsy: the new order-classifying focal cortical dysplasias. *Nat Rev Neurol*, 7,129-30.

Sisodiya, S.M., Fauser, S., Cross, J.H., Thom, M. (2009). Focal cortical dysplasia type II: biological features and clinical perspectives. *Lancet Neurol*, 8,830-43.

Spreafico, R., Blumcke, I. (2010). Focal Cortical Dysplasias: clinical implication of neuropathological classification systems. *Acta Neuropathol*, 120,359-67.

Tassi, L., Colombo, N., Garbelli, R., et al. (2002). Focal cortical dysplasia: neuropathological subtypes, EEG, neuroimaging and surgical outcome. *Brain*, 125,1719-32.

Tassi, L., Garbelli, R., Colombo, N., et al. (2010). Type I focal cortical dysplasia: surgical outcome is related to histopathology. *Epileptic Disord*, 12,181-91.

Tassi, L., Meroni, A., Deleo, F., et al. (2009). Temporal lobe epilepsy: neuropathological and clinical correlations in 243 surgically treated patients. *Epileptic Disord*, 11,281-92.

Tassi, L., Pasquier, B., Minotti, L., et al. (2001). Cortical dysplasia: electroclinical, imaging, and neuropathologic study of 13 patients. *Epilepsia*, 42,1112-23.

Urbach, H., Scheffler, B., Heinrichsmeier, T., et al. (2002). Focal cortical dysplasia of Taylor's balloon cell type: a clinicopathological entity with characteristic neuroimaging and histopathological features, and favorable postsurgical outcome. *Epilepsia*, 43,33-40.

Warren, C.P., Hu, S., Stead, M., Brinkmann, B.H., Bower, M.R., Worrell, G.A. (2010). Synchrony in normal and focal epileptic brain: the seizure onset zone is functionally disconnected. *J Neurophysiol*, 104,3530-9.

Wehner, T., Luders, H. (2008). Role of neuroimaging in the presurgical evaluation of epilepsy. *J Clin Neurol*, 4,1-16.

Wong, M. (2009). Animal models of focal cortical dysplasia and tuberous sclerosis complex: recent progress toward clinical applications. *Epilepsia*, 50 Suppl 9,34-44.

Wong, M. (2010). Mammalian target of rapamycin (mTOR) inhibition as a potential antiepileptogenic therapy: From tuberous sclerosis to common acquired epilepsies. *Epilepsia*, 51,27-36.

18

Vagus Nerve Stimulation in Refractory Epilepsy: State of the Art

Berhouma Moncef
Department of Neurosurgery B – Minimally Invasive Neurosurgery Unit, Pierre Wertheimer Hospital – Lyon, France

1. Introduction

Even if the notion of refractory epilepsy is difficult to define precisely, it is widely admitted that it corresponds to the failure of two or more drugs and occurrence of one or more seizures per month over 18 months. Approximately 30 to 35% of epileptic patients will experience refractory epileptic periods in their lifetime despite maximal antiepileptic medications or they will suffer from serious side effects of their medical treatments. Indeed neurosurgical resection procedures including cortectomies and temporal lobe surgeries may result in a dramatic improvement of seizure frequency in selected patients, but these procedures carry a non-negligible rate of potentially serious risks with a mortality rate reaching more than 3% in some centers.

Another surgical option with less risks and reversible action for these patients is represented by vagus nerve stimulation (VNS), mainly in those patients that are not candidates for a surgical resection. VNS consists in the chronic and intermittent stimulation of the tenth cranial nerve (vagus nerve) in its extracranial cervical segment. Even if the pathophysiology of VNS in the treatment of refractory epilepsy is not yet clearly understood, the procedure has shown its efficacy in terms of quality of life improvement since the end of the 1990's in many types of epilepsy. The United States Food and Drug Administration (FDA) have approved the technique in 1997 as an adjunct to pharmacotherapy for adults and adolescents (more than 12 years). The VNS device has been developed by Cyberonics, Inc (Houston, TX).

In this review, we describe the state of the art of VNS including technical considerations, possible mechanisms of action, main clinical studies and future trends.

2. Technical considerations

Initially, the FDA approved the use of the VNS system as an adjunctive therapy in adults and adolescents with partial onset seizures, but lately extended the use of the VNS device for children and in seizures other than partial onset. The placement of the device is performed either by neurosurgeons or ENT surgeons after rigorous selection of patients by specialized neurologists. The surgical procedure is simple but requires special skills to identify the vagus nerve in the neck and carries complications and potentially lethal risks (Santos 2004).

2.1 Vagus nerve anatomy and VNS device

The vagus nerve or tenth cranial nerve is composed for up to 80% of its fibers by afferent ones originating from the viscera while 20% of its fibers are efferent and dedicated to the innervation of the larynx but also to the parasympathetic management of the heart, lungs and digestive tract. During VNS, the procedure will involve the mid paralaryngeal skeleton portion of the vagus nerve just behind the carotid sheath between and posterior to the common carotid artery and internal jugular vein. It is important to avoid using the device on the vagus nerve before the birth of its cardiac superior and inferior branches.

The VNS device consists in a generator and a lead. This generator delivers an intermittent electrical stimulation with precise and adjustable characteristics including output current, pulse width, frequency and stimulation on and off time. These parameters are adjusted postoperatively depending on therapeutic response and clinical tolerance. Initially the output current is usually set to zero mA for the first 2 to 3 postoperative weeks. Normalized parameters have been found to be the more effective at the beginning of the adjustments and have been found to be the more valuable in double-blind controlled studies: 500 µs pulse width, 30 Hz signal frequency, 30 seconds on-time and 5 minutes off-time. Further incremental increases in output current may be necessary depending on therapeutic effects. A hand-held magnet is given to patients with VNS (or to their caregivers) to activate directly the generator trans-cutaneously in case of auras or partial fits in order to reduce the incidence of severe seizures.

2.2 Surgical procedure

Many variations of VNS placement techniques have been described until now. In the majority of cases, the left vagus nerve has been used because of potentially higher risks of bradycardia and cardiac rhythm anomalies with the right vagus nerve. There is no clear evidence for this last data, resulting in the placement of VNS devices on either side.

Preoperative consent must be obtained and signed either by the patient or his guardian, after explaining attending risks and benefits of the procedure. The patient should be informed of the scarring lines in the neck and the preaxillary region as well as the voice changes possibilities during the stimulation cycles of the device. The patient and/or guardian should also be informed of the limited duration of the battery that will have to be replaced within a 7 to 10 years period depending on parameters set.

Under general anaesthesia and orotracheal intubation, the patient is placed supine with the head turned to the right side for a left-sided VNS placement. A 3 cm transverse incision is performed at the level of the cricothyroid membrane parallel to the anterior edge of the sternocleidomastoid muscle. This latter is dissected medially until one reaches the common carotid artery and the internal jugular vein. The vagus nerve is usually found on the posterior wall of the carotid sheath. Nearly 25 to 35 mm of the nerve are carefully dissected without any tearing or injury to the nerve. The vagus nerve adventitia and vasa nervorum must be preserved. The choice of the lead model is adapted to the nerve diameter before being delicately placed around the vagus nerve. An ipsilateral infraclavicular subcutaneous pocket is dissected to receive the generator, while the lead connector is tunnelled subcutaneously and connected to the helical electrodes. Proper placement of helical lead (distal to superior laryngeal nerve and cardiac cervical branches) and electrodes orientation is mandatory before peroperative testing of the device. The surgical and anaesthetic teams must be aware of the potentially serious cardiac rhythm anomalies that may occur during VNS testing including cardiac arrest (2-3%). Various complications and side effects are actually very well documented (Table 1) (Spuck et al. 2010).

Complications	Infection (3-8%) requiring generally device explantation Vocal cord paralysis 0,7% (transient or permanent) that can be avoided with careful dissection of the nerve and rigorous choice of the size of the lead Hematoma, seroma Nausea and vomiting Paresthesia Bradycardia Cardiac arrest (1/400 to 1/800) Device malfunction Lead fracture Pneumothorax Facial paralysis Horner's syndrome
Stimulation cycle related side effects	Coughing Laryngismus Voice alteration Local strap sensation Neck muscle contractures and spasms Dyspnea Dyspepsia Dysphagia Local pain

Table 1. Complications and adverse effects of VNS

3. Rationale of VNS in refractory epilepsy

Pathophysiology and mechanisms of action of VNS in refractory epilepsy are still subject to discussions and debates (Barnes et al. 2003). As already said, vagus nerve is composed of 80 % of afferent fibers and 20 % of efferent ones. The afferent fibers of the vagus nerve are known to originate from nodose and jugular ganglia to innervate both nuclei tractus solitarius and projecting to different regions involved in epileptic activity. This afferent contingent of fibers is mainly composed of small diameter unmyelinated fibers (C) but also large diameter myelinated ones (A and B). It is hypothesized that the chronic and intermittent stimulation of these afferent fibers of vagus nerve are involved in the anti-epileptic effect of VNS, while the exact mechanism is still unclear. Initially, C fibers were thought to be responsible of this effect in animals, but human studies did not comfort this hypothesis. Elsewhere, it has been demonstrated that various thalamic nuclei contain thalamocortical relay neurons with large projections on cerebral cortex. VNS may therefore induce changes in the metabolism of these thalamic nuclei by the mean of trans-synaptic neurotransmission modulation, as shown by PET scan. This latter demonstrated an increase of the blood flow in both thalami secondary to VNS that correlates with anti-epileptic effect.

Many studies of neurochemical concentrations of aminoacids and neurotransmitters in CSF and brain samples during VNS have shown variations of ethanolamine in specific locations such as locus coeruleus, a region directly involved in seizure propagation. VNS is also involved in long stimulation of NTS, parabrachial nucleus, paraventricular nucleus of the hypothalamus, ventral bed nucleus of the stria terminalis, dorsal raphe nucleus and cingulated cortex. CSF aspartate level, an excitatory neurotransmitter, has also been shown to decrease significantly in chronic VNS.

On an electrical point of view, EEG studies have proven cortical synchronization or desynchronization depending on stimulation frequency and intensity, explaining the importance of rigorous stimulation parameters in VNS (Marrosu 2005).

4. Clinical outcome

Significant clinical data supports that chronic and intermittent VNS is actually considered as a valuable treatment of refractory epilepsy (Table 2). It is mandatory to present this therapeutic modality to patients and their family not as a curative treatment but as an adjunct to antiepileptic drugs. Additionally to the significant decrease of epilepsy frequency and severity according to Engel postoperative assessment (Table 3), VNS reduces antiepileptic drugs toxicity but also the frequency of epilepsy-related hospitalization which is a great financial issue. Efficacy and clinical tolerance of VNS may require a long period of parameters adjustments. After promising preliminary results of pilot studies in the 1990's, multicenter double-blinded randomized trials in adults with refractory epilepsy confirmed the efficacy of VNS in terms of reduction of frequency, severity and duration of seizures. It is now admitted that this efficacy may require several months or even years of VNS to be obvious. Patients are considered as responders to VNS if they experience more than 50 % of reduction in seizure frequency.

Series	N	Follow-up (months)	Mean age (years)	Change in seizure frequency from baseline
Salinsky et al (1996)	100	10-12	33,3	-32 %
Handforth et al (1998)	94	3-4	32	-27,9 %
Scherrmann et al (2001)	95	16	34,9	-30 %
Labar (2004)	269	12	32	-58 %
Saneto et al (2006)	43	18	8	-84 %
De Herdt et al (2007)	138	44	30	-51 %
Amar et al (2008)	3822	24	26	-66,7 %
Sherman et al (2008)	34	12	12,3	-51,2 %
Elliot et al (2011)	65	124,8	30	-76,3 %

Table 2. Selected published data on the efficacy of VNS in refractory epilepsy

In long-term follow-up studies, VNS has proven to have an excellent tolerability with continuation rates reaching 70 % at three years. These studies confirmed also the existence of an incremental and cumulative seizure suppression effect of VNS over time as a possible result of the optimization of parameters adjustments and/or antiepileptic medications changes.

Another benefit of VNS is the marked improvement of the overall quality of life in these patients, probably mediated by the reduction of antiepileptic drugs toxicity and treatment costs or epilepsy-related hospitalization reduction.

In the paediatric population, studies are less common even if they showed obviously better results of VNS on refractory epilepsy than adults, with reduction of 50 to 90% in seizure frequency at one-year follow-up. VNS have also shown evident efficacy in Lennox-Gastaud syndrome and tuberous sclerosis complex.

Class I No disabling seizures	A - Completely seizure-free since surgery B - Non-disabling simple partial seizures only C - Some disabling seizures after surgery but free of disabling seizures for at least 2 years D - Generalized convulsion with antiepileptic drug withdrawal only
Class II Rare disabling seizures	A - Initially free of disabling seizures but has rare disabling seizures now B - Rare disabling seizures since surgery C - More than rare disabling seizures since surgery but rare seizures for at least 2 years D - Nocturnal seizures only
Class III Worthwhile improvement	A - Worthwhile seizure reduction B - Prolonged seizure-free intervals but less than 2 years
Class IV No worthwhile improvement	A - Significant seizure reduction B - No appreciable change in seizure frequency C - Seizures are more frequent or worse

Table 3. Engel classification of postoperative outcome

5. Conclusion

Chronic and intermittent vagus nerve stimulation is actually considered as a safe and very effective complementary treatment for patients with refractory epilepsy. Initially indicated exclusively in adults, the technique is currently diffusing in paediatric patients. A cumulative incremental effectiveness of VNS has been demonstrated with an increasing efficacy over the years of stimulation. VNS is also considered as a very valuable technique for the improvement of the overall quality of life in patients with refractory epilepsy. VNS is moreover being used in a variety of other pathologies including major depression, Alzheimer disease, congestive heart failure or even bowel inflammatory disorders.

6. References

Amar AP. (2007). Vagus nerve stimulation for the treatment of intractable epilepsy.*Expert Rev Neurother* 7(12):1763-73.

Barnes A, Duncan R, Chisholm JA, Lindsay K, Patterson J, Wyper D. (2003). Investigation into the mechanisms of vagus nerve stimulation for the treatment of intractable epilepsy, using 99mTc-HMPAO SPET brain images. *Eur J Nucl Med Mol Imaging* 30(2):301-5. Epub 2002 Nov 29.

De Herdt V, Boon P, Ceulemans B, Hauman H, Lagae L, Legros B, Sadzot B, Van Bogaert P, van Rijckevorsel K, Verhelst H, Vonck K. (2007). Vagus nerve stimulation for refractory epilepsy: a Belgian multicenter study. *Eur J Paediatr Neurol* 11(5):261-9. Epub 2007 Mar 28.

Elliott RE, Morsi A, Tanweer O, Grobelny B, Geller E, Carlson C, Devinsky O, Doyle WK. (2011). Efficacy of vagus nerve stimulation over time: Review of 65 consecutive patients with treatment-resistant epilepsy treated with VNS >10years. *Epilepsy Behav* 20(3):478-83. Epub 2011 Feb 5.

Handforth A, DeGiorgio CM, Schachter SC, Uthman BM, Naritoku DK, Tecoma ES, Henry TR, Collins SD, Vaughn BV, Gilmartin RC, Labar DR, Morris GL 3rd, Salinsky MC, Osorio I, Ristanovic RK, Labiner DM, Jones JC, Murphy JV, Ney GC, Wheless JW. (1998). Vagus nerve stimulation therapy for partial-onset seizures: a randomized active-control trial. *Neurology*. 51(1):48-55.

Labar D. (2004). Vagus nerve stimulation for 1 year in 269 patients on unchanged antiepileptic drugs. *Seizure* 13(6):392-8.

Marrosu F, Santoni F, Puligheddu M, Barberini L, Maleci A, Ennas F, Mascia M, Zanetti G, Tuveri A, Biggio G. (2005). Increase in 20-50 Hz (gamma frequencies) power spectrum and synchronization after chronic vagal nerve stimulation. *Clin Neurophysiol* 116(9):2026-36.

Salinsky MC, Uthman BM, Ristanovic RK, Wernicke JF, Tarver WB. (1996) Vagus nerve stimulation for the treatment of medically intractable seizures. Results of a 1-year open-extension trial. Vagus Nerve Stimulation Study Group. Arch Neurol 53(11):1176-80.

Saneto RP, Sotero de Menezes MA, Ojemann JG, Bournival BD, Murphy PJ, Cook WB, Avellino AM, Ellenbogen RG. (2006). Vagus nerve stimulation for intractable seizures in children. *Pediatr Neurol* 35(5):323-6.

Santos P. (2004). Surgical placement of the vagus nerve stimulator. *Operative Techniques in Otolaryngology* 15, 201-209

Scherrmann J, Hoppe C, Kral T, Schramm J, Elger CE. (2001). Vagus nerve stimulation: clinical experience in a large patient series. *J Clin Neurophysiol* 18(5):408-14.

Sherman EM, Connolly MB, Slick DJ, Eyrl KL, Steinbok P, Farrell K. (2008). Quality of life and seizure outcome after vagus nerve stimulation in children with intractable epilepsy. *J Child Neurol* 23(9):991-8. Epub 2008 May 12.

Spuck S, Tronnier V, Orosz I, Schönweiler R, Sepehrnia A, Nowak G, Sperner J. (2010). Operative and technical complications of vagus nerve stimulator implantation. Neurosurgery 67(2 Suppl Operative):489-94